OSCE NEONATOLOGY
Survival Guide

Dr. Athar A Mujeeb
MBBS, MD, DM Neonatology, MRCPCH (UK)
Assistant Professor
Department of Neonatology
Seth G. S. Medical College and KEM Hospital
Mumbai, (India)

PEEPEE PUBLISHERS AND DISTRIBUTOR (P) LTD.®

OSCE Neonatology
Survival Guide

Published by
Pawaninder P. Vij and Anupam Vij
Peepee Publishers and Distributors (P) Ltd.
Head Office:
160, Shakti Vihar, Pitam Pura
Delhi-110034 (India)

Correspondence Address:
7/31, First Floor, Ansari Road, Daryaganj
New Delhi-110002 (India)
Ph: 41512412, 23246245, 9811156083
e-mail: peepee160@yahoo.co.in
e-mail: peepee160@gmail.com
www.peepeepub.com

First Edition: **2024**

ISBN: 978-81-9651-873-8

Preface

To become a neonatologist, everyone needs to pass an exit exam, whether he is a fellow, DM or DrNB student. Clearing the exit exam is tougher in a super specialty because of its vast study material, which brings unnecessary stress to the students. Those who have cleared the exam have always complained of mismanagement of time, especially in searching for study materials. You have to cover various topics in a short amount of time, especially in practicals. Any deviation or wastage of time or preparing from non-authentic source can be detrimental to your performance in practicals.

So keeping all these points in mind, this book was prepared to provide the basics of neonatology questions that are usually asked or have a probability of being asked, along with landmark evidence that is a must-know for any neonatology practical exam.

The information is presented in question-and-answer format, thus making it easy to remember.

Special chapters on how to approach a ventilation case, a developmental case, a growing preterm case, and a neonatal jaundice case are the special features of this book. All the possible questions and answers relevant to each of these cases are presented in an easy-to-remember manner.

All the major trials and other relevant evidence are given at the end of chapters, making your knowledge evidence-based and up-to-date so that your answers in the exam look perfect.

I hope that after going through this book, you will be able to answer the questions thoroughly, which can help you get good marks in practical exams. I wish you the best of luck in your exams.

All suggestions for the improvement of this book are most welcome.

Dr. Athar A Mujeeb

Acknowledgements

I want to express my gratitude to my teachers for teaching me the art of neonatology. I will always be thankful to those parents whose babies I cared for and treated. I will be thankful to Mr. Pawaninder Paul Vij (Managing Director), Mr. Anupam Vij (Director), and the entire publishing team of Peepee Publishers for making this book possible.

Contents

1 History of Neonatology

Pierre Budin (1846–1907), Professor of Obstetrics, Hospital de la Charite, Paris, France, the "Father of Neonatology

1834: James Blundell describes neonatal intubation.

1922: Hess First transport incubator for new-born's

1942: Terry First published description of Retrolental Fibroplasia (RLF)

1943: Alfred Blalock & Helen Taussig First "blue baby" operation for Tetralogy of Fallot (Blalock-Taussig or BT shunt)

1949: Dr. Hess and Evelyn C. Lundeen, RN, publish The Premature Infant: Medical and Nursing Care, which ushers in the modern era of neonatal medicine.

1952: Virginia Apgar reports on system of neonatal assessment that bears her name

1956: Jean Ward in 1956, with one of the first infants given phototherapy at Rochford General Hospital

1959: Mary Ellen Avery and Jere Mead Surfactant deficiency identified as the cause of respiratory distress syndrome (RDS)

1960: Alexander Schaffer First use of terms "neonatologist" and "neonatology" in textbook (Diseases of the New-born, Saunders, 1960). Dr. Alexander Schaffer [22] was the first one to coin the term Neonatology as the science of New-born medicine and Neonatologist as one practicing neonatal medicine in the preface to his book Diseases of the New-born (published by Saunders in 1960)

1963: Widely reported news item Patrick Bouvier Kennedy dies of respiratory distress syndrome, GA 34 weeks, BW 2100 grams. This led to increased public awareness of prematurity and its consequences, with increased funding for research for pediatric disorders.

1966: Victor Freda Prevention of maternal Rh sensitization (and erythroblastosis fetalis) by anti-Rh antibody (RhoGam).

1967: Northway, Rosan & Porter Bronchopulmonary dysplasia (BDP) described

1968: Amiel-Tison Neurological assessment of gestational age

1969: Forrest Bird Baby Bird, first time-cycled pressure-limited ventilator for infants

1970: Dubowitz Gestational age scoring method based on combined physical and neurological characteristics

1971: George Gregory Use of continuous positive airway pressure (CPAP) for respiratory distress syndrome (RDS), Columbia university

1971: Kirby and colleagues. Ayre's T-piece forms the mechanical basis of most neonatal ventilators currently in use

1972: Liggins Controlled trial: antenatal glucocorticoids for prevention of respiratory distress syndrome (RDS)

1979: Ballard Simplified gestational age scoring system (modified Dubowitz)

1980: Fujiwara First report of intratracheal administration of bovine surfactant in 10 preterm infants With RDS that showed dramatic improvement.

1981: Colin Morley who with Alec Bangham developed ALEC (or pumactant)

1984: Bengt Robertson (RO) and Tore Curstedt (CU) – the creators of the porcine surfactant – Curosurf, also known as poractant alfa. Together they produced a porcine surfactant, which they named after themselves – Curstedt – Robertson surfactant or Curosurf for short.

1991: Ballard New Ballard Score (NBS) for gestational age, extended for extremely premature infants <26 weeks gestation.

1992: (INSURE) technique first described more than by Verder et al.

2007: Less Invasive Surfactant Application (LISA) protocol developed by Angela Kribs et al.

2 Antenatal

What is the frequency of ideal antenatal visits?

- Done at interval of 4 weeks up to 28 weeks; at interval of 2 weeks up to 36 weeks and thereafter weekly until delivery.
- In the developing countries, as per WHO recommendation, the visit may be curtailed to at least 4; Around 16 weeks, second between 24–28 weeks, the third visit at 32 weeks and the fourth visit at 36 weeks.

Estimation of gestational age with Symphysio fundal height

It is measured as the distance over the abdominal wall from the top of the symphysis pubis to the top of the fundus in a centralised uterus along the long axis of the fetus.

Symphysio fundal height	Rough Gestational age in weeks
below umbilicus	20
above umbilicus	24
between xiphisternum and umbilicus-one third	28
between xiphisternum and umbilicus-two third (flanks free)	32
at xiphisternum	36
between xiphisternum and umbilicus-two third (flanks full)	40

What is the expected weight gain during pregnancy? As per BMI?

- 17% of pre-pregnancy weight of mother
- 1st trimester- 1-2 kg
- 2nd trimester - 5-6 kg
- 3rd trimester - 5-6 kg

Weight gain according to mother BMI- weight (kg)/ height^2 (meter)

- (Normal BMI- 18.5 - 24.9 Kg/m2)
- Underweight: < 18.5 – weight gain 12-18 kg
- Normal BMI: 18.5 - 24.9 - 11.5 - 16 kg
- Overweight: 25 - 29.9: 7 - 11.5 kg
- Obese: > 30 - 5 - 9 kg

Weight distribution during pregnancy:

- Uterus- 1 kg
- Amniotic fluid- 1 kg
- Fetus + placenta- 4 kg
- Blood volume - 2 kg
- Interstitial fluid- 2 kg
- New fat/ protein - 4 kg

What is the definition of anemia during pregnancy?

- ANEMIA : WHO DEFINITION Hb < 11 gm/dl and hematocrit < 30
- NFHS 4 - Incidence of anemia 50%
- ICMR classification of anemia severity in pregnancy:
- Mild: 10-10.9 g/dl
- Moderate anemia: 7.0 -10.0 g/dl
- Severe: < 7.0 g/dl
- Very severe: < 4 g/dl

What is the importance of maternal education?

- Maternal education < secondary school : suboptimal ANC care & therefore increased low birth weight, SGA & mortality

What is the importance of paternal age?

- Paternal age > 40 years : increase incidence of single gene and autosomal dominant disorders and schizophrenia

What are the various methods of Assessment of fetal pulmonary maturity?

- **Estimation of pulmonary surfactant** by Lecithin/ Sphingomyelin (L/S) ratio.

- o Amniotic fluid L/S ratio at 31–32 weeks is 1;
- o At 35 weeks L/S ratio is 2.
- o L/S ratio > 2 indicates pulmonary maturity.
- o In mother with diabetes L/S ratio > 3.5.

- **Shake test or Bubble test (Clement's):** The test is based on the ability of pulmonary surfactant to form a foam or bubble, on shaking which remains stable for at least 15 minutes. Amniotic fluid is mixed with 96 percent ethanol, shaken for 15 seconds and inspected after 15 minutes for the presence of **a complete ring of bubbles at the meniscus. If it is present, the test is positive and indicates maturity of the fetal lungs.**
- **Presence of phosphatidylglycerol (PG)** in amniotic fluid reliably indicates lung maturation.
- **Saturated phosphatidylcholine** > 500 ng/mL indicates pulmonary maturity.
- **Lamellar body** is the storage form of surfactant in the amniotic fluid. A lamellar body count > 30,000/µL indicates pulmonary maturity.

NORMAL LABOR (EUTOCIA):

Labor is called normal if it fulfils the following criteria.

- Spontaneous in onset and at term.
- With vertex presentation.
- Without undue prolongation.
- Natural termination with minimal aids.
- Without having any complications affecting the health of the mother and/or the baby.

What are the various Stages of Labor?

- **First stage:** It starts from the onset of true labor pain and ends with full dilatation of the cervix. Usual duration is 12 hours in primigravidae and 6 hours in multipara.
- **Second stage:** It starts from the full dilatation of the cervix (not from the rupture of the membranes) and ends with expulsion of the fetus from the birth canal. Usual duration is 2 hours in primigravidae and 30 minutes in multipara.
- **Third stage:** It begins after expulsion of the fetus and ends with expulsion of the placenta and membranes (after-births). Usual duration is 15 minutes in both primigravidae and multipara. The duration is, however, reduced to 5 minutes in active management.
- **Fourth stage:** It is the stage of observation for at least 1 hour after expulsion of the after-births.

What is the definition of abortion?

- Abortion is the expulsion or extraction from its mother of an embryo or fetus weighing 500 g or less when it is not capable of independent survival (WHO).
- This 500 g of fetal development is attained approximately at **22 weeks (154 days) of gestation**.
- **75% abortions occur before the 16th week and of these, about 75% occur before the 8th week of pregnancy.**

What is IUFD?

- IUFD-**Literally, intrauterine fetal death (IUD)** embraces all fetal deaths weighing 500 gram or more occurring both during pregnancy (antepartum death) and during labor (intrapartum).

What are the common causes of first trimester abortion?

- Genetic factors (50%). Most common abnormality is a balanced translocation
- Endocrine disorders (poorly controlled diabetes, luteal phase defect, presence of thyroid antibodies, polycystic ovarian disease).
- Immunological disorders (APLA, Autoimmune and Alloimmune).
- Infection
- Inherited thrombophilia
- Unexplained.

What are the common causes of second trimester abortion?

- Anatomic abnormalities—(a) Cervical incompetence (congenital or acquired). (b) Mullerian Fusion defects (Bicornuate uterus, septate uterus). (c) Uterine synechiae (d uterine fibroid.
- Maternal medical illness
- Inherited thrombophilia
- Unexplained.

What is recurrent miscarriage?

Recurrent miscarriage is defined as a sequence of three or more consecutive spontaneous abortion before 20 weeks.

What are the various types of placenta?

Circumvallate placenta - fetal membranes double back on the fetal side around the edge of the placenta.

Velamentous cord insertion - The umbilical cord inserts into the fetal membranes, and then travels within the membranes to the placenta. Normally, the umbilical cord inserts into the middle of the placenta as it develops.

- If the leash of blood vessels happens to traverse through the membranes overlying the internal os, in front of the presenting part, the condition is called vasa previa.

Marginal Insertion - The cord is located close to the edge of the placenta.

Battledore placenta - The cord is attached to the margin of the placenta. If associated with low implantation of the placenta, there is chance of cord compression in vaginal delivery leading to fetal anoxia or even death.

Bilobed placenta - A bilobed placenta is a placenta separated into two near equal lobes. Occurs in about 4% of pregnancies

What is placenta previa and its various types?

When the placenta is implanted partially or completely over the lower uterine segment (over and adjacent to the internal os) it is called placenta previa.

Type—I (Low-lying): The major part of the placenta is attached to the upper segment and only the lower margin encroaches onto the lower segment but not up to the os.

Type—II (Marginal): The placenta reaches the margin of the internal os but does not cover it.

Type—III (Incomplete or partial central): The placenta covers the internal os partially (covers the internal os when closed but does not entirely do so when fully dilated).

Type—IV (Central or total): The placenta completely covers the internal os even after it is fully dilated.

ABRUPTIO PLACENTA

It is one form of antepartum hemorrhage where the bleeding occurs due to premature separation of normally situated placenta.

How to confirm a diagnosis of rupture of membrane

To examine the collected fluid from the posterior fornix (vaginal pool) for:

- **Detection of pH** by litmus or Nitrazine paper. The pH becomes 6–6.2 (Normal vaginal pH during pregnancy is 4.5–5.5 whereas that of liquor amnii is 7–7.5). Nitrazine paper turns from yellow to blue at pH > 6;
- To note the **characteristic ferning pattern** when a smeared slide is examined under microscope;
- Centrifuged cells stained with 0.1% **Nile blue sulfate** showing orange blue coloration of the cells (exfoliated fat containing cells from sebaceous glands of the fetus).

3 Antenatal Scan/Screening

What is the purpose of first trimester antenatal scan examination?

- Confirmation of intrauterine pregnancy.
- Gestational sac size, location, and number
- Embryo and/or yolk sac identification
- Crown-rump length
- Fetal number, including amnionicity and chorionicity of multifetal gestations
- Embryonic/fetal cardiac activity
- Assessment of embryonic/fetal anatomy appropriate for the first trimester
- Evaluation of the maternal uterus, adnexa, and cul-de-sac
- Evaluation of the fetal nuchal region, with consideration of fetal nuchal translucency assessment
- To confirm viability, establish gestational age accurately, determine the number of fetuses and, in the presence of a multiple pregnancy, assess chorionicity and amnionicity.

Gestational age assessment and its variation per GA

- First trimester: CRL: accurate predictor of GA: 3-6 d
- Second trimester: BPD
- Third trimester: FL: accurate predictor of GA: 3-5 d
- At < 8 weeks and 6 days if the CRL and the LMP are

> 5 days different, the ultrasound is the best estimate for gestational age.

- From 9 0/7 to 15 6/7 weeks: CRL estimation of GA is expected to be within 7 days of the true GA.
- At 16 to 21 6/7 weeks GA: variation upto 10 days
- At 22 to 27 6/7 weeks GA: variation upto 14 days;
- At 28 weeks and beyond: variation upto 21 days.
  1. Double test - determination of PAPP – A and hCG – β (free) performed between 9 and 13 weeks' gestation
  2. Triple test - determination of hCG – β, α – fetoprotein and free estriol between 14and 19 weeks;
  3. Quadruple test – as above plus inhibin

CROWN RUMP LENGTH

- Developing embryo is measured end-to-end, distance from the top of head to bottom of the rump with embryo in neutral posture.
- Mean of three readings.
- 5 weeks 3 days to 13 weeks and 6 days of pregnancy

What's the purpose of SECOND TRIMESTER EXAMINATION?

- Fetal number, including amnionicity and chorionicity of multifetal gestations
- Fetal cardiac activity
- Fetal presentation
- Placental location, appearance, and relationship to the internal cervical os, with documentation of placental cord insertion site when technically possible
- Amniotic fluid volume
- Gestational age assessment
- Fetal weight estimation
- Fetal anatomical survey, including documentation of technical limitations presentation, cardiac activity, fetal biometry, amniotic fluid, placental characteristics and fetal organ anatomy

The sensitivity of specialized sonography in experienced centres is considered to be at least 80 percent (American College of Obstetricians and Gynecologists, 2011).

Missed anomalies such as microcephaly, anotia, choanal atresia, cleft palate, bile duct atresia, Hirschsprung disease, anal atresia, and congenital skin disorders.

Weight gain of fetus as per gestational age

- 15 weeks: 5 gms/d
- 24 weeks: 15 to 20 gms/d

- 34 weeks: 30 to 35 gms/d

What are the markers seen in 1st timester

- Nuchal translucency
- Ductus venosus flow
- Absent or hypoplastic nasal bone
- Tricuspid regurgitation

What are the markers seen in 2nd trimester

- Intracardiac echogenic focus
- Echogenic bowel
- Single umbilical artery
- Thickened nuchal fold
- Choroid plexus cyst
- Pylectasis
- Shortened long bones
- Ventriculomegaly (VM)
- Choroid plexus cysts (CPCs)
- Enlarged cysta magna
- Fifth finger clinodactyly

What is the significance of soft markers in antenatal scan?

SOFT MARKER significance = A priori risk × LR marker = Revised Risk

What is the implication of echogenic intracardiac focus in antenatal scan?

Echogenic intracardiac focus (EICF) is defined as a focus of echogenicity comparable to bone, in the region of the papillary muscle in either or both ventricles of the fetal heart. Seen in:

- 87 % LV
- 5% RV
- 7% are biventricular

The evidence is best for left or biventricular EICF as association with significant malformation.

Less frequent right-sided, biventricular, multiple EICF- higher risk of fetal aneuploidy compared to more common single LV EICF.

What is nuchal translucency and its implication?

- The nuchal space is a normal fluid-filled space behind the fetal neck that is present in all foetuses between 11 - 14 weeks of gestation.
- An increased NT has been associated with trisomy 21 (approximately 75% of trisomy 21), as well as trisomy 13, 18, Turner syndrome, as well as structural birth defects including CHDs, and GI, GU and musculoskeletal abnormalities.
- Value > 2.5 mm is significant
- NT over 3.5 mm is an indication for further- testing for aneuploidy, a detailed fetal anatomic survey by ultrasound, and/or fetal echo.
- Chromosomal abnormalities occur in 20-30% of fetuses with increased nuchal translucency (50% contributed by Down's syndrome).

What is normal nuchal translucency?

- Normal -1.2 to 2.1mm at 45mm - CRL 1.9 to 2.7 mm at 84 mm CRL

What is Nuchal FOLD?

- A thickened nuchal fold should not be confused with nuchal translucency, which is a specific measurement of fluid in the posterior aspect of the neck at 11 to 14 weeks' gestation.
- A nuchal fold measurement is obtained in a transverse section of the fetal head at the level of the cavum septum pellucidum and thalami, angled posteriorly to include the cerebellum.
- 5 mm = 16 – 18 weeks
- 6 mm = 18 – 24 weeks
- Thick nuchal fold of 6 mm or greater and showed that the risk for Down syndrome increased by approximately 17-fold

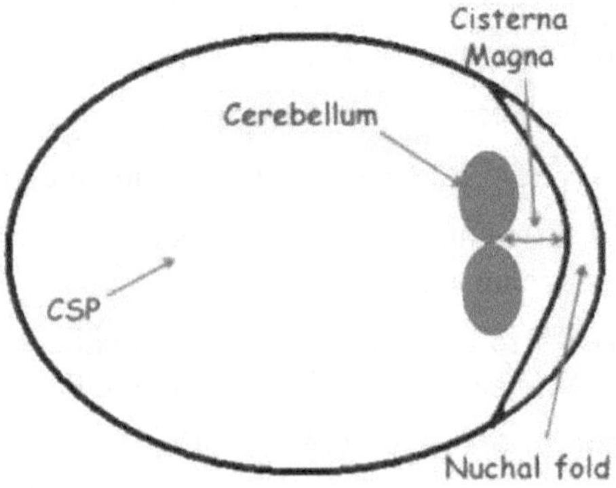

What is Nuchal index is the mean nuchal fold/mean biparietal diameter (BPD) × 100. A value of 11 or greater has a sensitivity of 50% and a specificity of 96% for downs syndrome.

What's the significance of Absence of nasal bone on antenatal scan?

- Nasal bones starting to appear at sixth week of gestation and seen at approximately 10 weeks gestation.
- Absent or hypoplastic nasal bone, defined nasal bone not visible in 1st trimester OR length of less than 2.5 mm in - 2nd trimester
- Absent or abnormally short nasal bone in cases of known trisomy 21 has been documented in 25–47% of cases reviewed.
- Overall likelihood ratio for Down syndrome is 51.

What is PYELECTASIS- dilatation of renal pelvis?

- 4 mm or more – second trimester
- 7 mm or more – third trimester
- 10 mm or more – hydronephrosis.

What is the significance of Single umbilical artery (SUA)?

- Incidence is in 0.5 to 5% of pregnancies.
- Isolated finding in 60-80% of cases
- Isolated SUA has not been found to be significantly associated with fetal aneuploidy.

Some studies have shown a higher risk of:

- Renal and cardiac abnormalities
- SGA, preterm birth
- Pregnancy-induced hypertension,
- Admission to the neonatal intensive care unit
- Perinatal mortality
- Higher rate of caesarean section due to non-reassuring fetal heart rate
- Higher rate of placenta or umbilical cord abnormalities

Echogenic bowel compared with surrounding bone or fetal liver.

- Compare to iliac wing

Causes of echogenic bowel are:

- Congenital viral infections (particularly CMV), toxoplasmosis, parvovirus, varicella, HSV.
- Aneuploidy
- Intra-amniotic bleeding
- Severe uteroplacental insufficiency
- Meconium peritonitis, Cystic fibrosis
- Anemia, and Fetal growth restriction (FGR)
- Cong bowel malformations (mainly upper GI malformations)

Cerebral ventriculomegaly is defined by atrial measurements 10 mm.

- Ventriculomegaly excess CSF within enlarged ventricles
- Mild (10-12 mm) 50-60 % normalizes
- Moderate (13 to 15 mm) 10-40 % normalizes
- 10-15 % of mild to moderate ventriculomegaly progress to severe
- Severe (> 15 mm)
  - Isolated ventriculomegaly refers to fetus with no other anomalies.
- Complex ventriculomegaly refers to cases with associated anomalies
- Hydrocephalus – ventriculomegaly secondary to imbalance between CSF production and absorption
- Large ventricles and a large head circumference suggest fetal hydrocephalus,
- While large ventricles and a small head are more suggestive of ex vacuo ventriculomegaly
- Measurements are obtained from an axial plane at the level of the thalamic nuclei just below the standard image to measure the BPD.

CHORIOD PLEXUS CYST

- CPC is a small sonographically discrete fluid-filled space ≥5 mm within the choroid plexus and it's seen as black echo-free areas.
- CPC typically regresses by 23 weeks regardless of karyotype
- In 50% of fetuses with trisomy 18.
- Isolated CPCs - no further investigation (in absence of any other risk factor).

Enlarged cisterna magna

The cisterna magna is measured as anterior/posterior diameter between the inferior/posterior surfaces of the vermis of the cerebellum to the inner surface of the cranium.

An enlarged cisternal magna is defined by anterior/posterior diameter 10 mm.

An enlarged cisterna magna is associated with:

- Other malformations

- Arachnoid cyst
- Dandy Walker malformation
- Dandy Walker variant
- Oro-facial–digital syndrome
- Meckel-Gruber syndrome

Short femur length

- Below the 2.5th percentile for gestational age
- Less than 0.9 of predicted by BPD. Causes -Down syndrome, skeletal dysplasia, fetal growth restriction

Short humerus length

- Below the 2.5th percentile for gestational age
- Less than 0.9 as predicted by BPD.
- Short humeral length- marker of fetal aneuploidy (trisomy 21).

What are the Soft markers for trisomy 21?

- Nuchal fold thickness (6mm or more)
- Short femur and humerus
- Renal pelvis dilatation (4mm or more)
- Echogenic bowel
- Echogenic intracardiac focus
- Hypoplastic/absent Nasal bone
- Aberrant Rt subclavian artery

What are the Soft markers for Edwards Syndrome

- Choroid plexus cysts -30-50% of Trisomy 18,
- Thick NT
- Cystic hygroma
- Ventriculomegaly

What are the Soft markers for Patau syndrome

- Nuchal thickening
- Ventriculomegaly

QUNITERO STAGING OF TTTS

STAGE	Findings	Management
STAGE I	oligo/ polyhydramnios	
STAGE II	bladder not visualized in donor	laser photocoagulation/ serial amniocentesis
STAGE III	critically abnormal Doppler in donor	laser photocoagulation
STAGE IV	hydropic changes in recipient (ascites/pericardial effusion)	laser photocoagulation
STAGE V	demise of one twin	

Two cranial signs in myelomeningocele.

- Scalloping of the frontal bones gives the head a lemon-shaped appearance ('lemon' sign). Due to reduction in intracranial volume due to herniation.
- The normally dumbbell-shaped cerebellum appears either absent or banana-shaped ('banana' sign). Results from downward herniation of posterior fossa contents.

Aneuploidy screening

First trimester screening

- At 11-14 weeks
- Maternal age
- B HCG
- PAPP-A
- NT
- OTHER USG FINDINGS

Turner syndrome, triploidies and sex chromosome anomalies – unrelated to maternal age

Risk of downs syndrome as per maternal age – 1:1000 below 30 yrs, 1:350 by 35 yrs and 1:100 after 40 yrs

Aneuploidy and congenital malformation

- Holoprosencephaly – trisomy 13
- CDH – trisomy 18
- Exomphalos- trisomy 18 (1:4), trisomy 13
- Megacystis- trisomy 18 or 13
- AV septal defect- trisomy 21

Second trimester serum testing

- At 15-20 weeks -
- Triple test- HCG, UE3, AFP
- Quadruple test- HCG, UE3, AFP + inhibin A
- Integrated test- NT + serum test (11-14wk) + quad test
- Step wise sequential screen

Invasive Prenatal Diagnostic Procedures

- Chorionic villus sampling
- Amniocentesis
- Cordocentesis

Non-invasive Prenatal Testing

- Cell-Free DNA -aneuploidy for chromosomes 13, 18, 21.

Chorionic villus sampling

- Transcervically – 10 to 13 weeks
- Transabdominally – 10 weeks to term
- Transcervical CVS – Adv: early genetic diagnosis • Disadv: Chromosome and enzyme composition is occasionally different from fetal cells
- Transabdominal CVS – minimal risk of infection
- Complication– fetal loss (1-2%), oromandibular limb deformities

Amniocentesis

- Puncture of amniotic sac per abdomen
- Early – 12-14 weeks
- Late – 15-20 weeks
- Risk factors – rh isoimmunisation in rh negative mothers, infection
- Complications – Pregnancy loss, amniotic fluid leakage, fetal trauma

Percutaneous Umbilical Cord Blood Sampling

- Diagnosis – of fetal anemia or thrombocytopenia, rapid karyotyping.
- Therapeutic tool – in utero transfusion of blood or platelets and, rarely, administration of anti-arrhythmic medications
- Procedure – under ultrasound guidance with a 22-gauge spinal needle into the umbilical vein beginning at 18 weeks' gestation
- Complications – Exsanguination (if the cord is lacerated), periumbilical vein hematoma in Wharton jelly, PROM, PTOL, or placental abruption.

4 Antenatal Doppler

What's the need of antenatal Doppler?

- Use of Doppler improves perinatal outcome, mainly by decreasing stillbirth and longer term neurologic impairments
- Minimize the morbidity by optimizing the timing of delivery
- Identify the foetuses at greater risk of hypoxia during labor
- The use of Doppler ultrasound in high-risk pregnancy was associated with a reduction in perinatal deaths (roughly 30 %)
- Fewer inductions of labour and lower rates of caesarean sections.
- No difference in operative vaginal births nor in Apgar scores <7 at five minutes.

Doppler indices

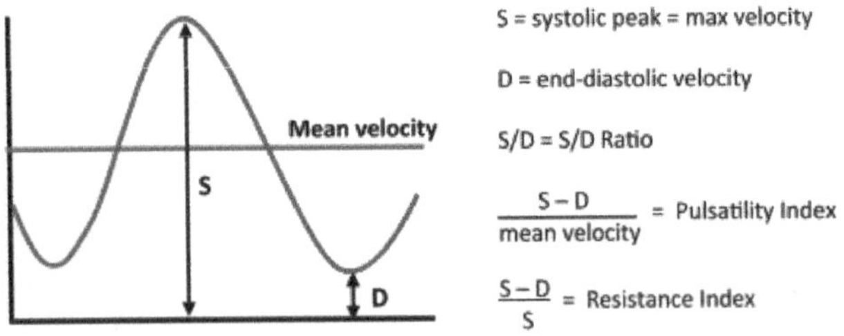

- Pulsatility index of Gosling
- Resistance index of Pourcelot
- S/D ratio
- D/A ratio

RI had the best discriminatory ability – than S/D and PI

The values of these ratios are not affected by the angle of insonation.

Common vessels for which Doppler is done antenatally

- Uterine artery
- Umbilical artery
- Middle Cerebral Artery
- Venous (UV, DV, IVC)
- Uterine artery – Maternal (resistance to uterus)
- Umbilical Artery – Placental (resistance to placenta)
- Arterial System (MCA) – Fetal (fetal adaptation to flow resistance change)
- Venous System – Fetal (fetal cardiac function)

Uterine artery Doppler

Uterine artery Doppler evaluation tool for identifying pregnancies that are at an increased risk for the development of pre-eclampsia and small fetus for gestational age.

High resistance with persistent notching may be normal in first trimester but not after that.

Umbilical cord artery	Pulsatility index Resistive index AEDF/REDF	Reduction in fetal mortality and in obstetric intervention
Fetal MCA	MCA PSV PI RI	Abnormal MCA PI was associated with greater perinatal morbidity
Ductus venosus	A wave and diastolic features	Determination of delivery by DV measures resulted in slight increase in mortality but reduction in morbidity

Umbilical Artery Doppler

- First fetal vessel to be evaluated by Doppler velocimetry
- Most easily measured parameter
- Assesses blood flow from the fetus to the placenta.
- Flow velocity waveforms from the umbilical cord have a characteristic saw-tooth appearance of arterial flow in one direction and continuous umbilical venous blood flow.
- Pulsatility index is known to be more resistant to changes in fetal heart rate variation, and is also the only index with a normal distribution.

UA Doppler studies have been found to be most useful in conditions of early-onset IUGR caused by uteroplacental insufficiency.

A normal systolic to diastolic ratio can be present despite a high pulsatility index or a very high resistance index and is indicative of decreased efficiency in the placental circulation.

In the growth-restricted fetus, A/REDF is often associated with fetal hypoxemia and acidemia, and increased perinatal morbidity and mortality.

The S/D ratio normally decreases from approximately 4.0 at 20 weeks to 2.0 at term, and it is generally less than 3.0 after 30 week

Because of downstream impedance to flow, more end-diastolic flow is observed at the placental end than at the fetal end. Thus A/REDF will appear first at the fetal cord end.

Umbilical artery Doppler measurements are made in a free loop of cord.

Fetal blood lactate level increases with increasing pulsatility index (i.e., increasing placental vascular resistance).

Fetal /neonatal death and diastolic flow in UA

- End diastolic flow present – 4 %
- AEDF – 40 %
- REDF – 75 %

REDF is associated with a risk of fetal compromise, perinatal mortality, neonatal neurological disturbances, and later neurodevelopmental disability.

Cochrane review with 18 studies and >10,000 pregnancies demonstrated that women with Doppler assessment had a significantly lower perinatal mortality (1.2%) compared with those without Doppler studies (1.7%) (RR: 0.67)

Perinatal outcome associated with AEDF/REDF

Perinatal Outcome	Mean
Perinatal mortality	45%
Gestational age	32 weeks
Birth weight	1050 g
Small for gestational age	65%
Caesarean section for fetal distress	75%
Apgar score at 5 min <7	25%
Admission to neonatal intensive care unit	85%
Congenital anomalies	10%
Aneuploidy	6.5%

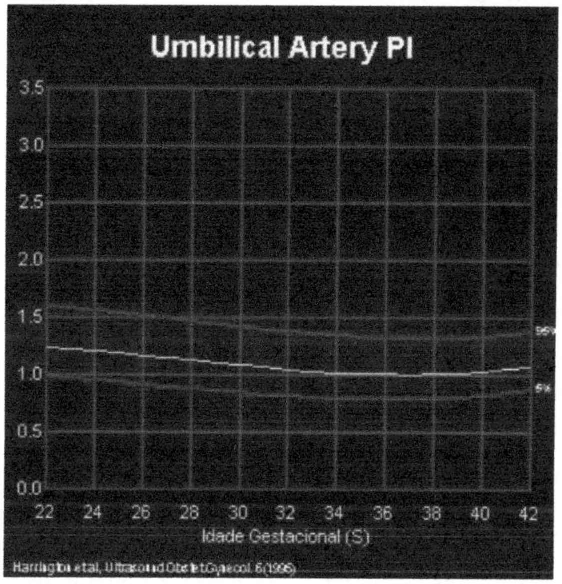

UA PI as per GA

Sequence of events in cases with increased placental resistance

Increased resistance in the placenta → ↓ diastolic blood flow velocity → Increasing S/D ratio & PI values. → Intermittently absent end-diastolic flow (EDF) → Persistently Absent EDF → Reversed EDF → Obliteration of >70% of placental tertiary villi.

- Rising index, even within the normal range (<95th percentile) -worsening fetal prognosis

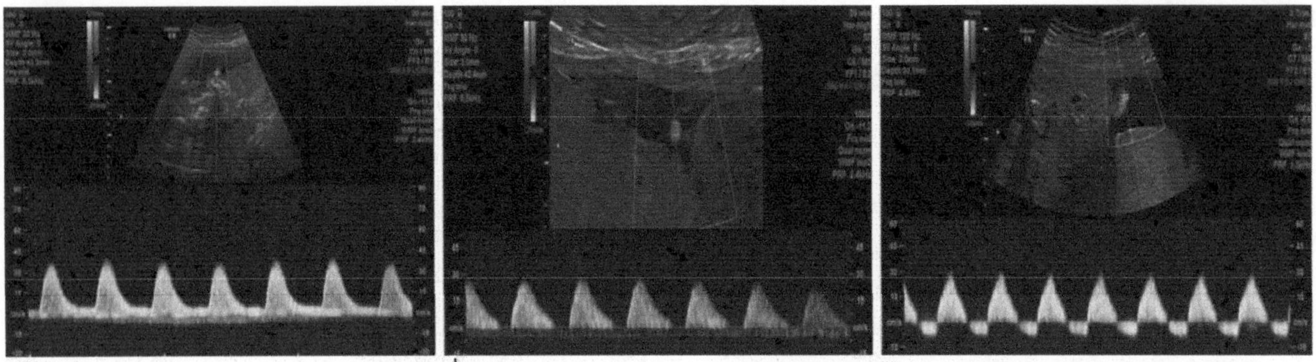

a b c

Positive end-diastolic flow (EDF) **AEDF** **REDF**

- Normal NST but abnormal S/D ratio had an outcome worse than those with an abnormal NST and a normal S/D ratio.
- Increased SD ratio- 30% fetal villous abnormal
- AEDF/REDF- 60-70 % fetal villous abnormal

Only the UA reverse end diastolic flow independently predicted poor neurodevelopment in FGR

Middle cerebral artery Doppler

Why MCA?

- Cerebral arteries respond rapidly to hypoxemia
- Easy to identify
- Low interobserver and intraobserver variability
- Early as 16-18 weeks, repeated 1-2 weeks interval

Doppler assessment of the MCA peak systolic velocity is considered to be the most effective monitoring tool for fetal anemia;

An increase in MCA velocities occurs with decreased fetal haemoglobin levels.

Normal middle cerebral artery (MCA) at term – normal peak systolic velocity (58 cm/s), high resistance, low end-diastolic velocity.

'Brain sparing' MCA – lower peak, much higher diastolic velocity suggests cerebrovasodilation

Anemic fetus with retained high resistance, elevated peak systolic velocity

Intrauterine hypoxemia leads to cerebrovascular dilation with an associated increase in diastolic flow and a decrease in the MCA pulsatility index.

A decrease in cerebroplacental ratio is indicative of fetal cerebral redistribution—a physiologic response to hypoxia.

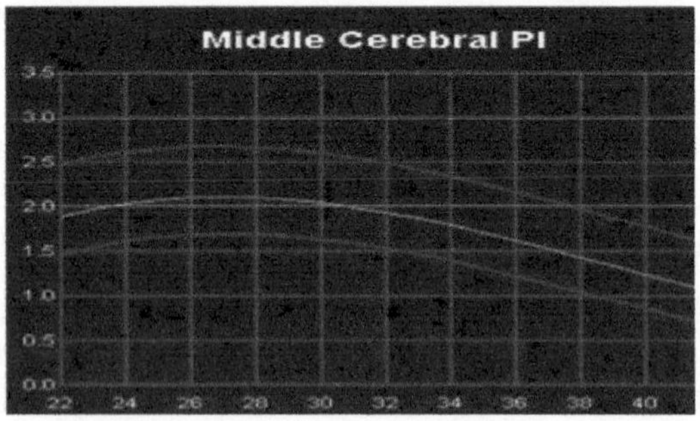

MCA PI as per GA

- Resistance in MCA decreases with advancing GA.
- IUGR with abnormal UA velocimetry, Elevated MCA PSV- **prediction of adverse outcome.**

<u>MCA DOPPLER IN FGR</u>

- Diastolic velocities in MCA rise due to redistribution of brain blood flow.
- **Brain-sparing”** – combination of sympathetic reflex-centralization of circulating blood volume, and altered cerebral autoregulation in the setting of lowered fetal blood oxygen content.
- Reduced MCA PI < 5th centile
- Reduced MCA PI/umbilical artery PI (Cerebroplacental Ratio)
- CPR (Cerebroplacental ratio) = MCA PI/ umbilical artery PI
- **Ratio of pulsatility index from cerebral circulation to index from umbilical artery; normal mean value is approximately 2.0**
- By expressing opposite-direction resistance changes as a ratio, the CPR magnifies them.
- CPR (<1) conferred an 11-fold increase in the risk of adverse perinatal outcome

Abnormal CPR is associated with:

- ↓ Gestational age at birth
- ↓ Mean birthweight
- ↓ Birthweight centile
- ↑ Rate of LSCS for fetal distress in labor
- ↑ Rate of Apgar scores less than 7 at 5 minutes
- ↑ Rate of neonatal acidosis
- ↑ Rate of NICU admissions
- ↑ Rate of adverse neonatal outcome/ perinatal death.

ROLE of MCA Doppler IN FETAL ANEMIA

- MCA PSV- monitoring of fetuses at risk of Rhesus disease or anemia due to parvovirus B19
- Peak systolic velocity (PSV) - 20-30 cm/s in early pregnancy AND 40-65 cm/s by the late third trimester.

Fetal anemia progresses (decreased viscocity)'!Right and left ventricular output increases by 45%, heart rate unchanged→Fetal blood vessel cross sectional area unchanged'→Poiseuille's law (velocity directly proportional to flow) (flow=velocity × cross sectional area)→ Increased velocity.

- Anemia- fetal chemoreceptor or baroreceptor stimulation →Redistribution of blood by dilation of the cerebral vessels →increasing substrate and oxygen supply to the brain

***Umbilical Vein- Protected* from the cardiac pressure-volume changes - has constant flow.**

Ductus Venosus Doppler

- Flow velocity pattern with several phases produced by atrial pressure-volume changes throughout the cardiac cycle.
- **S wave** - Initial antegrade peak- ventricular systole
- **V wave** - Brief post-systolic trough,
- **D wave** - Second antegrade peak- corresponds to early diastole,
- **A wave** - Second trough - atrial systole
- Hypoxia → DV becomes more dilated → Reduced flow during ventricular diastole, → Increased DV pulsatility index for veins (PIV), →Increasingly retrograde flow during atrial systole, seen as absent or reversed a-wave.
- PI >1 - DV dilatation and indicating poor outcome in severe FGR
- Absence or reversal of flow during atrial contraction (a wave) - failure of fetal circulatory compensation to supply well oxygenated blood to vital organ.
- Absent A wave-increased risk of fetal death in 1 week
- Reverse A wave ->7 days predicts stillbirth (100 %sensitivity, 80 % specificity)

Barcelona Center of Maternal-Fetal Medicine and Neonatology (BARCELONA GUIDELINES)

- **"True" FGR** – e/o abnormal fetoplacental function higher risk for fetal in utero deterioration, stillbirth and overall poorer perinatal outcome as compared with normally grown fetuses.
- **FGR is defined** - CPR <5th centile, UtA PI >95th centile and an EFW <3rd centile.
- **SGA** - subgroup of small fetuses that do not present the Doppler changes, EFW or BW <10th centile. No fetal adaptation to an abnormal environment and with perinatal outcomes similar to those of normally grown foetuses.

	Early onset FGR (<32 weeks)	**Late onset FGR (> 32 weeks)**
Problem	Management	Diagnosis
Placental Disease	Severe (UA Doppler abnormal, high association with preeclampsia)	Mild (UA Doppler normal, low association with pre-eclampsia)
Hypoxia	++ (systemic cardiovascular adaptation)	+/– (central cardiovascular adaptation)
Fetal maturity	Immature fetus = higher tolerance to hypoxia = natural history	Mature fetus = lower tolerance to hypoxia
Mortality and morbidity	High	Lower mortality (but common cause of late stillbirth); poor long-term outcome
Prevalence	Low	High

GRIT (Growth Restriction Intervention Trial)

- 587 babies, 24-36 weeks gestation with IUGR and abnormal Doppler.
- Early delivery vs late delivery based on Doppler
- Result: Median time-to-delivery interval - 0.9 days in immediate group and 4.9 days in delay group.
- Total deaths prior to discharge were 29 (10%) in the immediate group versus 27 (9%) in the delay group.
- Conclusion: At 2 years of age, there is a trend towards more disability in the immediate delivery group, but no overall difference in Griffiths DQ.

TRUFFLE trial

- Trial of Umbilical and Fetal Flow in Europe
- Women with a singleton fetus, 26–32 weeks, AC < 10th percentile and UA PI >95th percentile.
- Changes in the fetal ductus venosus Doppler waveform (DV) VS cardiotocography short-term variation (STV) to decide about delivery
- Group 1: control - Delivery based on CTG low STV
- Group 2a: Early ductus venosus changes (PI > 95th centile)
- Group 2b: Late ductus venosus changes (absent a-wave)
- Primary outcome: Survival without cerebral palsy or neurosensory impairment, or a Bayley III developmental score of less than 85, at 2 years of age
- The proportion of infants who survived without neurodevelopmental impairment between the three groups did not differ;
- Neurodevelopmental impairment was least frequent in survivors randomly assigned to the late ductus venosus group compared with those in the CTG STV group.
- Late ductus venosus changes - accompanied by a non-significant increase in perinatal and infant mortality and least neuro-impairment.
- Late changes in the DV waveform might produce an improvement in developmental outcomes at 2 years of age.

5 Amniotic Fluid

What are the contents of amniotic fluid?

- Contains water (99%), electrolytes, urea, creatinine, uric acid, fetal debris- lanugo, squamous cells, mucin, vernix, scalp hairs.

How amniotic fluid is formed

- Before 20 weeks of gestation amniotic fluid is an ultrafiltrate of maternal plasma.
- After 20 weeks of gestation fetal urine and lung liquid are the major contributors of AF with small contribution from fetal oro-nasal secretions.

At what gestation fetal kidney starts functioning

- Fetal kidneys start developing at 4-5 weeks of gestation and start secreting urine by 8-11 weeks of gestation.

What is the osmolality of amniotic fluid as per gestation?

- Osmolality of AF 290 mosm/kg (I trimester- isotonic with maternal serum)
- 255 mosm/ kg (near term- due to hypotonic fetal urine)

How much is the Volume of AF as per gestation week

- 10 weeks- 30 ml
- 16 weeks- 190 ml
- 32-35 weeks- 780 ml

Contributors of amniotic fluid

- Urine -800-1200
- Lung fluid -170 ml

Absorption of amniotic fluid

- Swallowing -500-1000 ml
- Lung fluid – 170 ml
- Intramembranous absorption – 200-500 ml
- Transmembranous absorption – 10 ml

How amniotic fluid is measured

- Maximum vertical pocket (in twin pregnancy)
- AFI

Maximum vertical pocket (MVP) as more predictive of poor outcome.

- MVP: >8- Polyhydramnios
- MVP <2 oligohydramnios

AFI

- The AFI is calculated as the mathematical sum of the deepest vertical fluid pockets from each of four quadrants of the uterus.
- The average AFI near term is 12 cm

Classification	**AFI**
• Polyhydramnios	• ≥25 cm
• Normal	• >8-<25 cm
• Moderate Oligohydramnios	• ≥5d≤8 cm
• Severe Oligohydramnios	• <5 cm

- Maximum volume of amniotic fluid is at roughly between 32-36 weeks of gestation

What are the functions of amniotic fluid?

- Allow room for fetal growth.
- Allow the freedom for fetal movement and permitting symmetrical musculoskeletal development
- Ingestion into GIT→ growth and maturation.
- Fetal pulmonary development.
- Protects the fetus and umbilical cord from trauma.
- Maintains temperature.
- As a barrier against infection.
- Aids dilatation of the cervix during labour.
- Indirect indicator of fetal well being

Perinatal mortality rate based on amniotic fluid volume

Normal AF volume	:	1.97/1000
Polyhydramnios	:	4.12/1000
Oligohydramnios	:	109.4/1000 (50 fold increase)

Causes of Oligohydramnios

- Spontaneous rupture of the membranes
- Premature rupture of the membranes
- Renal agenesis or obstructed uropathy
- Postmaturity syndrome
- Maternal Conditions
  - Antiphospholipid syndrome
  - Dehydration-hypovolemia
  - PIH
  - Uteroplacental insufficiency
  - Idiopathic

Causes of Polyhydramnios

- Central nervous system structural defects
- Obstruction or atresia of portions of the gastrointestinal tract
- Abdominal wall defects
- Aneuploidies
- Neuromuscular disorders
- Diabetes mellitus
- Combined Disorders
- Rh Isoimmunization
- Congenital infections (TORCH)
- Congenital anemias
- Idiopathic

Causes of nonimmune hydrops fetalis

1. Cardiovascular 15-35% - Increased central venous pressure
2. Chromosomal 5-15% - Cardiac anomalies, lymphatic dysplasia,
3. Hematologic 5-10% - Anemia, high output cardiac failure; hypoxia (alpha thalassemia)
4. Infectious 5-7% - Anemia, anoxia, endothelial cell damage, and increased capillary permeability
5. Thoracic 5 % - Vena caval obstruction or increased intrathoracic pressure with impaired venous return
6. Twin-twin transfusion 5-10% - Hypervolemia and increased central venous pressure
7. Urinary tract abnormalities 2-3% - Urinary ascites; nephrotic syndrome with hypoproteinemia
8. Gastrointestinal 0.5-5 % - Obstruction of venous return; gastrointestinal obstruction and infarction with protein loss and decreased colloid osmotic pressure
9. Lymphatic dysplasia 5% - Impaired venous return
10. Tumors, including 3% - Anemia, high output cardiac failure, hypoproteinemia
11. Skeletal dysplasia's 4% - Hepatomegaly, hypoproteinemia, impaired venous return
12. Inborn errors of metabolism 2% - Visceromegaly and obstruction of venous return, decreased erythropoiesis and anemia, and/or hypoproteinemia
13. Unknown 15-25%

6 Immune Hydrops

- Hydrops fetalis was first described by **Ballantyne in 1892.**
- In 1940, Rh blood group system was described by **Landsteiner and Wiener.**
- In **1961 Liley**, for the first time, described intrauterine transfusion into the abdominal cavity of the fetus as a preventive measure for immune hydrops.
- WHO recommends empirical use of anti-D Ig following any Rh sensitizing event.

What is the definition of Hydrops Fetalis?

Hydrops fetalis (HF) is defined as the presence of excessive fetal fluid in two or more of the following spaces on sonography:

• **Ascites**	Echolucent rim encompassing entire fetal abdomen in the transverse view.
• **Pleural effusions**	Unilateral or bilateral visualization of lung border
• **Pericardial effusion**	Non physiologic fluid ≥2 mm
• **Skin edema**	Subcutaneous edema ≥5 mm
• **Polyhydramnios**	Single deepest fluid pocket ≥8 mm or AFI ≥25 cm
• **Placentomegaly**	Placenta thickness ≥ 4 cm in first trimester ≥6 cm in second trimester

What is the Sequence of appearance of fluid in hydrops fetalis ?

- Firstly Polyhydramnios and placentomegaly seen on USG then Hepatomegaly and pericardial effusions
- Late findings are of ascites, scalp edema and pleural effusions.
- Finally, oligohydramnios.

What is the mortality of Untreated hydrops?

- Immune HF: 10%-24%.
- Non-immune HF: 76%-90%.

Basics of Immune hydrops

Immune hydrops occur in 1 in 2000 birth.

What are the Antigens responsible for immune hydrops?

- Rh antigen (D, C,c,E,e),
- ABO
- KELL
- Kidd
- MNS
- Duffy.

Discuss about Rhesus factor system

Rhesus factor system is the largest of all of the blood groups and has more than 50 different described antigens.

- **Most important antigens are** ____ D,C,c,E,e.
- The Rh proteins are encoded by two genes on chromosome 1
- Rh has dominant inheritance
- C and E have co-dominance type of inheritance.
- Rh positive person can be (small d means no antigen)
- Homozygous (DD) – 40%
- Heterozygous (Dd) – 60%.
- Rh negative can be – dd
- **Prevalence of Rh negative blood group in Indians 5 %**
- **Weak D type** : decreased number of intact D antigens on the surface of the red cells
- **Partial D type:** D antigens that are missing a portion, called epitopes.
- D antigen is expressed as part of the RBC membrane at day 38 of gestation.

What is direct coombs test (done in babies)?

Take blood sample from a patient (baby) with immune mediated hemolytic anemia – antibodies will be attached to antigens on the RBC surface.

The patient (baby) washed RBC will be incubated with antihuman antibodies. Antihuman antibodies form links between RBCs by binding to the human antibodies on RBCs causing agglutination.

What is Indirect coombs test (done in mother)?

Mother's serum which contains Rh antibodies (if she is sensitized) is added to RBCs. The antibodies get attached to antigen on RBCs. Now anti human antibodies are added which lead to agglutination.

Degree of Risk of Developing isoimmunization according to period of gestation

Gestational period	Percentage sensitization %
After 1st TM abortion	2 %
After MTP (mid trimester)	4-5%
At term after Delivery— Rh incompatibility	16% • 2% at the time of delivery, • 7% will develop anti D antibodies by the 6 months of delivery, • 7% get sensitized e.g. they develop anti D slowly and very low titer which becomes detectable and measurable in next pregnancy.
ABO incompatible	1.5 -2 %

Protection from Likelihood of Isoimmunization (D negative woman delivering D positive ABO compatible baby) after intervention or with associated ABO incompatibility

Condition/intervention	Percentage
Associated ABO incompatibility	1-2%
Following post-partum prophylaxis	1.5%
Antenatal prophylaxis in addition	0.18%

As the pregnancy progresses, the possibility of feto-maternal hemorrhage increases,

- 3% in first trimester
- 12% in the second
- 45% in the third
- 64% at the time of delivery

0.01 mL of antigen-positive blood is sufficient to cause sensitization.

- The risk of sensitization is related to the **volume of blood** that passes between the fetus and mother.
- For 0.1 mL of blood, the risk of sensitization is 3%
- For 0.4 mL, the risk rises to 22%.

Immunological Non responders – pregnancy induced suppression of immune system – 30%

What is Grandmother theory of Rh isoimmunization?

- Rh –ve (dd) fetus rarely may be exposed to maternal D antigen as result of materno fetal haemorrhage and may become sensitized in their intra uterine life.
- When such girl at her adult age has pregnancy with Rh +ve fetus, the very first fetus may suffer from haemolytic disease of new-born.
- This mechanism of isoimmunisation is called grand mother theory.

Fate of isoimmunized pregnancies

Severe Rh disease	30
Moderate Rh disease	30
Mild disease	40
Still birth	14

Pathophysiology of hydrops in general

Edema formation results from one of the following possible processes:

1. Anemia, resulting in high-output cardiac failure.
2. Elevated central venous pressure (CVP)
3. Decreased lymphatic flow
4. Capillary leak

Risk Factor	Risk of sensitization
Spontaneous abortion	2%-3%
Therapeutic abortion	4-5%
Ectopic pregnancy	2-5%
Chorionic Villous sampling	50%
Amniocentesis	10%
Percutaneous umbilical blood sampling	40%
Abruptio Placentae/Placenta Praevia/External cephalic Version/Trauma	Variable

Cont...

Pregnancy (28wks -	7-8% (First pregnancy)
<72 hours Postpartum)	15% (Second pregnancy)
Delivery	50%

Anti D prophylaxis for Rh negative pregnancy

Postpartum prophylaxis decreases risk of sensitization to 1-2%.

Antenatal plus postnatal prophylaxis decreases risk to 0.1-0.3 %.

A single 300 microgram dose contains sufficient anti-D to suppress the immune response to 15 mL of D-positive red cells (or 30 mL fetal D-positive whole blood).

10 microgram dose sufficient for ___ 1 ml of fetal whole blood (___ 0.5 ml of fetal RBC).

- **Half-life of anti D is :** mean – 24 days.

What is the Mechanism of action of anti D?

- **Antigen masking :** Ab cover the Ag sites + RBC rendering them unavailable to maternal lymphoid cells.
- **Clearance and antigen deviation** – Ag is directed away from the endothelial sys preventing production of antibodies.
- **Central inhibition :** Rh IgG in presence of fetal RBC generate immune complexes that induce suppressor T cells.
- **Co-inhibition by cross linking** : B cells may be co inhibited by cross linking of the heterologous receptors, thus the B cell may be inhibited before an immune response is established
- **Anti-idiotypic antibodies** : Monovalent anti idiotypic antibodies deliver weak inhibitory signals to B cells, thereby suppressing of the immune response

How to follow up of a Rh negative pregnancy during antenatal visits?

- All pregnant should be tested for Rh isoimmunization at registration and again at 28 weeks
- Those mothers who are Rh –ve non-immunized at 28 weeks: give 300µg of Rh IgG (in deltoid) (As the half-life of the Rh IgG is 21 to 30 days the injection is protective until term)
- Give 300µg of Rh IgG within 72 hours of delivery if cord blood reveals Rh D+
- **First trimester sensitization:** 50 microgram can be used for first-trimester events and protects against a feto-maternal bleed of 2.5 mL red cells
- **Second and third trimesters and postpartum** – The standard 300 microgram dose is recommended.
- An appropriate dose within 72 hours of delivery of a D-positive New-born
- Should be given as soon as possible after recognition of the omission.
- Partial protection is afforded with administration within 13 days of the birth or a potentially sensitizing event.
- Some experts recommend giving it as late as 28 days

Causes of failure of anti D prophylaxis

- Dose too small
- Dose too late >72 hours
- Patient already immunized, low titers not recognized
- Defective immune globulin
- Large FMH

What is kleihauer betke test?

- Done for quantification of fetomaternal haemorrhage
- Based on acid elusion technique.
- Fetal and maternal RBCs have different response to citrate acid phosphate buffer solution
- Maternal cells get eluded leaving behind only cell membrane and hence appear swollen round large GHOST CELLS against normal fetal cells whose Hb remain unaltered and hence look as red refractile round cells.
- Percentage of fetal cells are counted
- Fetal blood volume = MBV × maternal Hct × % fetal cells in KB /New-born Hct
- Volume of the feto-maternal bleeding = % fetal RBC in maternal blood × 50
- If in 50 low power fields of maternal peripheral blood 80 fetal RBC's are found- it is estimated that 4ml of fetomaternal hemorrhage has occurred

Evaluation of Rh sensitized mother

- Non invasive - USG
- USG Doppler- MCA PSV
- Invasive - Amniocentesis
- Cordocentesis

MCA PSV

As anemia progresses stroke volume increases and blood viscosity decreases, – If crossectional area remain same using Doppler velocity, – Flow can be calculated by

Poiseuille's equation and hence anemia can also be calculated

Why MCA selected

- Cerebral arteries respond rapidly to hypoxemia by increasing blood flow velocity to maintain cerebral perfusion
- MCA is easy to identify with low inter-observer and intra-observer variability.
  - Measurements of the MCA-PSV can be started as early as **16-18 weeks** and should be repeated at **1 to 2 week** intervals
  - **MCA-PSV > 1.5 MoMs for GA** ___ Moderate to severe fetal anemia.
  - 1.29 times the MOM for mild anemia,
  - 1.5 times the MOM for moderate anemia,
  - 1.55 times the MOM for severe anemia
  - Fetal hydrops is rare with a hemoglobin concentration greater than 5 gm/dL.

What are the Indications for fetal therapy in case of immune hydrops

- Delta OD 450 in zone 3 of liley curve (not used now)
- MCA peak systolic velocity >1.5 MOM
- Fetal anemia on cordocentesis
- Immature fetus

Types of Intrauterine fetal transfusions

- Intravascular transfusion.
- Intraperitoneal Transfusion - Usually performed before 18 weeks when an intravascular transfusion is technically impossible because of small umbilical vessels, fetal position or the location of the umbilical vessels.

LOTUS study

The LOTUS study evaluated the neurodevelopment of children with haemolytic disease treated with an intrauterine transfusion.

291 children were evaluated at a median age of 8.2 years (range, 2-17 years)

Cerebral palsy was detected in 2.1%

Severe developmental delay in 3.1%

Bilateral deafness in 1.0%

Overall incidence of NDI was 4.8%

The only risk factor that could be linked with neurodevelopmental delay was severe fetal HF. The very high rate of intact survival in these at-risk pregnancies complicated by severe anemia is reassuring and confirms the relative safety of the treatment with intrauterine transfusions even in the fetus with severe haemolytic disease.

Indications for Exchange Transfusion

- Features of Hydrops
- Cord Hb < 10g/dL and/or cord TSB> 5mg/dL
- Serum bilirubin in exchange range zone as per Modified AAP charts for near term and term babies
- Rise in TSB >1 mg/dL/hr despite PT
- Rise of TSB > 0.5mg/dL/hr despite PT if Hb 10-12g/dL
- Any TSB > 12mg/dL in first 12 hour
- Consider early if neurological sings are present

Volume calculation for DVET

- 2 × baby's blood volume
- Baby's blood volume= 80-90 ml/kg (term) and 90-100 ml/kg (preterm)

KELL ANTIGEN

3rd most common cause of Haemolytic disease of New-born

- The Kell antigen is the first RBC - specific blood group antigen to be expressed during the burst-forming unit erythroid stage of RBC development.
- Maternal anti Kell antibodies can target early erythroid progenitors
- Features as Hypoproliferative SEVERE anemia without Reticulocytosis and Hyperbilirubinemia
- In Kell alloimmunization, early suppression of fetal RBC synthesis results in less bilirubin being released during hemolysis.

What is Mirror syndrome

- If placental hydrops is significant, an additional life-threatening complication has been described — Ballantyne's syndrome (also known as mirror syndrome, triple edema, and pseudotoxemia).
- The mother develops preeclampsia along with severe edema that is similar to that of the fetus
- Caused by vascular changes in the swollen, hydropic placenta, this likely related to antiangiopenic factors produced by hyperplacentosis

- Reversal of maternal symptoms has been reported with the resolution of fetal hydrops after in utero treatment

Role of IvIG in isoimmunisation

- The use of exchange transfusion decreased significantly in the immunoglobulin treated group (typical RR 0.35, 95% CI 0.25 to 0.49)
- The mean number of exchange transfusions per infant was also significantly lower in the immunoglobulin treated group (MD 0.34, 95% CI 0.50 to 0.17)

DCC IN ALLOIMMUNIZED WOMEN

- Tanushree sahoo et al evaluated the outcome of delayed versus early cord clamping in 70 Rh alloimmunized Infants at 28 to 41 weeks of gestation and found DCC group had a **higher mean PCV at 2 h of life**
- However, incidence of DVET and PET, duration of PT, echocardiography parameters, and BT until 14 weeks of postnatal age were similar between the groups.

7 Antepartum and Intrapartum Assessment

1. Fetal movement - Detection by maternal perception or by real-time ultrasonography
2. Fetal heart rate
   - Nonstress test: response of fetal heart rate to movement
   - Contraction stress test: response of fetal heart rate to stimulated (oxytocin and nipple stimulation) or spontaneous uterine contraction
3. Fetal biophysical profile - Combination of fetal breathing, movement, tone, heart rate reactivity, and amniotic fluid volume
4. Fetal growth - Detection of intrauterine growth retardation
5. Fetal blood flow velocity - Detection by the Doppler technique of flow velocity in umbilical and fetal systemic and cerebral vessels

Fetal movements

Commences at 7 weeks gestation becomes organized by 20 to 30 weeks and by 36 weeks behavioral states are established.

- **A "count to 10" method by the mother** is the only approach to fetal movement, which has been validated as a screening test.
- The same time of day is chosen, fetal movements are noted with the expectation of 10 fetal movements achieved within 2 hours.
- Lack of attaining 10 movements prompts evaluation.
- Approx. 10 fetal movements in 2 hours are considered normal but sleep cycle of fetus may range from 20 mins to 75 mins.

Non Stress Test (NST)

- Principle: Fetal activity results in a reflex acceleration in HR by 32 weeks of GA.
- FHR variability and accelerations are not present before 24 weeks of gestation
- Between 24 to 32 weeks, they are present but not as term pregnancy, accelerations are discreet & not more than 10 bpm
- 24-28 weeks, up to 50% of NST are nonreactive
- At 28-32 weeks, 15% nonreactive

The inhibitory influence on the heart rate is conveyed by the vagus nerve, whereas excitatory influence is conveyed by the sympathetic system.

Interpretation of NST

- Normal NST (Reactive)
- Atypical NST (Equivocal)
- Abnormal NST (Non reactive)

Predictability of fetal well being based on NST

- High sensitivity >90%
- Low specificity 45 - 55% – thus better at predicting the absence of fetal compromise than its presence.
- Negative predictive value is better
- Positive predictive value of non-reactive NST- 25-50%

What is a Reactive NST?

- HR between 110 and 160 bpm
- Normal beat-to-beat variability
- Two accelerations of at least 15 bpm lasting for not < 15 seconds each within a 20-minute period.

What do you mean by a Nonreactive NST?

- Less than two accelerations in 40 minutes.
- Absence of these accelerations in a fetus who previously demonstrated them may indicate that hypoxia has sufficiently depressed the CNS to inactivate the cardiac reflex.
- Testing reflexes the current fetal state and cannot predict future events or precisely the neonatal outcome.

What is Inadequate NST?

- Adequate fetal heart tracing cannot be obtained for any reason

Contraction Stress Test

- Used in the past as a follow-up evaluation after a nonreactive stress test
- A negative stress test is defined as absence of any late decelerations with the contractions
- A positive (abnormal) result is indicated by persistent late decelerations over several or more contractions

What is Biophysical Profile (BPP)?

- NST with other parameters determined by USG
- A score of 0 or 2 is assigned for the absence or presence of each of the following:
  - Reactive NST - ≥2 FHR accelerations lasting ≥15 s over 20min
  - Adequate Amniotic fluid volume (≥1 pocket of amniotic fluid measuring ≥2 cm in two perpendicular planes
  - Fetal breathing movements -≥1 episode of breathing movements lasting 30 s
  - Fetal activity- ≥3 discrete body or limb movements
  - Fetal musculoskeletal tone - ≥1 episode of active extension and flexion of limbs or trunk

What is the Sequence of fetal Response to Hypoxia?

Healthy foetuses exhibit the BPP's constituent components in a regular order:

1) Foetal tone develops between 7.5 and 8.5 weeks,
2) Foetal movement between 9 and 20 weeks,
3) Foetal breathing between 22 and 24 weeks, and
4) FHR reactivity between 24 and 28 weeks.

They disappear in the presence of antepartum hypoxia, they typically do so in the reverse sequence in which they first appeared (for example, FHR reactivity is gone first, then foetal breathing, foetal movements, and finally foetal tone) (See Table).

Modified Biophysical Profile

- Nonstress test performed twice weekly and combined with amniotic fluid index (<5cm). Requires only 10 mins to perform.
- ACOG and AAP conclude the use of this modified BPP as an excellent antepartum survelliance method for fetal wellbeing.

Intrapartum Assessment of the Fetus

- Fetal heart rate
- Fetal acid-base status

Intrapartum monitoring - Systematic approach - four aspects:

- Baseline heart rate
- Baseline heart rate variability
- Presence of accelerations
- Presence of decelerations

Interpretation and Management of Biophysical Profile

Score	N/Abnormal	Perinatal mortality within 1 week if no intervention done	Management
10/10	N	<1/1000	No action
8/8	N		NO ACTION
8/10 (ABN NST)	N		NO ACTION
8/10 (ABN AFI)	ABN	89/1000	Rule out ROM, delivery/observation
6/8	Asphyxia possible	Variable	Repeat in 4-6 hrs
6/8 (Abn AFI)	Asphyxia suspected	89/1000	Repeat – consider delivery
4/8	Asphyxia suspected	91/1000	>36 weeks immediate delivery /repeat
2/8	High likelihood of asphyxia	125/1000	Delivery stat
0/8	High likelihood of asphyxia	600/1000	Stat delivery

Baseline HR: 110 and 160 bpm.

Fetal bradycardia: <110 beats/min for >10min -CHB a/w congenital heart malformation or maternal SLE.

Other Causes of fetal bradycardia • Prolonged cord compression • Cord prolapse • Tetanic uterine contractions • Paracervical block • Epidural and spinal anesthesia • Maternal seizures • Rapid descent •

Baseline tachycardia: >160 beats/min for >10min

Causes of fetal tachycardia • Fetal hypoxia • Maternal fever, hyperthyroidism • Maternal or fetal anemia • Parasympatholytic drugs • Sympathomimetic drugs like tocolytics • Chorioamnionitis • Fetal tachyarrhythmia • Prematurity

Fetal dysrhythmias: FHR >200 bpm.

In isolation, tachycardia is poorly predictive of fetal hypoxemia or acidosis unless a / w reduced beat-to-beat variability or recurrent decelerations.

Beat-to-beat variability

- Calculated of each RR interval.
- Measured by the difference between two lines drawn through the highest and lowest point of the trace in any one-minute segment.
- Moderate 6–25 beats/min
- Minimal Undetectable to ≤5 beats/min
- Marked >25 beats/min

Causes of Reduced beat-to-beat variability: Depression of the fetal CNS

- Immaturity,
- Hypoxia,
- Sleep,
- Maternal medications: narcotics, sedatives, β-blockers, and IV MgSO4.

What are fetal Decelerations?

- Decelerations are drops in FHR by > 15 beats/min from the baseline lasting for > 15 sec
- They can be further classified as:
  - Early decelerations
  - Variable decelerations
  - Late deceleration

Early decelerations

- Gradual decrease onset to nadir ≥30 s with contraction
- Symmetric in shape
- Mirrors uterine contractions in time of onset, duration, and termination.
- Benign and usually accompanied with good beat-to-beat variability.
- Seen in active labor: fetal head compressed in pelvis, → parasympathetic effect.

Late decelerations

- Gradual decrease onset to nadir ≥30 s; nadir of deceleration occurring after peak of contraction
- Decreases in the FHR associated with uterine contractions.
- Onset, nadir, and recovery of the deceleration occur after the beginning, peak, and end of the contraction respectively.
- **A fall in the heart rate of only 10 to 20 bpm below baseline (even if still within the range of 110 to 160 bpm) is significant.**

Causes of Late decelerations:

- Excessive uterine contractions (usually caused by oxytocin)
- Abruptio placentae
- Severe maternal anemia or hypoxemia uteroplacental insufficiency and possible fetal hypoxia.

Mechanisms of late decelerations

Decreased fetal PO2 (hypoxemia) during a uterine contraction is detected by Chemoreceptors

↓

Chemoreceptors signal the medullary vasomotor center

↓

Sympathetic outflow results in peripheral vasoconstriction to redistribute oxygenated blood away from the extremities, gut and kidneys

↓

Blood flow to the brain, heart, adrenal glands and placenta is preserved or increased

↓

Peripheral vasoconstriction causes the blood pressure to rise

↓

Rising blood pressure is detected by baroreceptors

↓

Baroreceptors signal the medullary vasomotor center

↓

Parasympathetic (vagal) stimulation of the heart causes a gradual slowing of the FHR to reduce cardiac output and maintain normal blood pressure.

What are Variable decelerations?

- **Variable Abrupt decrease onset to nadir <30 s; decrease ≥15 beats/min lasting ≥5 s to <2min**
- Vary in shape & timing relative to contractions.
- Result from fetal umbilical cord compression.
- Moderate to severe variable decelerations (defined as decelerations to 70 to 80 beats/minute for >60 seconds with three contractions or to a rate of <70 beats/minute for 30 to 60 seconds), severe variable decelerations (decelerations to a rate of <70 beats/minute for ≥60
- Variable decelerations are a **cause for concern if**
  - Severe (down to a rate of 60 bpm)
  - Lasting for 60 seconds or longer
  - Associated with poor beat to beat variability,
  - Mixed with late decelerations.

As the uteroplacental insufficiency/hypoxia worsens:

- Beat-to-beat variability reduced and then lost
- Decelerations last longer, Begin sooner following onset of a contraction, Take longer to return to baseline,
- Rate to which the fetal heart slows → lower.

Recurrent Occur with ≥50% of uterine contractions in any 20-min window

Intermittent declaration Occur with <50% of uterine contractions in any 20-min window

Repetitive late decelerations demand action.

Prolonged deceleration

Prolonged deceleration is > 15 bpm and lasts > 2 minutes but < 10 minutes from onset to return to baseline.

A prolonged deceleration that lasts > 10 minutes is considered a change in baseline.

Three (3) Tier System for intraprtum monitoring

Category I

Category II

Category III

Category 1 considered a "normal" tracing with:

- Baseline FHR 110-160 bpm
- Moderate variability
- No late or variable decelerations
- Strongly predictive of normal fetal acid-base status
- No intervention required

Category II

Category II is also known as an *"indeterminate"* tracing because it does not meet criteria for Category I or III.

- Covers a wide range of FHR patterns
- Some patterns are concerning for fetal acidosis
- Some patterns require intrauterine resuscitation
- Requires continued monitoring and re-evaluation

Baseline rate

- Bradycardia not accompanied by absent baseline variability
- Tachycardia

Baseline FHR variability

- Minimal baseline variability
- Absent baseline variability with no recurrent decelerations
- Marked baseline variability

Accelerations

- Absence of induced accelerations after fetal stimulation

Periodic or episodic decelerations

- Recurrent variable decelerations accompanied by minimal or moderate baseline variability
- Prolonged deceleration more than 2 minutes but less than 10 minutes
- Recurrent late decelerations with moderate baseline variability
- Variable decelerations with other characteristics such as slow return to baseline, overshoots, or shoulders

Category III

Category III patterns are considered abnormal.

- Predictive of abnormal fetal acid-base status
- Require prompt evaluation

Characteristics:

Absent variability *and* recurrent late decelerations

OR

Recurrent variable decelerations

OR

Bradycardia

OR

Sinusoidal pattern

Criteria for identifying a sinusoidal FHR

1. A stable baseline FHR of 120~160 bpm with regular sine wave-like oscillations
2. An amplitude of 5 to 15 bpm
3. A frequency of 2 to 5 cycles/min
4. Fixed or absent short-term variability
5. Oscillation of the sine wave above and below the baseline

Fetal scalp blood sampling:

- An intrapartum scalp pH >7.20 with a base deficit < 6 mmol/L is normal.

Normal values of umbilical artery blood gas

- pH 7.26
- Partial pressure of oxygen 15 mm Hg
- Oxygen saturation 25%
- Partial pressure of carbon dioxide 48 mm Hg
- Base deficit 5 mmol/L

Deficits less than 12 mmol/L very rarely resulted in moderate or severe neurological signs

Base deficit – reflects - accumulation of metabolic acids (tell about severity and duration of hypoxic-ischemic insult)

Umbilical Artery pH and Neonatal Outcome (OR)

pH < 7.00 - perinatal mortality 6.1, perinatal morbidity - 12.5 (6.1–25.6)

8 Antenatal Steroid (ANS)

- Liggins and Howie observed that Lambs who received glucocorticoids and delivered prematurely had lungs that remained partially expanded
- 1972 —>Liggins and Howie performed a landmark RCT; Betamethasone given to mother antenatally → decreased RDS and mortality in there preterm babies.
- In pregnancies at risk for premature delivery, when treated with corticosteroids infants demonstrated a decreased risk of respiratory distress syndrome (RDS) compared with those not treated with steroids.3 Additionally, they found that early
- Neonatal mortality was 3.2% in the antenatal corticosteroid treated group and 15.0% in the controls (P 5 .01).
- From these early studies, Liggins 3 hypothesized that glucocorticoids caused premature liberation of surfactant into the alveoli, by induction of an enzyme related to the biosynthesis of surfactant.

EFFECTS OF ANS

1. ANS accelerates the effect of endogenous corticosteroids
2. induction of type II alveolar cells that increases surfactant production
3. Surfactant proteins A, B, C, and D are all increased
4. Increases enzymes necessary for phospholipid synthesis
5. Also stimulates lung structural development
6. Increase fetal pulmonary beta-receptors: releases surfactant & helps in absorption of alveolar fluid
7. Increase ENaC expression: facilitates perinatal lung liquid clearance

Effect of Antenatal Corticosteroid overall at different levels

- Thinning of the mesenchyme of the alveolar capillary structure
- Increased saccular an alveolar gas volume
- Decreased alveolar septation
- Increased surfactant
- Increase compliance
- Improved gas exchange
- Decreased epithelial permeability
- Improved surfactant treatment response
- Decreases inactivation of surfactant
- Decrease RDS
- No effect on BPD directly
- Decreased mortality

NICE guidelines for use of ANS

- 24- 34 weeks
- Consider – 23-24 weeks and 34-36 weeks
- Rescue dose not routinely given

ACOG guidelines for use of ANS

- 24-36/6
- Consider 23-24
- Single repeat course

RANZOG liggins institute guidelines for use of ANS

- 24-35 weeks
- Upto 39 weeks
- A maximum of 3 single repeat doses of ANS

WHO guidelines for use of ANS

- 24- 34 weeks
- Single repeat dose

How ANS reduces IVH

- Antenatal corticosteroids promote circulatory stability in the vulnerable vascular germinal matrix
- The precise molecular mechanism of action of how antenatal corticosteroids reduce IVH is unclear.
- Vascular endothelial growth factor promotes angiogenesis in the germinal matrix, which in rabbit

models has been thought to contribute to increased vascular fragility and hemorrhage.

- In vitro, the downregulation of vascular endothelial growth factor is accomplished by glucocorticoids, resulting in the suppression of angiogenesis in various disease models.
- Additional growth factors, as upregulated by glucocorticoids, have been found to play a key role in maturation of the vasculature in immature blood vessels

What is the ACOG recommendation for antenatal corticosteroid?

The American College of Obstetricians and Gynecologists recommends a single course of corticosteroids for women between 24 0/7 weeks' and 33 6/7 weeks' gestation, and recently extended this recommendation to include late preterm pregnancies (34 0/7–36 5/7 weeks' gestation). Antenatal steroids may also be considered for pregnant women as early as 23 0/7 weeks' gestation, who are at risk of preterm delivery within 7 days.

Role of antenatal corticosteroid in periviable period. (NICHD)

22 weeks GA – less death and NEC

23, 24, 25 weeks GA – less death and neurodevelopmental outcome, IVH, PVL, NEC

The Antenatal Steroids for Term Caesarean Section (ASTECS) randomized trial

They found significantly decreased rates in their primary outcome of RDS requiring admission to the neonatal intensive care unit (0.051 in the control group vs 0.024 in the treatment group; RR, 0.46; 95% CI, 0.23–0.93).

The ideal therapeutic window after administration is when delivery occurs 24 hours to 7 days after a complete course of treatment.

Dexa vs Betamethasone

- In a 2000 Consensus Panel convened by the NICHD, no significant scientific evidence supported the preferential benefit of betamethasone over dexamethasone.
- The American College of Obstetricians and Gynecologists notes the inconsistency of these data, and that no sufficient evidence supports the recommendation of one corticosteroid regimen over the other.

Doses

The standard treatment dose should consist of either (i) two 12-mg doses of betamethasone given intramuscularly 24 hours apart or (ii) four 6-mg doses of dexamethasone administered intramuscularly every 12 hours.

Compared with intramuscular dexamethasone, neonates given oral dexamethasone had a significantly increased incidence of neonatal sepsis (RR, 8.48; 95% CI, 1.11–64.93); no statistical differences were seen for other outcomes

When to give Rescue dose of antenatal steroid

The American College of Obstetricians and Gynecologists recommend a single repeat course of antenatal corticosteroids should be considered if:

(i) the patients is less than 34 0/7 weeks' gestation,

(ii) she is at imminent risk of delivery within the next 7 days, and

(iii) her prior course of antenatal corticosteroids was administered more than 14 days ago

Repeat administration reduced the risk of

- RDS (RR, 0.83; 95% CI, 0.75–0.91), and
- Composite serious infant outcome (RR, 0.84; 95% CI, 0.75–0.94).

When evaluating long-term childhood outcomes, no significant harm or benefit was observed with rescue course. Rescue corticosteroids could be considered as early as 7 days from the prior dose if the second course will be completed at less than 34 weeks' gestation.

Fetal side effects of antenatal corticosteroid

- Transient decreases in variability on external fetal heart rate monitoring
- Occasionally reduced scores on the biophysical profile for fetal breathing and body movements.
- Body movements were reduced on day 2 by 50% and breathing movements were largely absent on day 2; all values returned to baseline on day 4.
- Additionally observed was a transient improvement in umbilical artery end-diastolic flow, lasting up to 3 days.

Effect of multiple courses of antenatal steroid

- Infants exposed to multiple courses of steroids weighed less at birth were shorter and had a smaller head.
- increase in the number of small-for-gestational age infants

Features of Betamethasone:

- Half-life is - 72 hours with large volume of distribution
- Betamethasone (betamethasone sodium phosphate & betamethasone acetate): 2 doses of 12 mg im, 24 hours apart.
- Acetate is a long acting salt (not available in india)
- More costly
- Less stable at high temperatures
- Preparation available in India is Betamethasone phosphate —> short acting- Requires more frequent administration

Features of Dexamethasone:

- Half-life is - 60 hrs thus more frequent dosing
- Dose of Dexamethasone: 4 doses of 6 mg im,12 hours apart
- Substantially cheaper
- More readily available
- Can be stored at room temperature
- Less likely to decrease fetal breathing movements and fetal heart rate variability Compared to betamethasone

Dexamethasone Sodium Phosphate available in India

- Is available in 4 mg per ml strength.
- Dose 6 mg each every 12 hourly for 4 doses Four doses (equivalent to 24 mg total
- Deep Intramuscular
- Preferably anterolateral aspect of thigh
- 2 ml disposable syringes and 22/23 gauge needles
- No need to refrigerate

Why betamethasone & dexamethasone is preferred compared to other steroid?

- Have identical biologic activity, and readily cross the placenta. They are devoid of mineralocorticoid activity.
- Have relatively weak immunosuppressive actions.
- Have longer duration of action in comparison with cortisol and methylprednisolone. (**Betacode trial)**
- They are less extensively metabolized by the placental enzyme 11-beta hydroxysteroid dehydrogenase type 2

Higher dose – doubling the dose of betamethasone to 24 mg per day was not associated with increased efficacy.

Shorter dosing interval – Shortening the dosing interval been proposed to increase the probability of completing the steroid course before delivery. The safety and effectiveness of this approach are unclear as it is supported by limited low-quality evidence.

Why Intravenous steroid not given for lung maturity?

- The clinical efficacy has not been studied in human pregnancy.
- Intravenous administration results in rapid peaks and troughs in maternal and fetal steroid concentrations.
- This produces less sustained fetal exposure to corticosteroid stimulation and thus may not be as effective as intramuscular administration.

Cochrane review 2017, 30 studies (7774 women and 8158 infants)

1. Reduction in: **perinatal death (RR 0.72**, 95% CI 0.58 to 0.89; participants = 6729; moderate-quality)
2. **Neonatal death (RR 0.69**, 95% CI 0.59 to 0.81; participants = 7188; studies = 22)
3. RDS (average RR 0.66, 95% CI 0.56 to 0.77; participants = 7764; studies = 28; -quality)
4. **Moderate/severe RDS (average RR 0.59,** 95% CI 0.38 to 0.91; participants = 1686; studies = 6;
5. **IVH (average RR 0.55**, 95% CI 0.40 to 0.76; participants = 6093; studies = 16; moderate-quality)
6. **NEC (RR 0.50**, 95% CI 0.32 to 0.78; participants = 4702; studies =10)
7. **Need for mechanical ventilation (RR 0.68,** 95% CI 0.56 to 0.84; participants = 1368; studies = 9)
8. **Systemic infections in the first 48 hours of life (RR 0.60,** 95% CI 0.41 to 0.88; participants = 1753; studies = 8)

COCHRANE 2020 EMMA GOLDRICK

- 27 studies (11,272 randomised women and 11,925 neonates) from 20 countries. Ten trials (4422 randomised women) took place in lower or middle resource settings.
- In 19 trials the women received a single course of steroids. In the remaining eight trials repeated courses may have been prescribed
- **Perinatal death** (risk ratio) **(RR) 0.85,** 95% confidence interval (CI) 0.77 to 0.93; 9833 infants; 14 studies; high certainty evidence;
- **Neonatal death** (RR 0.78, 95% CI 0.70 to 0.87; 10,609 infants; 22 studies; high certainty evidence);

- **Respiratory distress syndrome** (RR 0.71, 95% CI 0.65 to 0.78; 11,183 infants; studies = 26; high certainty evidence).
- **Antenatal corticosteroids probably reduce the risk of IVH (RR 0.58**, 95% CI 0.45 to 0.75; 8475 infants; 12 studies; moderate certainty evidence),
- little to no effect on birthweight (mean difference (MD) 14.02 g, 95% CI 33.79 to 5.76; 9551 infants; 19 studies; high certainty evidence).
- **Antenatal corticosteroids probably lead to a reduction in developmental delay in childhood (RR 0.51, 95% CI 0.27 to 0.97; 600 children; 3 studies; moderate certainty evidence; 3.8% fewer, 95% CI 0.2% to 5.7% fewer).**

Maternal outcomes

- Antenatal corticosteroids probably result in little to no difference in **maternal death** (RR 1.19, 95% CI 0.36 to 3.89; 6244 women; 6 studies; moderate certainty evidence),
- **Chorioamnionitis** (RR 0.86, 95% CI 0.69 to 1.08; 8374 women; 15 studies; moderate certainty evidence),
- **Endometritis** (RR 1.14, 95% CI 0.82 to 1.58; 6764 women; 10 studies; moderate certainty;)

ACS in late preterms Antenatal Late Preterm Steroids Trial (ALPS trial) 2016 by Gyami-Bannerman C et al:

- Administration of betamethasone led to significant decrease in need for respiratory support in first three days of life (RR 0.67)
- Reduction was only significant for TTN and BPD

Antenatal Steroids for Term Caesarean Section (ASTECS) trial

- Corticosteroids significantly decreased the rate of admission to the special care nursery for respiratory distress (RR, 0.46; 95% CI, 0.23-0.93)
- Rates of both RDS and TTN appeared to be reduced to an equivalent extent

ACS in LMIC- ACT Trial Althabe et al (2015)- The Antenatal Corticosteroids Trial (ACT)

- Conducted in six LMICs: Argentina, Guatemala, India, Kenya, Pakistan and Zambia
- Assessed the feasibility, effectiveness, and safety of use of ACS in mothers at risk of preterm birth at all levels of care in low and middle-income countries.
- But in all the births (all weights) - increased risk of neonatal mortality , increased still birth, increased maternal infection
- Intervention was associated with an increased OR of suspected maternal infection

ASTEROID TRIAL - Incidence of survival without neurosensory disability at age 2 years did not differ between dexamethasone and betamethasone.

(WHO ACTION-I) Trial

- Aimed - The safety and efficacy of antenatal glucocorticoids in women in low-resource countries who are at risk for preterm birth
- RCT, pregnant women between 26 weeks 0 days and 33 weeks 6 days
- n= 2852, Bangladesh, India, Kenya, Nigeria, and Pakistan
- Neonatal death occurred in 278 of 1417 infants (19.6%) in the dexamethasone group and in 331 of 1406 infants (23.5%) in the placebo group (relative risk, 0.84; 95% confidence interval [CI], 0.72 to 0.97; P=0.03).
- Stillbirth or neonatal death occurred in 393 of 1532 fetuses and infants (25.7%) and in 444 of 1519 fetuses and infants (29.2%), respectively (relative risk, 0.88; 95% CI, 0.78 to 0.99; P=0.04);
- The incidence of possible maternal bacterial infection was 4.8% and 6.3%, respectively (relative risk, 0.76; 95% CI, 0.56 to 1.03).
- There was no significant between-group difference in the incidence of adverse events.
- Among women in low-resource countries who were at risk for early preterm birth, the use of dexamethasone resulted in significantly lower risks of neonatal death alone and stillbirth or neonatal death than the use of placebo, without an increase in the incidence of possible maternal bacterial infection.

ACTION-II trial

- A double blind, randomized trial in four hospitals in India between 26 December 2017 to 21 May 2020. Pregnant women at risk of imminent preterm birth between 34 weeks 0 days and 36 weeks 0 days of gestation were recruited. Women were randomly assigned (1:1) to a course of 6 mg intramuscular dexamethasone or an identical placebo.
- Randomized 782 women, 391 to each arm.
- Neonatal death occurred in 11 of 412 liveborn babies (2.7%) in the dexamethasone group and 12 of 425

liveborn babies (2.8%) in the placebo group (RR 0.95; 95% CI 0.42–2.12).

- Any baby death occurred in 16 of 417 infants (3.8%) in the dexamethasone group and 19 of 432 infants (4.4%) in the placebo group (RR 0.87; 95% CI 0.45–1.67).
- Severe neonatal respiratory distress was infrequent in both groups (0.8% vs 0.5%; RR 1.56; 95% CI 0.26–9.29).
- Possible maternal bacterial infection did not differ between groups (2.3% vs. 3.8%, RR 0.60; 95% CI 0.27–1.35).
- Fewer neonates in the dexamethasone group required resuscitation at birth (RR 0.38, CI 0.15–0.97).
- Other secondary outcomes were similar in the two arms. The trial was stopped due to lower than expected prevalence of primary outcomes and slow recruitment
- Interpretation Antenatal dexamethasone did not result in a reduction in neonatal death, stillbirth or neonatal death, or severe neonatal respiratory distress in this trial. The overall trend of effects suggests that potential benefit of dexamethasone in late preterm cannot be excluded, and further trials are required.

WHO action III trial (result awaited)

The aim of this trial is to assess the benefits and possible harms of two regimens of antenatal corticosteroids, dexamethasone phosphate 4 × 6mg IM q12h and betamethasone phosphate 4 × 2mg IM q12h, compared to placebo, when given to pregnant women in the late preterm period (gestation age of 34 + 0 to 36 + 5 weeks) when they are at risk of preterm birth.

Government of India recommendation for ANS

Single course of injection of Dexamethasone to be administered to women with preterm labour (between 24 and 34 weeks of gestation) at all levels of health facilities in the public as well as the private sector.

WHO ACTION TRIAL

- Multicountry, randomized trial involving pregnant women between 26 weeks 0 days and 33 weeks 6 days of gestation who were at risk for preterm birth.
- 2852 women (and their 3070 fetuses)
- Intramuscular dexamethasone or identical placebo
- Neonatal death occurred in 278 of 1417 infants (19.6%) in the dexamethasone group and in 331 of 1406 infants (23.5%) in the placebo group (relative risk, 0.84; 95% confidence interval [CI], 0.72 to 0.97; P=0.03).
- Stillbirth or neonatal death occurred in 393 of 1532 fetuses and infants (25.7%) and in 444 of 1519 fetuses and infants (29.2%), respectively (relative risk, 0.88; 95% CI, 0.78 to 0.99; P=0.04);
- The incidence of possible maternal bacterial infection was 4.8% and 6.3%, respectively (relative risk, 0.76; 95% CI, 0.56 to 1.03). There was no significant between group difference in the incidence of adverse event

CONCLUSIONS

- Among women in low-resource countries who were at risk for early preterm birth, the use of dexamethasone resulted in significantly lower risks of neonatal death alone and stillbirth or neonatal death than the use of placebo, without an increase in the incidence of possible maternal bacterial infection

Antenatal Betamethasone for Women at Risk for Late Preterm Delivery (ALPS)

- Singleton pregnancy at 34 weeks 0 days to 36 weeks 5 days of gestation who were at high risk for delivery during the late preterm period (up to 36 weeks 6 days)
- Two injections of betamethasone or matching placebo 24 hours
- Neonatal composite of treatment in the first 72 hours (the use of continuous positive airway pressure or high-flow nasal cannula for at least 2 hours, supplemental oxygen with a fraction of inspired oxygen of at least 0.30 for at least 4 hours, extracorporeal membrane oxygenation, or mechanical ventilation) or stillbirth or neonatal death within 72 hours after delivery - in 165 of 1427 infants (11.6%) in the betamethasone group and 202 of 1400 (14.4%) in the placebo group (relative risk in the betamethasone group, 0.80; 95% confidence interval [CI], 0.66 to 0.97; P=0.02)
- Severe respiratory complications, transient tachypnea of the New-born, surfactant use, and bronchopulmonary dysplasia also occurred significantly less frequently in the betamethasone group.
- There were no significant between-group differences in the incidence of chorioamnionitis or neonatal sepsis.
- Neonatal hypoglycemia was more common in the betamethasone group than in the placebo group (24.0%

vs. 15.0%; relative risk, 1.60; 95% CI, 1.37 to 1.87; P<0.001).

- CONCLUSIONS
- Administration of betamethasone to women at risk for late preterm delivery significantly reduced the rate of neonatal respiratory complications

ANTENATAL CORTICOSTEROIDS FOR LATE PRETERM GESTATION IN LOW-RESOURCE COUNTRIES (ACTION-II)

(P) In women at risk of imminent late-preterm delivery between 340/7 to 360/7 weeks' gestation,

(I) Does intramuscular dexamethasone sodium phosphate to a maximum of four doses

(C) Compared to placebo,

(O) Reduce the risk of stillbirth, neonatal death, or severe neonatal respiratory distress in low resource countries?

Inclusion criteria: Pregnant women at 34 weeks 0 days to 36 weeks 0 days of gestation, who were at risk for delivery within the upcoming 48 hours

Primary outcome: Neonatal death within 28 days, any death (stillbirth/ neonatal death), severe respiratory distress and suspected or confirmed maternal bacterial infection.

No statistically significant difference was noted between the studied groups as regard any of primary outcome items:

(1) Neonatal mortality was reported in 2.7% of the dexamethasone group versus 2.8% in the placebo group (RR 0.95; 95% CI 0.42–2.12; P = 0.89),

(2) Any baby death occurrence rates was 3.8% in the dexamethasone group compared to 4.4% in the placebo group (RR 0.87; 95% CI 0.45–1.67; P = 0.89),

(3) Few neonates exhibited severe neonatal respiratory distress within the whole cohort (0.8% vs 0.5%; RR 1.56; 95% CI 0.26–9.29; P = 0.89).

(4) Possible maternal bacterial infection was 2.3% in dexamethasone group versus 3.8% in placebo group (RR 0.60; 95% CI 0.27–1.35; P = 0.002 for non-inferiority).

Neonates in dexamethasone group had significantly less need for resuscitation at birth compared to placebo (1.5% vs 3.8%; RR 0.38, 95% CI 0.15–0.97; P = 0.043)

No statistically significant difference between both arms regarding any of maternal or neonatal adverse events, including neonatal hypoglycemia.

CONCLUSION:

The authors conclude that antenatal dexamethasone use, compared with placebo, was not associated with reduced neonatal mortality or severe respiratory distress rates, however, it resulted less need for resuscitation at birth. Clinical benefits of antenatal steroid use cannot be excluded and further trials in low-resource countries are warranted.

ANTENATAL DEXAMETHASONE REDUCES MORTALITY IN PRETERM INFANTS IN LOW RESOURCE COUNTRIES

Oladapo, OT, et al. (2020). "Antenatal Dexamethasone for Early Preterm Birth in Low-Resource Countries" The New England Journal of Medicine. PMID: 33095526

(P) Premature infants born to mothers at risk for preterm delivery who are given

(I) Antenatal dexamethasone compared to

(C) Placebo have

(O) Reduced neonatal mortality and combined stillbirth and neonatal mortality, without resulting an increased maternal infection risk?

Primary outcome:

1. The incidence of neonatal death was significantly lower in the dexamethasone group compared to the placebo group (19.6% vs 23.5%; RR 0.84; 95% confidence interval [CI], 0.72 to 0.97; P=0.03).
2. The incidence of stillbirth or neonatal death was also significantly lower in the dexamethasone group compared to the placebo group (25.7% vs 29.2; RR 0.88; 95% CI 0.78 to 0.99, P=0.04).
3. Possible maternal bacterial infection was not higher in the dexamethasone group compared to the placebo group (4.8% vs 6.3%; RR 0.76; 95% CI 0.56 to 1.03; P=0.002 for non-inferiority).

Secondary outcome: The incidence of early neonatal death, severe respiratory distress syndrome 24 hours after birth, neonatal hypoglycemia 6 hours after birth, the use of CPAP, and the duration of oxygen therapy were all significantly lower in the dexamethasone group compared to the placebo group

CONCLUSION

Authors conclude that using antenatal dexamethasone for women at risk for imminent preterm birth in low resource settings significantly reduces the risks of neonatal death, and stillbirth or neonatal death, without increased harm to women or New-borns. Authors advocate for dexamethasone use in hospital settings where obstetric physicians can confirm the gestational age and identify women at risk for imminent preterm birth, and where resources for providing minimum standard neonatal care for premature New-borns are available, including access to CPAP and oxygen.

Effects of repeat prenatal corticosteroids given to women at risk of preterm birth: An individual participant data meta-analysis PLOS Medicine | https://doi.org/10.1371/journal.pmed.1002771 April 12, 2019

The primary outcomes for the infants were serious outcome, use of respiratory support, and birth weight z-scores; for the children, they were death or any neurosensory disability; and for the women, maternal.

Trials were eligible for inclusion if they randomised women considered at risk of preterm birth who had already received an initial, single course of prenatal corticosteroid seven or more days previously and in which corticosteroids were compared with either placebo or no placebo.

Eleven trials, conducted between 2002 and 2010, were identified as eligible:

1. There was no significant difference in the proportion of infants with a serious outcome (relative risk [RR] 0.92, 95% confidence interval [CI] 0.82 to 1.04, 5,893 infants, 11 trials, p = 0.33 for heterogeneity).
2. There was a reduction in the use of respiratory support in infants exposed to repeat prenatal corticosteroids compared with infants not exposed (RR 0.91, 95% CI 0.85 to 0.97, 5,791 infants, 10 trials, p = 0.64 for heterogeneity).
3. The number needed to treat (NNT) to benefit was 21 (95% CI 14 to 41) women/fetus to prevent one infant from needing respiratory support.
4. Birth weight z-scores were lower in the repeat corticosteroid group (mean difference í0.12, 95%CI í0.18 to í0.06, 5,902 infants, 11 trials, p = 0.80 for heterogeneity).

No statistically significant differences were seen for any of the primary outcomes for the child (death or any neurosensory disability) or for the woman (maternal sepsis

- Infants exposed to between 2–5 courses of repeat corticosteroids showed a reduction in both serious outcome and the use of respiratory support compared with infants exposed to only a single repeat course.
- However, increasing numbers of repeat courses of corticosteroids were associated with larger reductions in birth z-scores for weight, length, and head circumference

Antenatal betamethasone and incidence of neonatal respiratory distress after elective caesarean section: pragmatic randomised tria Antenatal Steroids for Term Elective Caesarean Section (ASTECS) Research Team

Objective: To test whether steroids reduce respiratory distress in babies born by elective caesarean section at term.

Interventions: The treatment group received two intramuscular doses of 12 mg betamethasone in the 48 hours before delivery. The control group received treatment as usual.

Outcome measures

The primary outcome was admission to special care baby unit with respiratory distress. Secondary outcomes were severity of respiratory distress and level of care in response

1. Of the 35 babies admitted to special baby units with respiratory distress, 24 were in the control group and 11 in the intervention group (P = 0.02).
2. The incidence of admission with respiratory distress was 0.051 in the control group and 0.024 in the treatment group (relative risk 0.46, 95% confidence interval 0.23 to 0.93).
3. The incidence of transient tachypnoea of the New-born was 0.040 in the control group and 0.021 in the treatment group (0.54, 0.26 to 1.12).
4. The incidence of respiratory distress syndrome was 0.011 in the control group and 0.002 in the treatment group (0.21, 0.03 to 1.32).

CONCLUSIONS

Antenatal betamethasone and delaying delivery until 39 weeks both reduce admissions to special care baby units with respiratory distress after elective caesarean section at term.

9 Maternal Medical Disease (PIH and GDM)

Pregnancy induced hypertension is defined as an increased BP first detected after 20 weeks of gestation. It usually returns to normal within 12 weeks post partum.

Pre-eclampsia is PIH + proteinuria or end organ dysfunction.

Chronic hypertension is hypertension detected before 20 weeks of gestation or persistent after 12 weeks post delivery.

Diagnosis is made by 2 elevated BP readings taken 4 hours apart

Anti-hypertensives commonly used in PIH.

- α methyl Dopa
- Labetolol
- Hydralazine
- Nifedipine

MgSO4 – used for prophylaxis for seizures

- Pritchard regime - the loading bolus dose of 4 g of MgSO4 is given slowly intravenously over 5-10 min and this is followed by 10 g given intramuscularly (5 g in each buttock).
- Zuspan regime - Loading dose 4 g magnesium sulfate intra- venously 20% over 20 minutes and maintenance dose 1 g/hour intravenously in infusion pump till 24 hours of delivery or last seizure whichever is later.

GDM

The WHO and FIGO recommendation for screening of GDM

Universal screening for GDM at 24-28 weeks

Fasting ≥126 mg/Dl OR 75gm 2hr BS ≥140 mg/dL. Suggestive of GDM.

The American & Canadian guidelines universal screening by two step approach.

50g one hour blood sugar test >140 mg/dL (screen positive)

If positive then 100gm OGTT 2 or more abnormal values GDM.

GDM

Def: Impaired Glucose Tolerance (IGT) with onset / first recognition during pregnancy.

National guideline:

Single step test (WHO recommendation)- 75gm glucose OGTT, irrespective of the last meal if BS >140 mg/dL after 2 hours. Suggestive of GDM

Universal screening at first antenatal contact if first test is negative repeat at 24-28 weeks of gestation.

If first time of contact is beyond 28 weeks, only one test.

Postpartum period, OGTT should be repeated at 6 weeks after delivery, if BS<140 mg/dL, refer to NCD clinic for Post Prandial Blood Sugar testing annually.

75 gm glucose in 300 ml water irrespective of the last meal given within 5-10 minutes evaluates BS after 2 hours.

If vomits within 30 minutes of intake, repeat the next day/ refer to a facility. If vomits after 30 minutes continue the test.

Criteria for the Diagnosis of Type 2 Diabetes Mellitus

Symptoms of diabetes (polyuria, polydipsia, and unexplained weight loss)

+

Random plasma glucose level >200 mg/dL (11.1 mmol/L). (Irrespective of last meal)

OR

Fasting glucose level >126 mg/dL (7.0 mmol/L). (Fast for atleast 8 hrs)

Two-hour plasma glucose >200 mg/dL (11.1 mmol/L) during a 75-g OGTT.

Pathogenesis of malformations in fetus of mothers with GDM

- Reduced levels of arachidonic acid and *myo*-inositol and accumulation of sorbitol and trace metals in the embryo.
- Fetal hyperglycemia promotes excessive formation of

oxygen radicals in the mitochondria of susceptible tissues leads to formation of hydroperoxides which inhibit prostacyclin. The resulting overabundance of thromboxanes and other prostaglandins may then disrupt vascularization of developing tissues.

- Any elevation of the HbA1c above normal increases the risk of teratogenesis proportionately.

After 24 weeks, growth velocity of the IDM fetus abdominal circumference typically begins to rise above normal

Head growth and femur growth were similar to those of normal fetuses; abdominal circumference growth significantly exceeded that of controls beginning at 32 weeks' gestation

This central depositing of fat is a key characteristic of diabetic macrosomia and underlies the pathology associated with vaginal delivery in these pregnancies.

Pedersen (1952) hypothesized that maternal hyperglycemia stimulates fetal hyperinsulinemia, which in turn mediates acceleration of fuel utilization and growth.

10 Chorioamnionitis

Infection is associated directly or indirectly with 40% to 60% of preterm birth.

Intraamniotic infection has been shown to be commonly associated with preterm PROM, especially at earlier gestational ages.

How is premature rupture of membranes diagnosed?

- The visualization of amniotic fluid passing from the cervical canal and pooling in the vagina.
- A basic pH test of vaginal fluid (The normal pH of vaginal secretions is generally 4.5–6.0, whereas amniotic fluid usually has a pH of 7.1–7.3).
- Arborization (ferning) of dried vaginal fluid, which is identified under microscopic evaluation.

Among women with preterm PROM, clinically evident intraamniotic infection (chorioamnionitis) occurs in approximately 15–25%.

Chorioamnionitis complicates 1% to 5% of all pregnancies

When characteristic clinical signs are present, the condition is usually termed 'clinical chorioamnionitis'.

Histologic chorioamnionitis (inflammation of the chorion and amnion) is three times as common as clinical chorioamnionitis confirmed by amniotic fluid culture.

Two main varieties of chorioamnionitis can be identified:

- Acute chorioamnionitis
- Subclinical chorioamnionitis

Chorioamnionitis is almost always polymicrobial.

Ureaplasma urealyticum and *Mycoplasma hominis* are the most common organisms recovered (47% and 30%, respectively) in culture-proved chorioamnionitis

Other cultivable organisms include anaerobes, such as *Gardnerella vaginalis* (25%) and bacteroides (30%), and aerobes, including GBS (15%) and *Escherichia coli* (8%).

Diagnosis requires presence of the following:

- Maternal fever (≥100.4°F) plus two other findings
- Maternal leukocytosis,
- Maternal and fetal tachycardia,
- Uterine tenderness,
- Foul-smelling or purulent amniotic fluid

In ORACLE I study, a total of 4827 women with pPROM were divided into 4 groups.

In the Erythromycin vs placebo group- Among the 2260 singletons in this comparison, erythromycin group had significantly fewer neonatal deaths, CLD, and abnormal usg at discharge. (125 of 1111 [11.2%] vs 166 of 1149 [14.4%], p=0.02).

There was no difference between co amoxiclav and placebo groups in terms of primary outcomes or between co amoxiclav and erythromycin vs placebo.

In the ORACLE 2 study for preterm labour with intact membranes, there was no difference between antibiotics and placebo in terms of mortality, abnormal USG or CLD.

In the ORACLE study 7 year follow up, in the pPROM group there was no long term adverse outcomes including functional impairment or cerebral palsy.

But in preterm labour with intact membranes there was a higher incidence of cerebral palsy and functional impairment with erythromycin and co-amoxiclav.

Cochrane review for antibiotics in pprom was published in 2013.

- It included 22 trials, involving 6872 women and babies.
- There was a statistically significant reduction in abnormal cerebral ultrasound scan prior to discharge from hospital (RR 0.81, 95% CI 0.68 to 0.98).
- Co-amoxiclav was associated with an increased risk of neonatal necrotising enterocolitis (RR 4.72, 95% CI 1.57 to 14.23).
- There is no statistical difference between erythromycin and co amoxiclav in terms of the primary outcomes studied in this review except NEC.

Intrauterine Inflammation, Infection or both (Triple I)

Under the new proposal, Triple I is diagnosed when fever is present with one or more of the following:

1. Fetal Tachycardia (> 160 bpm for 10 minutes or longer)
2. Maternal WBC > 15,000 in absence of corticosteroids
3. Purulent fluid from the cervical os (cloudy or yellowish thick discharge confirmed visually on speculum exam to be coming from the cervical canal)
4. Biochemical or microbiologic amniotic fluid results consistent with microbial invasion of the amniotic cavity

The panel also recommended that the diagnosis of fever be standardized as follows:

- Maternal temperature ≥39.0 °C or 102.2 °F on one reading constitutes a fever.
- If the temperature is ≥38.0 °C or 100.4 °F but less than 39.0 °C or 102.2 °F, the temperature should be re-taken in 30 minutes for confirmation.
- A repeat temperature ≥38.0°C or 100.4°F constitutes a documented fever.19,20 For the diagnosis of fever, temperature should be measured orally

In order to be confirmed, Triple I should be accompanied by objective laboratory findings of infection in amniotic fluid (AF) (e.g. positive gram stain for bacteria, low AF glucose, high WBC count in the absence of a bloody tap, or positive AF culture results) or histopathological evidence of infection or inflammation or both in the placenta, fetal membranes or the umbilical cord vessels (funisitis). Cases can thus be categorized as follows:

1. Isolated maternal fever (not Triple I)
2. Suspected Triple I
3. Confirmed Triple

Suspected triple I

Fever without a clear source plus any of the following

- Fetal tachycardia > 160 for 10 minutes or longer
- Maternal wbc >15000 in absence of corticosteroid
- Definite purulent fluid from the cervical os

Confirmed triple I

All of the above plus

- Amniocentesis positive gram stain
- Low glucose or positive amniotic fluid culture
- Placental revealing infection

Broad-spectrum antibiotics for preterm, prelabour rupture of fetal membranes: the ORACLE I randomised trial

- 4826 women with pPROM were randomly assigned
  - o 250 mg erythromycin (n=1197),
  - o 325 mg co-amoxiclav (250 mg amoxicillin plus 125 mg clavulanic acid; n=1212),
  - o Both (n=1192),
  - o Or placebo (n=1225)
  - o Four times daily for 10 days or until delivery

Primary outcome measure was a composite of neonatal death, chronic lung disease, or major cerebral abnormality on ultrasonography before discharge from hospital

- Women allocated erythromycin only or placebo, fewer had the primary composite outcome of neonatal death, chronic lung disease, or major cerebral abnormality on ultrasonography before discharge from hospital in the erythromycin group (151 of 1190 [12·7%] vs 186 of 1225 [15·2%], p=0·08) than in the placebo group
- Co-amoxiclav only and co-amoxiclav plus erythromycin had no benefit over placebo with regard to this outcome in all infants or in singletons only.
- Use of erythromycin was also associated with prolongation of pregnancy, reductions in neonatal treatment with surfactant, decreases in oxygen dependence at 28 days of age and older, fewer major cerebral abnormalities on ultrasonography before discharge, and fewer positive blood cultures
- co-amoxiclav only and co-amoxiclav plus erythromycin were associated with prolongation of pregnancy, they were also associated with a significantly higher rate of neonatal necrotising enterocolitis

Broad-spectrum antibiotics for spontaneous preterm labour: the ORACLE II randomised trial

6295 women in spontaneous preterm labour with ***intact membranes and*** without evidence of clinical infection were randomly assigned

- 250 mg erythromycin (n=1611),
- 325mg co-amoxiclav (250 mg amoxicillin and 125 mg clavulanic acid; n=1550),

- Both (n=1565),
- Or placebo (n=1569)

Four times daily for 10 days or until delivery, whichever occurred earlier

The primary outcome measure was a composite of neonatal death, chronic lung disease, or major cerebral abnormality on ultrasonography before discharge from hospital

None of the trial antibiotics was associated with a lower rate of the composite primary outcome than placebo

This trial provides evidence that antibiotics should not be routinely prescribed for women in spontaneous preterm labour without evidence of clinical infection.

11 Periviable Birth

Periviable birth is currently defined as delivery occurring from 20 0/7 through 25 6/7 weeks of gestation

Newborn outcome specific descriptions of eraly preterm birth	
Previable	Not sufficiently developed to survive outside the uterus
Marginal viability	23 0/7 through 26 6/7 wk of gestation
Threshold of viability	At or before 25 wk of gestation or < 750g, 23–25 wk of gestation
Periviable	20 0/7 through 25 6/7 wk of gestation

A consensus statement by the American College of Obstetricians and Gynecologists and the Society for Maternal-Fetal Medicine

Provision of ANS, caesarean delivery for fetal indication, and neonatal assessment for resuscitation

- At 20 to 21 weeks: are not recommended
- At 22 weeks: Clinicians may consider
- At 23 weeks: active treatment; but do not give a firm recommendation for any of them
- At 24 weeks: caesarean delivery should be considered and all active measures recommended
- At 25 weeks: caesarean delivery and all other active treatment recommend

Interventions Available Before a Periviable Birth

Surgical Interventions:

- Cerclage (greatest impact specific to periviable outcomes)
- Amniocentesis

Medical Interventions:

- Progesterone
- Corticosteroids
- Magnesium sulphate
- Tocolysis

2017 consensus of ACOG and Society of Maternal-Fetal Medicine on Pre-viable birth recommends

- 24 0/7 weeks onwards: Resuscitation to be done
- 22 0/7 to 23 6/7 weeks: Considers resuscitation
- Below 22 weeks: resuscitation is not recommended

IMA/IAP/NNF policy

- 20-24 weeks: not viable and no resuscitation
- 24-28 weeks: case to case basis decision to be taken

12 Placenta

Events after fertilization

- 1st day : Fertilization
- 2nd day : 2 cell zygote blastomere
- 3rd day : Morula:16 cells

The morula consists of two groups of cells: • Inner Cell Mass (Central Cells) • Outer Cell Mass (Peripheral Cells)

At 9th day Implantation: Blastocysts: 2 layers • Embryoblast derived from Inner Cell Mass • Trophoblast derived from Outer Cell Mass: the invading cells

Trophoblast differentiation • Syncytiotrophoblast: outer multinuclear • Cytotrophoblast: inner mononuclear

Stages in formation of placenta

- Implantation day 6-7
- Prelacunar period day 7-8
- Lacunar day 8-9
- Primary villus day 12-15
- Secondary villus day 15-21
- Tertiary villus day 18-term

Maternofetal barrier-components contains following layers

- Syncytiotrophoblast
- Cytotrophoblast
- Trophoblastic basal lamina
- Connective tissue
- Fetal endothelial basal lamina
- Fetal endothelium

The mean maternofetal diffusion distance decreases from 50-100 μm to 4-5 μm at term

Mechanisms of placental transfer

- Diffusion
- Facilitated diffusion
- Active transport
- Receptor mediated endocytosis

Endocrine functions of placenta

- Human chorionic gonadotrophin
- Progesterone
- Human placental lactogen/human chorionic
- Somatomammotrophin
- Hypothalamic-like releasing and inhibiting
- Peptides: CRH, GnRH, TRH et

Human chorionic gonadotrophin

- Secreted by syncytiotrophoblasts
- Detected in maternal circulation 24 hours after implantation
- Peaks by 9-10 weeks
- Doubling time: 2.11 days
- Stimulates formation of corpus luteum • Placental steroidogenesis • Facilitate implantation • Progesterone secretion • Immunosupressive function

Human chorionic somatomammotrophin (hCS)

- In maternal circulation
  - Mobilizes Free fatty acids
  - Insulin resistance
- Affect fetal growth by
  - Regulating IGF-1
  - Placental nutrient transport

Macroscopic Features of normal Placenta

- 90% of the cases, a disk-like, flat, round to oval
- 10% it has abnormal shapes, such as – Placenta bilobata, placenta duplex, placenta succenturiata, and placenta membranacea.
- The average diameter is 22 cm,
- Thickness in the center is 2.5 cm, & Weight 470 g
- The fetal surface of the mature placenta is "bosselated" by presence of tiny white elevations underneath the chorion, giving the surface a mosaic, irregular pattern

- The amnion has no blood vessels, so it's transparent.

Maternal Surface of placenta

Cotyledons are is subdivision of the maternal surface of the placenta. – Divided by septa made up of infolding of decidua and extravillous trophoblast. – Normally 10 to 40 in numbers

Causes of Low weight placenta:

- Low maternal weight
- Low wt gain
- High maternal Hb
- PIH

Causes of Placentomegaly

- Immune haemolytic anemia
- Hydrops
- Non immune chronic anaemia
- Cardiac failure
- Fetal hypoproteinemia
- Placental tumours
- IDM

Amnion nodosum

The amnion is rough and shows numerous fine granules which are whitish, opaque, raised lesions of uniform (around 5 mm) size

Nodules can be easily dislodged • Histologically, consists of granular material containing fetal cells and debris with occasional hair fragments

The presence of amnion nodosum accompanies oligohydromnios, which can be secondary to urinary tract obstruction or renal agenesis

It signifies probable presence of pulmonary hypoplasia.

Meconium-containing macrophages present within the amnion within 1 hour of meconium exposure and within the chorion within 3 hour

Placenta in Chorioamnionitis

In chorioamnionitis the fetal surface appears dull and opaque with an obscure vascular pattern. • The amniotic fluid is cloudy, and the placenta, membranes, and amniotic fluid may have a foul odour

Functions of placenta

- Gas exchange
- Nutrient transfer
- Neuroendocrine organ
- Metabolism
- Barrier function

Gross examination of placenta

- Odour
- Shape, size
- Colour, consistency
- Accessory lobe
- Membrane (invert them)

- Site of tear
- Insertion
- Colour :opaque , green
- Squamous metaplasia, amnion nodosom
- Amniotic band

Examination of Cord

- Length ,Coiling
- Attachment
- Knot, Constriction, Swelling
- Thrombosis,
- Umbilical Vessel

Examination of Fetal surface of placenta

- Colour & contour
- Vessels
- Thrombus

Examination of Maternal surface of placenta

- Abruption (fresh /old)
- Infarction
- Calcification
- Cotyledons, subdivisions of placenta
- Cut surface
- Color : dark red vs pale
- Intervillous thrombi & infarcts
- Chorioangiomas
- On histologic examination some infarcts" may turn out to be Choriocarcinoma

Amniotic band syndrome

Amnion rupture sequence, Amniotic deformity, adhesion and mutilation (ADAM) complex

- The abnormalities range from constriction rings,

amputations, and syndactyly, fusion defects of the cranium and face, and clefts caused by either mechanical vascular effect

- On histopathology amnion is absent from fetal surface

Umbilical cord anomaly: cord length

- Cord length is dependent on the stretch provided by fetal intrauterine motor activity
- Normal length: 54 and 61 cm at term.
- An abnormally short cord is defined as being less than 35 cm, and long cord more than 86 cm or more than 2sd from mean (national collaborative perinatal study, Naeye et al.)
- Normal length needed for vertex vaginal delivery is 32 cm
- Boys have slightly longer cord than girl

Features of Short cords

- Incidence of short cords is 0.4% to 0.9%.
- Can be found in maternal ingestion of beta-blockers, twin pregnancy, uterine abnormalities, or reduced amniotic fluid volume, infants with decreased limb movement and down syndrome.
- Short cord are associated with SGA, fetal distress, placental separation, or cord rupture

Features of Long cords

- Incidence is 0.5% to 3.7%
- Long cord can cause entanglement, formation of knots, strangulation, prolapse, difficult delivery, blood volume shift

Coiling /twisting of umbilical cord

- Most of the times twisting of cord are counter clockwise.
- The coiling index, as measured by counting the number of coils (coils/cm) is about 0.20. Range is 0.17 to 0.49 for placental 0.72 for the fetal end.
- Complete absence of coiling is found in 4.3% of cords.
- It is associated with abnormal karyotypes, single umiblical artery, twinning & adverse perinatal outcome
- Abnormally low twisting have high incidence of fetal heart rate disturbances.
- High twisting is seen with preterm birth & maternal cocaine use.

Velamentous insertion of the cord

- The cord inserts into the membranes
- The vessels run unprotected in the membranes predisposing them to compression & danger of vessel rupture
- Found in 2% of cases
- If associated with vasa previa the perinatal mortality 75 to 100%

Single umbilical artery (SUA)

- This anomaly is present in 0.7 to 1.0% of single placentas and in 3 to 7.0% of multiple birth placentas.
- Perinatal autopsy series the incidence varied from 2.7% to 12%.
- Female have more incidence of of SUA
- The incidence is increased in infant with associated congenital malformations.
- It is associated with maternal diabetes and maternal smoking
- Also with LBW, PT & IUGR
- An increase in fetal malformation is reported in association with single umbilical artery in between 20% and 50% of cases
- Frequently associated malformations are sirenomelia sequence, VACTERL complex and anorectal atresia and esophageal atresia
- A significant proportion of asymptomatic infants born with a single umbilical artery have occult renal anomalies
- SUA is seen more frequently in trisomy 13, trisomy 18, and Zellweger syndromes. (not in trisomy 21)
- Further investigation is recommended if a single umbilical artery is associated with one other major anomaly

Placenta in multiple pregnancy

- A dichorionic septum usually has a small ridge where it turns up from the placental surface (USG delta sign)
- The membrane is lift up from surface and observed
- Dichorionic membrane looks opaque whereas,
- Monochorionic membrane looks transparent.
- Ideally the layers should be divided & counted.

13 Preterm Birth

Definition of Preterm labour

- Regular uterine contraction accompanied by progressive dilatation and cervical effacement before 37 weeks
  - At least 6 contractions/ hr
  - cervical dilatation > 3 cm
  - effacement at least 80%
  - Ruptured membranes +/- bleeding.

Conditions leading to preterm birth-

1. **Spontaneous preterm birth**
   - Idiopathic (45-50%)
   - Preterm prelabour rupture of membrane (30%)
2. **Provider initiated preterm birth**
   - Medical indication (maternal or fetal) (15 – 20%
   - Preeclampsia – 43%
   - Fetal distress – 28%
   - Intrauterine growth restriction – 10%
   - Abruption – 7%
   - Fetal demise – 7%

Factors leading to preterm birth

1. Decline in progesterone action
2. Cervical disease
3. Uterine overdistension
4. Decidual senescence
5. Breakdown of maternal fetal tolerance
6. Stress
7. Vascular disorders
8. Infection
9. Unknown

Endocrinology of Parturition

- Progesterone
- Estrogen
- Corticotropin releasing harmone
- Oxytocin

Placental CRH acts as a clock controlling the length of pregnancy.

Elevated CRH levels and fall in CRH binding protein in pregnancy in mothers with Preterm labour

Adrenal steroids, Prostaglandins and oxytocin have a direct positive feedback on placental CRH

No increase in circulating oxytocin with onset of labor and normal parturition observed in pituitary gland dysfunction also.

Oxytocin receptors are upregulated and OTR m RNA concentrations upregulated in OT binding sites.

Acts via Inositol triphosphate and cyclic AMP pathway

Fetal Brain growth in last trimester of pregnancy

- Cerebral surface area triples between 25 & 40 weeks due to gyrification.
- Crucial development (24 to 32 weeks): neurogenesis, proliferation of axons in periventricular regions, development of the oligodendrocytes (OL), astrocytes and microglia, synaptogenesis, and myelination.
- OL: myelinating cells in the brain play a critical role in the maturation of white matter.
- Microglia: synaptogenesis and tissue repair.
- Cerebellum: 5-fold increase in volume between 24 & 40 weeks of GA

A total of 40 - 60% of survivors born at < 28 weeks of gestation still develop moderate or severe NDI in form of cerebral palsy (CP), intellectual disability, deafness, and blindness.

Incidence of CP with GA

• 22–27 weeks of GA:	• 14.6%
• 28–31 weeks GA:	• 6.2%
• 32–36 weeks GA:	• 0.7%
• Term:	• 0.1%

Morbidities associated with prematurity

- Increased risk of cognitive impairment 10-35%,
- Emotional disturbances 25%,
- Socio-adaptive and behavior disorders 35%
- (Autism Spectrum Disorder 20%,
- Attention Deficit Hyperactivity Disorder10- 20%)

The hallmark of preterm brain injury includes

- Periventricular WMI: ranges from focal cystic necrosis to diffuse non-necrotic lesions.
- Diffuse microcystic WMI is more common currently.
- Dysmaturation and maturational arrest are emerging as key factors in preterm encephalopathy.
- Cerebellar injury, secondary to cerebellar hemorrhage, is now recognized as the important complication of preterm birth leading to NDI. Cerebellar atrophy can be seen as early as 2 months after hemorrhage.
- Cerebellar injury: cognitive deficits, language impairment, and autism spectrum disorder

Antenatal interventions to improve perinatal outcome

- Antenatal steroid
- MgSO4
- Antibiotic prophylaxis
- Tocolysis
- Mode of delivery
- Others: Progesterone, DHA, Choline, NAC

Delivery room interventions to improve perinatal outcome

- Optimal management of preterm delivery
- DCC / UCM
- Plastic wraps
- CPAP in DR

Postnatal interventions

- Prevention & management of acute illnesses of prematurity
- Aggressive nutrition and human milk feeding
- Developmentally Supportive Care (DSC)
- Family Centered Care (Kangaroo Mother care)
- Pain management
- Pharmacotherapy

Magnesium sulphate for antenatal neuroprotection

- Meta-analysis (11 observational studies)- MgSO4 significantly reduces mortality (RR 0.73; 95% CI 0.61-0.89) and cerebral palsy (OR 0.64; 95% CI 0.47-0.89
- Recommended (strong- moderate quality evidence) to use in less than 32 weeks GA

MOA OF MGSO4

- Noncompetitive NMDA receptor antagonist
- Decreases extracellular glutamate under ischemic conditions
- Limits calcium influx through voltage gated channel-limits apoptosis

Reduced IL 6 and TNF alpha (See Table)

- **25% of all cases of CP are in infants born < 34 weeks of gestation.**

Cochrane

- Concluded that antenatal magnesium sulphate therapy

MagNET (Magnesium and neurological Endpoints Trials)	Increased mortality in MgSO4 group. Stopped prematurely.
ACTOMgSO4 (Australasian colloborative trial of MgSO4)	CP rates similar (RR 0.85; 95 CI 0.55-1.31)Motor dysfunction decreased in MgSO4 group (RR 0.53; CI 0.3-0.92)
PREMAG trial	White matter injury similar (RR 0.78; CI 0.47-1.31)Death/ motor dysfunction less with MgSO4 (RR 0.62; CI 0.41-0.93)
BEAM (Beneficial Effects of Antenatal MgSO4)	Pediatric mortality- no impactModerate to severe CP reduced in MgSO4 (RR 0.55; CI 0.32-0.95)
MAGPIE (MgSO4 for prevention of Eclampsia	Pediatric follow up showed no difference in neurological outcome or mortality at 18 months

Magnesium Sulphate to Prevent Cerebral Palsy following Preterm Birth

given to women at risk of preterm birth substantially **reduced the risk of cerebral palsy in their children with a relative risk of 0.68 (95% CI 0.54–0.87).**

- There was also a significant **reduction in the rate of substantial gross motor dysfunction** (RR 0.61; 95% CI 0.44–0.85).
- When only those trials using magnesium sulphate for neuroprotection were analysed as a subgroup, a similar magnitude of reduction was seen (RR 0.71; 95%CI 0.55-0.91).

All used a **loading dose of magnesium sulphate that varied between 4 and 6 g. Not all trials administered a maintenance infusion and in those that did, the dose varied: 1 g/hr, 2 g/hr or 2–3 g/hr**

Vaginal progesterone prophylaxis for preterm birth (the OPPTIMUM study): a multicentre, randomised, double-blind trial

Double-blind, randomised, placebo-controlled trial of vaginal progesterone, 200 mg daily taken from 22–24 to 34 weeks of gestation, on pregnancy and infant outcomes in women at risk of preterm birth.

Vaginal progesterone was not associated with reduced risk of preterm birth or composite neonatal adverse outcomes, and had no long-term benefit or harm on outcomes in children at 2 years of age.

14 Care in Delivery Room

Apgar score and other important information at birth

- Score at 1 and 5 minutes for all infants, and if the score is less than 7, keep scoring at every 5 minutes until 20 minutes have passed or until two successive scores of 7 or greater are obtained
- Among all components colour correlates the least with umbilical pH, arterial carbon dioxide and base excess
- Low Apgar scores are not diagnostic of asphyxia.
- A term fetus swallows approximately 450 ml of amniotic fluid each day
- Gastric emptying of a term baby 20 ml/hour.
- Aspiration > 15 ml is abnormal
- >25 ml is always abnormal and suggests an obstruction at the pylorus or duodenum.
- Immediately after birth, healthy term infants are awake for 30 to 60 minutes start breastfeeding in this period
- After initial wakefulness, infants sleep for several hours.
- Infants who remain alert, stare, or fail to go into a quiet sleep are likely demonstrating neurologic irritability.
- Premature infants may not demonstrate this period of alertness followed by sleep.
- Crown-rump/ total length ratio the mean value is 0.653 at 27 weeks to 0.673 at 40 weeks.

Ensure strict asepsis at birth & follow 7 cleans strictly:

What are the 7 cleans?

Clean hands, clean surface, clean scissor / blade, clean tie, clean gauze (for eyes), clean umbilical cord and clean perineum.

Recommended delivery room temperature

NRP DR temp -23 to 25 ^{O}C

Indian NRP DR temp – 25 to 27 ^{O}C

Delay the cord clamping for at least 30 – 60 seconds for vigorous term and preterm neonates.

Clamp the cord immediately if placental circulation is not intact, e.g. placental abruption, bleeding placenta previa or cord avulsion.

Use sterile disposable cord clamp instead of cord ties. Length: 2-3 cm proximal and 2-3 cm distal to clamp/tie. Inspect the cord every 15-30 minutes for initial few hours after birth for early detection of any oozing from the cord.

Resuscitate if required as per NRP guidelines.

Assess vital signs.

Wipe the infant dry with pre-warmed sheets. Remember to dry the infant's body except hands. Leave amniotic fluid on hands as it is helpful in facilitating Breast Crawl. Remove wet sheets & wrap with a fresh pre-warmed sheet.

Skin-to-skin (STS) contact with the mother immediately after birth: Place the infant in chest-to-chest contact with the mother, covering them both with a warm sheet or cover. In addition to maintaining normal temperature of the neonate, STS promotes early breastfeeding and decreases the pain and bleeding in the mother.

Delay, minimize or eliminate postpartum procedures that interfere with first contact. Minimize suctioning & do gently if needed. Infants who cry immediately and do not have significant oral secretions do not need routine suctioning. Delay Vitamin K injection until after first contact

Collect cord blood sample as directed under following situations:

1. All infants requiring resuscitation: umbilical arterial sample for cord ABG.
2. Rh Negative mothers: blood group, bilirubin, DCT & Hb and PCV.
3. Mothers with O blood group: blood group, DCT.
4. For Infant of a diabetic mother: cord sugar.

Do a brief examination of the infant to ensure the following as described below:

1. Infant has achieved early transition.
2. To assess weight and gestational age to determine

whether the infant can be kept with mother or needs transfer to the neonatal unit.

3. To detect life threatening congenital anomalies at the earliest.
4. To initiate early Skin to Skin contact, Breast Crawl and Breastfeeding
5. To detect other problems if any

Do not attempt to remove vernix as it can result in trauma to skin and chances of infection.

Do not give routine baby bath. Wipe with warm, moist gauze if the infant is smeared with blood or meconium. Be sure to dry the area to avoid hypothermia.

Do not give routine stomach wash after birth. If the infant is born through meconium stained liquor, aspirate the stomach and give stomach wash.

Vitamin K

- Administer Vit. K (K1 preferably) 1mg IM to all term and 0.5 mg IM to all preterm infants to prevent Vitamin K Deficiency Bleeding (VKDB).
- To prevent hemorrhagic disease of the New-born (see Haematology) caused by insufficient prenatal storage of Vitamin K and Vitamin K in breastmilk
- Oral Vitamin K is inferior to IM

Administer vaccines (as per policy): zero dose polio, hepatitis B and BCG in DR Complete the formalities of infant identification including showing the infant to the mother / relative, even for infants who are to be transferred for specialized care.

Perform detailed head to toe examination once the infant is stable & breastfeeding is established.

Confirming whether the infant has achieved early transition:

- Note vital signs. When the infant cries well immediately after birth, it suggests that transition from the intra uterine to the extra uterine environment has occurred satisfactorily. Yet check that the respiratory rate is normal 40-60 breaths per minute, heart rate is above 100 and that the infant is pink.
- The respiratory rate during early transition ranges from 60 to 100 bpm & then slows to 50 to 60 bpm. This is particularly true for infants born of an elective caesarean section.
- Healthy infants may continue to breathe well above 60 bpm; they do not appear distressed & can slow their rate enough to feed successfully. Infants with hyperventilation to compensate for metabolic acidosis, to increase O2 intake or to eliminate CO2 are unlikely to slow their rate enough to feed successfully.
- Observe for alertness. Healthy term infants are generally awake for 30 -60 mins immediately after birth with intermittent gross body movements and then asleep for several hours. Such movements are indicative of a healthy infant.
- Term infants without period of wakefulness before sleep may be lethargic and term infants who fail to go into quite sleep may be neurologically irritable. Preterm infant may not demonstrate above states

Weigh the baby, assign sex & assess gestational age:

Assessment of weight & gestational age helps to decide whether infant can be roomed in with mother or needs observation in the neonatal unit.

Initiation of Breastfeeding

Initiate breastfeeding within the first hour after birth. This stimulates the prolactin reflex, initiates lactation, and promotes bonding. Secretion of oxytocin enhances expulsion of the placenta & limits the post-partum blood loss.

Breast Crawl:

1. Placed the infant prone on mother's abdomen immediately after cutting the cord if the baby is vigorous and becoming pink.
2. Allow the infant to crawl to breast to latch onto the nipple to initiate breastfeeding. Smell of amniotic fluid preserved on hands facilitates successful breast crawl. Not to wipe the hand of the baby.
3. Let the baby take lead & avoid take over behaviour.
4. Breast crawl generally occurs within 50 - 60 mins after birth.
5. Do not leave the mother and infant unattended during this period.

FBNC guidelines for New-born care corner

- New-born Care Corner (NCC) is a space (20-30 sqft) within delivery room (DR) and maternity operation theatre where immediate care is provided to all New-borns
- This area is mandatory for all health facilities where deliveries take place in order to provide acceptable environment to all infants after birth.

Preterm Infant Outcomes after Randomization to Initial Resuscitation with FiO2 0.21 or 1.0 Ola D. Saugstad

To determine rates of death or neurodevelopmental impairment (NDI) at 2 years corrected age (primary outcome) in children

Initial resuscitation of infants <32 weeks' gestation with initial FiO2 0.21 had no significant effect on death or NDI compared with initial FiO2 1.0.

Further evaluation of optimum initial FiO2, including SpO2 targeting, in a large randomized controlled trial is needed

Resuscitation with room air

Preterm (less than 35 weeks of gestation)

- Meta-analysis of 7 randomized trials
- Initiating resuscitation: high oxygen ≥ 65% and low oxygen (21% to 30%)
- **No improvement in survival to hospital discharge with the use of high oxygen.**
- No benefit was seen for the prevention of BPD, IVH, or ROP.

When oxygen targeting was used as a cointervention, the oxygen concentration of resuscitation gas and the preductal oxygen saturation were similar between the high- oxygen and low oxygen groups within the first 10 minutes of life

Delivery Room Interventions for Hypothermia in Preterm Neonates: A Systematic Review and Network Meta-analysis *Thangaraj Abiramalatha*

Objective: To identify the delivery room thermal care intervention that can best reduce neonatal hypothermia and improve clinical outcomes for preterm neonates born at 36 weeks' gestation or less.

Compared with routine care alone, plastic bag or wrap with a thermal mattress (mean difference [MD], 0.98 °C; 95% credible interval [CrI], 0.60-1.36 °C),

- cap (MD, 0.83 °C; 95% CrI, 0.28-1.38 °C),
- bag or wrap with heated humidified respiratory gas (MD, 0.76 °C; 95% CrI, 0.38-1.15 °C),
- bag or wrap with a plastic cap (MD, 0.62 °C; 95% CrI, 0.37-0.88 °C),
- mattress (MD, 0.62 °C; 95% CrI, 0.33-0.93 °C), plastic bag or wrap (MD, 0.56 °C; 95% CrI, 0.44-0.69 °C), associated with greater core body temperature.

When compared with routine care alone, a plastic bag or wrap with heated humidified respiratory gas was associated with less risk of major brain injury (risk ratio, 0.23; 95% CrI, 0.03-0.67; moderate certainty of evidence),

A plastic bag or wrap with a plastic cap was associated with decreased risk of mortality (risk ratio, 0.19; 95% CrI, 0.02-0.66; low certainty of evidence).

Conclusions and relevance:

Results of this study indicate that most thermal care interventions in the delivery room for preterm neonates were associated with improved core body temperature (with moderate certainty of evidence).

Specifically, use of a plastic bag or wrap with a plastic cap or with heated humidified gas was associated with lower risk of major brain injury and mortality (with low to moderate certainty of evidence).

Maintaining normothermia immediately after birth in preterm infants <34 weeks' gestation: A systematic review and meta-analysis 2023

V.V. Ramaswamy, J.A. Dawson, M.F. de Almeida et al., Maintaining normothermia immediately after birth in preterm infants<34 weeks' gestation: A systematic review and meta-analysis, Resuscitation

DR temperature of ≥ 23C, radiant warmer in manual mode, use of a plastic bag or wrap and a head covering is suggested for preterm New-born infants <34 weeks' gestation.

Heated humidified gases and thermal mattresses could be considered in addition to plastic bag or wrap provided if resources allow, in settings where hypothermia incidence is high. Careful monitoring to avoid hyperthermia is needed.

DR temperature 24–26 C versus 20–23 C. A higher DR temperature possibly resulted in higher mean body temperature (CoE: very low) and a lower rate of moderate hypothermia CoE: very low)

Comparison of devices for New-born ventilation in the delivery room

Objective: To evaluate the effectiveness and safety of a T-piece resuscitator compared with a self-inflating bag for providing mask ventilation to New-borns at birth

- There was no statistically significant difference in the incidence of HRe"100 bpm at 2 minutes after birth between the T-piece and self-inflating ba,
- Total of 86 New-borns (17%) in the T-piece group and 134 New-borns (26%) in the self-inflating bag group were intubated in the delivery room (OR, 0.58;

95% CI, 0.4-0.8; P=.002). The mean±SD maximum positive inspiratory pressure was 26±2 cm H2O in the T-piece group vs 28±5 cm H2O in the self-inflating bag group (P<.001). Air leaks, use of drugs/chest compressions, mortality, and days on mechanical ventilation did not differ significantly between groups.

Conclusion

There was no difference between the T-piece resuscitator and a self-inflating bag in achieving an HR of ≥100 bpm at 2 minutes in New-borns ≥26 weeks gestational age resuscitated at birth. However, use of the T-piece decreased the intubation rate and the maximum pressures applied.

15 Delayed Cord Clamping

Delayed umbilical cord clamping (not earlier than 1 min after birth) is recommended for improved maternal and infant health and nutrition outcomes.

Placental Transfusion- Transfer of residual placental blood (~30-40%) to the baby during the first few minutes of age

What are the various Methods of Placental Transfusion?

- Delayed cord clamping (DCC)-> 30 SEC
- Physiology based cord clamping
- Umbilical cord milking (UCM) -Intact UCM AND Cut UCM (Rare)

What are the factors which affect PLACENTAL TRANSFUSION?

- Timing of cord clamping
- Breathing efforts
- Uterine contraction
- Spasm of umbilical artery
- Gravity NO MAJOR ROLE

What is ACOG recommendation for DCC?

The American College of Obstetricians and Gynecologists now recommends a delay in umbilical cord clamping in vigorous term and preterm infants for at least 30–60 seconds after birth.

First 30 seconds of DCC - blood volume increases by 12 mL/kg

Cochrane database systemic review 2013 of DCC in term babies

- Increases Hb concentration at 24- 48 hrs
- Improves iron stores at 3- 6 months
- Marginally increases need for phototherapy
- Does not increase maternal PPH

Cochrane systemic database review 2019

Effect of timing of umbilical cord clamping and other strategies to influence placental transfusion at preterm birth on maternal and infant outcomes.

DCC VS ECC

Outcomes	aRR, 95% CI
Primary outcomes	
Mortality before discharge	**0.73 (0.54-0.98)**
IVH (any grade)	**0.83 (0.70-0.99)**
IVH (severe grades)	**0.94 (0.63-1.39)**
Death or NDI	**Not reported**
Chronic lung disease	**1.04 (0.94- 1.14)**
Secondary outcomes	
IVH grade 1-2	**0.72 (0.51-1.02)**
need for inotropes	**0.37 (0.17-0.81)**
need for blood transfusion	**0.66 (0.50-0.86)**

- There are insufficient data for reliable conclusions about the comparative effects of UCM compared with delayed or early clamping (mostly low or very low certainty).

Umbilical Cord Milking

- Increased placental transfusion in a rapid time frame (10–15 seconds)
- Applied when immediate infant resuscitation is needed or maternal hemodynamic instability occurs
- The cord is pinched between the fingers and the hand then moved towards the baby before releasing the cord.
- Approximately 20 cm of the umbilical cord is vigorously milked towards the umbilicus 2-3 times before clamping the cord.
- The speed of milking is approximately 20 cm per two seconds
- Position of the baby in relation to the placenta: for most studies the baby lies on the mother's thigh.

– At this time, there is not sufficient evidence to recommend for or against DCC- FOR TWIN GESTATION

– The umbilical cord not is clamped earlier than 1 minute after birth in term or preterm infants who do not require positive pressure ventilation.

Physiological based cord clamping

- Involves deferring umbilical cord clamping until the New-born has commenced breathing or respiratory support has started and the lung has aerated
- Receiving placental transfusion at birth is more beneficial for the depressed neonate
- Prevents hypovolemia and by providing better perfusion to all organs
- Allows lung aeration
- Pulmonary gas exchange initiated
- Increase pulmonary blood flow, cardiac output sustained
- Smoother transition

What is Nepcord 3 trial

New-born infants in the intervention (intact cord) group started to breathe and establish regular breathing earlier than in the immediate cord clamping group

Resuscitation Platforms for intact cord resuscitation (ICR)

- Life Start Trolley
- FDA approved
- Nooma cart
- Inspire Bed

– UCM should not be practiced in < 28 weeks

– PBCC and I-UCM are alternative proposed methods for depressed & hemodynamically unstable neonates

DCC vs ECC

Rabe H, Gyte GML, Díaz-Rossello JL, Duley L. Effect of timing of umbilical cord clamping and other strategies to influence placental transfusion at preterm birth on maternal and infant outcomes. Cochrane Database of Systematic Reviews 2019

- Fewer babies died before discharge (20 studies, 2680 babies) (aRR 0.73, 95% CI 0.54- 0.98)
- Fewer babies had any grade IVH (15 studies, 2333 babies) (aRR 0.83, 95% CI 0.70- 0.99)
- No effect on CLD (6 studies, 1644 babies) (aRR 1.04, 95% CI 0.94- 1.14)
- Insufficient data on PVL (4 studies, 1544 babies) (aRR 0.58, 95% CI 0.26- 1.30)

Effects of delayed versus immediate umbilical cord clamping in reducing death or major disability at 2 years corrected age among very preterm infants (APTS): a multicentre, randomised clinical trial

Infants (<30 weeks gestation) were randomly assigned before birth (1:1) to have clinicians aim to delay clamping for 60 s or more or clamp within 10 s of birth, both without cord milking.

The primary outcome was death or major disability (cerebral palsy, severe visual loss, deafness requiring a hearing aid or cochlear implants, major language or speech problems, or cognitive delay) at 2 years corrected age

1. Death or major disability was determined in 1419 (93%) infants and occurred in 204 (29%) of 709 infants who were assigned to delayed clamping versus 240 (34%) of 710 assigned to immediate clamping, (relative risk [RR]) 0·83, 95% CI 0·72–0·95; p=0·010)
2. 60 (8%) of 725 infants in the delayed clamping group and 81 (11%) of 720 infants in the immediate clamping group died by 2 years of age (RR 0·70, 95% CI 0·52–0·95);
3. Among Survivors major disability at 2 years occurred in 23% (144/627) versus 26% (159/603) of infants, respectively (RR 0·88, 0·74–1·04).

Conclusion

Clamping the umbilical cord at least 60 s after birth reduced the risk of death or major disability at 2 years by 17%, reflecting a 30% reduction in relative mortality with no difference in major disability

Umbilical cord milking in preterm infants: a systematic review and meta-analysis Haribalakrishna Balasubramanian, 1 Anitha Ananthan, 2 Vaibhav Jain, 1 Shripada C Rao, 3 Nandkishor Kabra

Main outcome measures Mortality and morbidities in preterm neonates

Results

Nineteen studies (2014 preterm infants) were included.

Five studies (n=922) compared cord milking with delayed cord clamping, whereas 14 studies (n=1092) compared milking with immediate cord clamping.

1. Cord milking, as opposed to delayed cord clamping, significantly increased the risk of intraventricular haemorrhage (grade III or more) (risk ratio (RR): 1.95 (95% CI 1.01 to 3.76), p=0.05).
2. When compared with immediate cord clamping, cord

milking reduced the need for packed RBC transfusions (RR:0.56 (95% CI 0.43 to 0.73),

Conclusion

1. Umbilical cord milking, when compared with delayed cord clamping, significantly increased the risk of severe intraventricular haemorrhage in preterm infants, especially at lower gestational ages.
2. Cord milking, when compared with immediate cord clamping, reduced the need for packed RBC transfusions but did not improve clinical outcomes

Umbilical cord milking in nonvigorous infants: a cluster-randomized crossover trial (minvi) Anup C. Katheria, MD Published: August 12, 2022

In (P) non-vigorous New-borns born between 35 and 42 weeks' gestation, does (I) umbilical cord milking (UMC) versus (C) early cord clamping (ECC) reduce (O) admission to the neonatal intensive care unit in the (T) first 24 hours of life.

Inclusion criteria:

- New-borns delivered at 35 – 42 weeks' gestation who were non-vigorous at birth.
- The frequency of NICU admission **(primary outcome)** between the UCM (199/872 = 23%) and ECC (239/858 = 28%) groups was different, however, after accounting for study design by site, it was not statistically significant (OR, 0.69; 95% CI, 0.41-1.14).
- The most common cause for NICU admission was respiratory distress (UCM 19% vs ECC 22%)

Effect of cut umbilical cord milking (C-UCM) as compared to early cord clamping (ECC) on hematological and clinical hemodynamic parameters in non-vigorous preterm neonates of 30–35 weeks gestation. European Journal of Pediatrics 2023

The mean Hct at 48 h was higher in the C-UCM group.

Significantly higher was the mean Hct at 12 h, 6 weeks and mean serum ferritin At 6 weeks of age in the milked group (p<.0001).

Mean blood pressure at 1 h and 6 h was also significantly higher in the milked arm.

Need for transfusion and inotropes was less in the milked group but not statistically significant.

Conclusion: C-UCM stabilizes initial blood pressure and results in higher hematocrit and improved iron stores. It can be an alternative to DCC in non-vigorous preterm neonates of 30–35 weeks' gestation

Association of Umbilical Cord Milking vs Delayed Umbilical Cord Clamping With Death or Severe Intraventricular Hemorrhage Among Preterm Infants 23-31 weeks' gestation) Anup Katheria, MD JAMA. 2019

Interventions: Participants were randomized to umbilical cord milking (n = 236) or delayed umbilical cord clamping (n = 238).

The primary outcome was a composite of death or severe intraventricular hemorrhage

- Twelve percent (29/236) of the umbilical cord milking group died or developed severe intraventricular hemorrhage compared with 8% (20/238) of the delayed umbilical cord clamping group (risk difference, 4% [95% CI, -2% to 9%]; P = .16).

There was no statistically significant difference in death

- Severe intraventricular hemorrhage was statistically significantly higher in the umbilical cord milking group than in the delayed umbilical cord clamping group (8% [20/236] vs 3% [8/238], respectively; risk difference, 5% [95% CI, 1% to 9%]; P = .02)
- Among infants born at 23 to 27 weeks' gestation, severe intraventricular hemorrhage was statistically significantly higher with umbilical cord milking than with delayed umbilical cord clamping (22% [20/93] vs 6% [5/89], respectively; risk difference, 16% [95% CI, 6% to 26%]; P = .002).
- UCM in the near-term/term non-vigorous New-born was not associated with a reduction in NICU admissions compared with ECC.

UCM was associated with a reduction in cardiorespiratory support in the delivery room, fewer cases of moderate-to-severe HIE, lower use of therapeutic hypothermia, and higher hemoglobin.

There was no evidence of harm associated with UCM compared with ECC.

Bell EF, Acarregui MJ. Restricted versus liberal water intake for preventing morbidity and mortality in preterm infants. Cochrane Database of Systematic Reviews 2014,

Restricted water intake:

- ↑ Postnatal weight loss
- ↓ PDA (RR 0.52, 95% CI 0.37 to 0.73); NNT 7
- ↓NEC (RR 0.43, 95% CI 0.21 to 0.87); NNT 20
- Trends toward (not statistically significant)

  ↑ Dehydration

  ↓ BPD, IVH and death

16 Birth Injury

Risk factors for birth injury are:

- Prematurity
- Small maternal stature
- Maternal pelvic anomaly
- Prolonged labor
- Unusual rapid labor
- Oligohydramnious
- Malpresentaion of the fetus
- Use of forceps or vaccum
- Versions and extractions
- Very low birth weight
- Extreme prematurity
- Fetal macrosomia
- Fetal anomaly
- Maternal obesity: BMI > 40 kg/m^

STERNOCLEIDOMASTOID INJURY
Congenital or muscular torticollis
Most likely the cause – muscle compartment syndrome from intrauterine positioning
Can also arise during delivery as the muscle is hyperextended and rupture- hematoma- fibrosis - shortening
Might present as a palpable mass 1-2cm
Head tilt to the side of the lesion
Mostly noted at 1-2 week
Facial asymmetry, hemihypoplasia

BRACHIAL PLEXUS INJURY

- 1-4 per 1000 live births
- It is most commonly Unilateral
- Right side is more commonly involved

Risk factors for brachial plexus injury

1. Vertex deliveries with shoulder dystocia
2. Breech deliveries
3. Macrosomic baby
4. Vaginal deliveries (it is rare in Caesarean sections)
5. Instrumentation

What is Naraka's Grades of brachial plexus injury?

1. Grade I – Erb's palsy (C5,C6) – most common (50% cases)
2. Grade II – (C5 , C6,C7) injury – 33% cases
3. Grade III – total plexus lesions – 17 %cases
4. Grade IV – lesions of Grade 3 with Horner's syndrome (cervical sympathetic chain)
5. Klumpe's paralysis(C8,T1) is extremely rare

Prognosis of brachial plexus injury

- Return of biceps function by 3 months is the most important indicator of recovery.
- When combined with shoulder abduction, wrist extension and finger extension – 95% chance of normal function
- When biceps recovers later than 3 mo chance of complete recovery is unlikely

What is the Scope in brachial plexus injury?

Brachial plexus exploration with intraoperative EMG – neurolysis, nerve repair, nerve graft and nerve transfer - with subsequent reconstruction (tendon transfer using lat. Dorsi and T. major to rotator cuff)

Timing – between 3 to 6 month age

Indication –

1. Global injury
2. Horner's syndrome
3. No return of Biceps function till 3 months

Subgaleal haemorrghae

A 1-cm increase in the depth of subgaleal space may hold up to 260 mL of blood.

Anticipate a 40-mL blood loss for every 1-cm increase in occipitofrontal circumference.

17 Assessment of Gestational Age

Based on Uterine Size:

- 12 weeks – palpable just above pubic symphysis
- 16 weeks – fundus of the uterus - midpoint b/w umbilicus & pubic symphysis
- 20 weeks – fundus -palpable at umbilicus
- >20 weeks – pubic symphysis to fundal height in cm should correlate with wk of gestation

Based on appearance of epiphysis

Femoral epiphyseal ossification center	32 weeks
Proximal tibial ossification centres	35 weeks
Calcaneal	first visible ossification center, appearing at end of 24th week
Talar ossification center	from 26 weeks
Distal Femoral Epiphysis	1 or 2 mm - 33 weeks in 87.0% of fetuses,equal to 3 mm greater than 37 weeks in 85% of foetuses.
Proximal Tibial Epiphysis	PPV of 83% for 37 weeks gestation
Proximal humeral epiphysis	100% PPV for ≥38 weeks

Name some other criteria's for GA assessment

1. Robinson's criteria, "gestational assessment by neurological examination" 1966.
2. Konigsberger, 1966, "Judgement of fetal age by neurological examination"
3. Farr, 1966, "some external characteristics used in GA":
4. Ameil-Tisons, "neurologic assessment of maturity" 1968:
5. Dubowitz score, 1970, "clinical assessment of GA"
6. Parkins criteria, 1976, "Rapid assessment of ga": arc of diseases of childhood.
7. Hittners eye exam, 1977, "assessment of ga by examination of anterior vascular capsule of lens":
8. Cappuro score 1978 : a simplified method of diagnosis of ga in New-born infant"
9. Ballards maturational score (revised dubowits score)1979: "a simplified score of assessment of fetal maturation of newly born infants"
10. Narayans 1982 : paediatrics "a simple method of assessment of ga in New-born infants, paediatrics"
11. New ballards score, 1991 : "new ballards score expanded to include extremely premature infants

Based on neurological criteria	Robinson Amiel-Tison
Based on Physical characteristics	Farr Hittner Parkin Narayanan Eregie
Combination of physical & neurological	Dubowitz score Konigsberger cappuro Ballards maturational score New ballards score

PARKINS CRITERIA used when NBS is not feasible to do due to sickness of baby

It has 4 components

- *Skin texture:*

0- very thin, gelatinous
1- thin & smooth
2- smooth & medium thickness
3- slight thickening & stiff feeling, cracking & peeling esp. on hands & feet
4- thick & parchment like with deep cracking

• *Skin color: quite*
0- dark red
1- uniformly pink
2- pale pink
3- pale, nowhere pink except ears, lips, palms & soles

• *Breast size:*

0- no breast tissue palpable
1- palpable 1 or both sides ≤ 0.5 cm
2- 1or both sides 0.5-1cm
3- both sides > 1cm

• *Ear firmness: palpate & fold upper pinna:*

0- pinna soft & easily folded in bizarre positions, no recoil
1- soft along edge, easily folded but recoils slowly
2- cartilage felt at the edge of the pinna, springs back readily
3- firm, cartilage at the periphery & springs back immediately

SCORE	GA IN WEEKS
1	27
2	30
3	33
4	34.5
5	36
6	37
7	38.5
8	39.5
9	40

- can be performed in an ill baby without manipulation or movement
- GA estimated within ± 15 days (95% CI)
- at any time in first 2 days of life

Hittner Eye examination for GA assessment

- Grade 4- 27-28 weeks, centre of the lens
- Grade 3- 29-30 weeks, spares the centre, 3/4th
- Grade 2- 31-32 weeks, half of lens is involved
- Grade 1- 33-34 weeks, periphery of lens
- Technique –simple, needs an ophthalmoscope only
- Can be adopted by a resident doctor with little experience.
- sick babies not exposed much in this procedure
- useful in limp babies
- Gestational assessment - even after death (up to 4-6 hrs) - importance in medico legal cases where age is disputed

NARAYANAN GA estimation

1. Ant vascular capsule
2. Plantar creases
3. Ear firmness
4. Breast nodule

- 95% CI of 11 days,
- Applicable to New-born infants, including sick babies, at any time within the first 2 DOL

Gestational age has strong correlation with foot length

Foot length of 73.7mm -cut- off point for differentiating between term and preterm babies. Foot length measurements-easily used by peripheral health workers to differentiate term & preterm babies.

NEW BALLARDS SCORE – you have to read it in detail

Ballard Maturational Score (revised Dubowitz). Six neurological and six external features from original Dubowitz: posture, square window, arm recoil, popliteal angle, scarf sign, heel to ear, skin, lanugo, plantar creases, breast development eyelid/ ear firmness and genitalia.

LSCS decreases neurological maturity score

Difference between old and new Ballard score

Old Ballard score given in 1979

1. Scores ranged from 5 to 50
2. 26-44 weeks
3. Score starts with 0
4. Inaccurate in extremely preterm
5. Best assessment between 30-42 hrs of life
6. Eyes not included
7. Old-overestimated the age of extremely premature & under estimated post mature with deviation of >2wks
8. It was more inaccurate in very low birth weight infants with a deviation of over 2 weeks

NBS revised in 1991

1. -10 to 50
2. 20-44 wk
3. Starts with -1
4. More accurate
5. Assessment upto 96 hrs of life
6. Eyes included
7. NBS accuracy is <1wk

POSTURE

The foetus gradually assumes increasing passive flexor tone as development goes along in a centripetal orientation, with lower extremities developing somewhat before upper extremities.

Sequence ankle, knees, wrist, hip flexion, hip adduction, elbow flexion last shoulder girdle flexion.

Position – supine wait till infant settles in a relaxed posture.

The figure that most closely depicts the infant's preferred posture is selected.

Square window

Measures wrist flexibility and/or resistance to extensor stretching

Straighten the infant's fingers and apply gentle pressure on the dorsum of the hand near the fingers

Angle between the palm of the infant's hand and forearm is measured

Arm recoil

Asses the passive flexor tone of the biceps muscle

Supine,

One hand beneath the infant's elbow for support. Hold the forearms flexed against the arms for 5 seconds.

Flex the elbow briefly then momentarily extends the arm before releasing the hand.

The angle of recoil to which the forearm springs back into flexion is noted

Extremely pre-term infant - no arm recoil.

Don't hold the arm in the extended position for a prolonged period, as this causes flexor fatigue and results in a falsely low score due to poor flexor recoil.

Popliteal angle

Assesses maturation of passive flexor tone about the knee join

Supine, diaper removed

Thigh is placed gently on the infant's abdomen with the knee fully flexed.

Grasp the foot at the sides with one hand while supporting the side of the thigh with the other. Don't exert on hamstrings

Extend leg till you get a definite resistance to extension

ÿþMeasure the angle from the back of the leg to the thigh .

Frank breech position will interfere with popliteal angle in first 24 to 48 hours of age due to prolonged intrauterine flexor fatigue.

The test should be repeated once recovery has occurred; alternately, a score similar to those obtained for other items in the exam may be assigned.

Scarf sign

Passive tone of the flexors about the shoulder girdle.

The point on the chest to which the elbow moves easily prior to significant resistance is noted. Landmarks noted in order of increasing maturity are: full scarf at the level of the neck (-1); contralateral axillary line (0); contralateral nipple line (1); xyphoid process (2); ipsilateral nipple line (3); and ipsilateral axillary line (4).

Heel to Ear

Passive flexor tone about the pelvic girdle

The infant is placed supine and the flexed lower extremity is brought to rest on the mattress alongside the infant's trunk. The infant's thigh laterally alongside the body with the palm of one hand. The other hand is used to grasp the infant's foot at the sides and to pull it toward the ipsilateral ear.

Fetal neonatal conditions affecting NBS

- Obesity-hydrops & IDM
- Hydrops-chest wall edema
- IUGR
- Orthopaedic anomalies-arthrogryposis, hip dislocation, amputation,phecomelia
- Neuropathy affecting tone: post asphyxial depression, deep sleep, coma, anomaly
- Intrauterine compression: twin, oligohydramnios

Fetal & neonatal conditions associated with hypotonia

1. CCF
2. Severe anemia
3. Hypoglycaemia

4. Hypoxia
5. Acidosis
6. Chromosomal anomalies with tonal deviation e.g., Down's syndrome
7. Restraining devices e.g., splints
8. Race
9. Delivery conditions
10. Fetal presentations
11. Birth injuries: fracture clavicle, humerus, femur; brachial plexus injury
12. Route of delivery

Maternal conditions affecting Apgar score

1. Maternal medications: beta blockers, MgSo4
2. Sedation
3. Uterine malformation: bicornuate, septate
4. Uterine tumor: myoma

18 Fluid and Electrolyte

Perinatal Changes in TBW - Isotonic contraction of ECF - physiological transition

Term babies don't get dehydrated because postnatal there will be shifting of extra vascular fluid into intravascular space which maintain fluid status of baby despite low milk intake.

The same causes postnatal diuresis as intravascular volume increases and so blood in atrium increases which cause anp release, which causes postnatal diuresis

Hormones that regulate volume status anp bnp vasopressin prolactin and angiotensin renin system

Effect of DCC on blood volume in a neonate

- 30 sec delay increase blood volume to 75 ml per kg
- 60 sec to 85 ml per kg and 90 sec to 90 ml per kg

Weight loss in 1st week of life

- Term: 5 to 10% - regain 7-10 days
- Preterm: 10 to 15% - regain 14-21 days

Average IWL of Premature Infant (ml/kg/d)

Age in days	750-1000 gms	1000-1500 gms	1500-2000 gms	>2000
0-7	60-70	40-50	20-30	15-20

Insensible water losses:

- < 1000 grams: 60- 80 ml/ kg/ day,
- 1000- 1500 grams:40- 60 ml/ kg/ day,
- 1500 grams: 20 ml/ kg/ day

Factors affecting IWL

- Radiant warmer Increased - 50%
- Phototherapy Increased - 50%
- High humidity Decreased - 30%
- Plastic heat shield Decreased - 30%

Urine sp gravity: not helpful in infants on diuretics

Plasma osmolarity: < 280 mOsm/L s/o SIADH

What is FENa: (U Na × Pl Cr / U Cr × Pl Na0 × 100

- < 1%: ↓ RBF
- 2.5%: ARF
- 2.5%: PTs < 32 weeks

NORMAL Urine specific gravity 1.008 to 1.012

16 WKS GA – TBW -94 %

TERM TBW 75 % (1/2 ECF, ½ ICF)

Physiology of fluid Changes during labour & delivery,

- Few days prior to delivery - ↑ catecholamines, vasopressin, and cortisol – Rise in arterial BP.
- Translocation of blood from placenta to fetus.
- Intrapartum hypoxia leads to ↑capillary permeability
- Shift of fluid from intravascular into interstitium

Postnatally,

- ↑ oxygenation + changes in vasoactive hormone production restore capillary membrane integrity
- Absorption of interstitial fluid into intravascular compartment
- Aids in maintaining intravascular volume during first 24-48 hours postnatally, when oral fluid intake is limited

Delayed cord clamping allows 25-50 ml/kg transfer to neonate (i.e 25-50% increase in total blood volume)

Changes in post natal period

- Postnatal ↑capillary membrane integrity favour absorption of interstitial fluid into intravascular compartment
- ↑circulating blood volume
- Stretching of atrial walls
- Release of ANP
- Sodium & water excretion
- Term – upto 10% weight loss
- Preterm – 15-20% weight loss

IUGR babies (term or preterm) – smaller initial weight loss, regain birth weight earlier

Antenatal steroids accelerate renal maturation Better capacity to regulate their postnatal ECF volume

Urine Concentration capacity:

- Adults - 1500 mOsm/kg
- Term - 800 mOsm/kg
- Preterm - 600 mOsm/kg

Limited by structural immaturity of renal medulla, ↓ urea generated osmotic gradient in medulla, preferential blood flow through vasa recti, decreased transcription & protein synthesis of AQ2 water channels.

Diluting capacity:

- Adult - 50 mOsm/kg
- Term - 50 mOsm/kg
- Preterm - 70 mOsm/kg

Atrial Natriuretic Peptide

- Stretch of atrial wall – most potent stimulus
- Direct inhibitory effect on RAAS
- Vasodilatory and renal natriuretic action
- Reduced ANP secretion, increased vasopressin - Oliguric effects of PEEP

Brain (or B type) Natriuretic Peptide

- Released from ventricular myocardium in response to increase in wall tension
- Direct inhibitory effect on RAAS, Natriuresis, diuresis, vasodilatation
- Levels increase rapidly after D1 (× 20 times that at birth), postnatal diuresis

Term neonates – FENa <1% (transient ↑in diuretic phase)

Premature infant – FENa 5-6% (inversely proportional to GA)

Onset of diuresis heralds the resolution of RDSSurfactant causes early onset of diuresis

Sensible water loss: Urine Stools

Insensible water loss: skin (2/3), respiratory tract (1/3)

Among environmental factors, ambient humidity has greatest effect on IWL

Replace Gastric aspirates: ½NS

Replace Bilious aspirates: NS

Third spacing

- Phenomenon by which fluids and electrolytes accumulate in static body fluid compartments
- Occurs in sepsis, hydrops, hypoalbuminemia, intra-abdominal infections, after abdominal or cardiac surgeries
- NEC: fluid in mucosal and sub-mucosal tissues

(HIDDEN EDEMA!) Does not contribute to effective arterial volume and circulatory balance. Patient may appear edematous even though their intra vascular volume is decreased. Rx with colloid/ crystalloid.

Causes of hyponatremia

- An inability to excrete a water load
- Excessive sodium losses
- Inadequate sodium intake

- Acute-onset hyponatremia – Duration of < 48 hours
- Chronic hyponatremia– Duration of > 48 hour

Isotonic hyponatremia (280–295mOsm/L) : is extremely rare and is generally due to laboratory errors like hyperlipidemia & hyperproteinemia.

Hypertonic hyponatremia (>295 mOsm/L) may be found occasionally, particularly in premature infants in the case of hyperglycemia.

Hypotonic hyponatremia (<280 mOsm/L) is frequent in the New-born and may be classified into 3 subtypes according to the patient's ECF volume status: hypovolemic, euvolemic and hypervolemic.

HYPONATREMIA

Causes of Hyponatremia due to ECF volume depletion

Renal

- Diuretic use
- VLBW with renal water and Na wasting
- Adrenal or renal tubular salt losing disorder

Prerenal

- Gastrointestinal losses (vomiting, diarrhea)
- Third- space losses of ECF

Urine excretion of sodium may be <20 mEq/L in prerenal and >20 mEq/L in renal

Causes of Hyponatremia due to ECF volume excess

Pre- renal cause

- Edema-forming states:
  - Congestive heart failure
  - Liver failure/cirrhosis
  - Nephrotic syndrome
  - Indomethacin therapy

Renal failure:

- Acute
- Chronic

Causes of Hyponatremia with normal ECF volume

- This is a dilutional form without signs suggesting hypervolemia or hypovolemia
- Weight gain usually occurs without edema
- Predisposing factors
  - Excess fluid administration
  - Syndrome of inappropriate antidiuretic hormone (SIADH) secretion

What is SIADH

- Predisposing Factors
- Pain
- Opiate administration
- Intraventricular hemorrhage (IVH)
- Asphyxia
- Meningitis
- Pneumothorax and positive-pressure ventilation.

Diagnosis of SIADH.

- Weight gain usually occurs without edema
- Decreased urine output
- Hypotonic hyponatremia
- Increased urine osmolality > serum osmolality
- Increased sodium excretion and specific gravity
- Normal renal, adrenal and thyroid function

Chronic hyponatremia

- Preterms with mild to moderate chronic hyponatremia may experience poor growth and development retardation
- Represent a risk factor of adverse outcome : sensory neural hearing loss,cerebral palsy, behaviour and memory disturbance, cerebral haemorrhage and mortality

Formulae for calculating Na+ Deficit (mEq) = 0.7 × Body Weight (kg) × ([Na+] desired " [Na+]) current

Asymptomatic hyponatremia: 2/3rd of replacement sodium should be provided in first 24 hours and remaining 1/3rd in next 24 hour

Serum sodium should not increase by more than 8–10 mEq/L in the 24 hours so as to avoid both cerebral edema and the risk of myelinolysis

Symptomatic or serum sodium <120meq/lit:

Calculate sodium deficit to raise serum sodium to 120meq/lit and give as 3% Nacl over 3-6 hours with once serum Na+ reaches 120meq/lit then correct the remaining deficit over next 48 hours

Mean sodium content of breast milk

- Colostrum (<5d) : 22 (+12) mmol/l
- Transitional milk (5d-10d) : 13 (+3) mmol/l
- Mature milk (>15d) : 7 (+2) mmol/l

Why are New-borns vulnerable for hypernatremia?

- Lesser ability and the maturity of the ADH system to trigger the concentration of urine for the compensation of selective water loss
- The compensation by the thirst mechanism is not possible
- The ISWL in the neonates and especially the preterm may be very high in the first 15 days of life.

Babies usually look deceptively well hydrated, as the IVF is maintained very well at the expense of the ICF

Absence of classic signs of dehydration with weight loss of 10-15% of the body weight and absence of circulatory impairment – suspect hypernatremia dehydration.

Disturbed neurology as a predominant feature

Hyper irritability to stimuli despite extreme lethargy when undististurbed- characteristic feature.

Classify dehydration based on excessive weight loss into mild (5%), moderate (10%) and severe (15%); Deficit replacement will be 50 ml/kg, 100 ml/kg and 150 ml/kg respectively

Each ml of 3% NaCl contains 0.5 mEq of Na

Start with dextrose free fluid if there is no hypoglycaemia as dextrose further increases osmolarity, and hypernatremia is mostly associated with hyperglycemia.

Do not give insulin infusion to correct hyperglycemia as it increases idiogenic osmoles formation in brain.

Start with potassium free fluid till good urine output established or if hypokalaemia is present then add potassium 2 mEq/kg/day

Give IV calcium if hypocalcaemia is present

19 Fetal Growth

Human fetal growth happens in three stages

- Phase of cellular hyperplasia-first 16 weeks (5g/day)
- Phase of cellular hyperplasia and hypertrophy-17 to 32 weeks (15 to 24 g/day)
- Phase of cellular hypertrophy-after 32weeks (30 to 35 g/day

***Features of IUGR*:**

- It defined as being below the 10% percentile of the recommended gender-specific birth weight for GA reference curves
- FGR and SGA are not synonymous; not all FGR are SGA
- 50-70 % of SGA are constitutionally small but not FGR
- A third variety seen in developing countries, mixed IUGR, characterized by both reduction in cell number & cell size with clinical features of both symmetrical & asymmetrical IUGR. This occurs when early IUGR is affected further by placental causes in late pregnancy
- FGR -Second leading cause of perinatal morbidity and mortality after prematurity

Symphysio fundal height in FGR

Between 20-34 weeks, SFH in cms corresponds to gestational age in weeks.

Difference >3cm, Single value below 10th centile, static slow or crossing centile on serial measurement important

FETAL ULTRASOUND in FGR

- CRL - most accurate indicator of gestational age in the first trimester.
- Parameters: BPD, FL, EFW, AC; HC/AC and FL/AC ratio: >2SD in case of asymmetric FGR

BIPARIETAL DIAMETER

- BPD is measured from the outer edge of the proximal skull to the inner edge of the distal skull. It is measured at the level of the thalami and cavum septum pellucidum.
- BPD is most accurate from 14-26 weeks (with a variation of 7-10 days)

ABDOMINAL CIRCUMFERENCE

- It is measured in a transverse view of the fetus, at the level of fetal stomach and portal vein (including skin and subcutaneous tissue).
- It has the widest variation of 2-3 weeks since it involves soft tissue.
- It is most affected by fetal growth(most sensitive indicator of intrauterine fetal growth restriction
- AC<5th percentile is highly suggestive of IUGR

Scanning for FGR

- Routine dating scan is done at 9-11 weeks and anomaly scan at 16-20 weeks whereas sonography for routine fetal growth assessment is done at 32-34 weeks.Estimated fetal weight < 10th percentile for GA (sensitivity 68%, specificity 89%) for FGR
- When using 2 measurements of AC or EFW to estimate growth velocity, at least 3 weeks apart to minimise false–positive rates; more frequent measurements in severe cases
- Reported mean growth rates for AC and EFW after 30 weeks of gestation 10 mm/14 days and 200 g/14 days.
- Change in AC of < 5mm over 14 days suggestive of FGR.

Early onset FGR (< 32 weeks)

Effective fetal weight or abd cir < 3 rd centile

OR

UA with AREDV

OR

EFW or AC < 10th combined with one or more of following

- UA PI > 95th
- Ut A PI > 95th

Late onset FGR (> 32 weeks)

EFW or AC < 3rd

OR

2 or more of the following 3

- EFW or AC < 10th
- EFW or AC crossing >2 centiles
- CPR < 5th or UA PI > 95th

Stage based management of FGR

- Stage 1 – mild placental insufficiency – only PI changes – 37 weeks
- Stage 2 – severe placental insufficiency – UA AERDV or REVERSE AOI – 34 weeks
- Stage 3 low suspicion of metabolic acidosis – UA REDV DV PI > 95th – 30 weeks
- Stage 4 High suspicion of fetal acidosis – DV reverse A FLOW, FHR deceleration – 26 weeks

COCHRANE 2017 compared use of Doppler USG of the umbilical artery with no Doppler or with CTG

1. In high-risk pregnancy, fewer perinatal deaths (RR 0.71)
2. For stillbirths, no clear difference
3. Fewer inductions of labour
4. Fewer caesarean sections
5. No difference in Apgar scores less than seven at five minutes

Postnatal diagnosis of IUGR

1. Clinical examination
2. Anthropometry
3. Ponderal index
4. Clinical assessment of nutrition (CAN) score
5. Cephalization index- Ratio of the head circumference (HC) to body weight Higher cephalization index: greater degree of brain vulnerability & increased likelihood of cerebral palsy & severe psychomotor retardation
6. Mid-arm/head circumference ratios

Normal value of MAC/HC: 0.32–0.33 & in term IUGR, a value < 0.27 is considered features of fetal malnutrition

CAN <25- poor nutrition of fetus

GA assessment using the Ballard is not accurate, as physical components are underscored or over scored. No such problem with the neurological component

1. Decreased blood flow, low estradiol level & low subcutaneous fat
2. Less mature appearing female genitalia (due to reduced fat deposit in the labia majora)
3. Skin is continuously exposed to amniotic fluid due to decreased vernix > cracked & peeled skin
4. Mature sole crease pattern, less well-formed ear cartilage.

Developmental origin of Health and disease

- Barker, in his observational studies, showed that infants, who were born in the 1920s and 1930s with low weight, had high incidence of CAD, DM, hyperinsulinemia, and hypercholesterolemia in adulthood.
- Thrifty phenotype (Barker hypothesis)- MOST ACCEPTABLE theory for DOHAD
- Various adult diseases the IUGR infant is prone to develop in his adulthood as per "developmental origin of health and diseases (DOHAD)".
- IUGR infants undergo epigenetic modification in-utero and postnatally have abnormal nutrition and growth leading to various disease of adulthood in these infants.

Thrifty Phenotype (Barker Hypothesis

- Proposed that early-life environment has long-term effects on the latter life.
- Adverse antenatal environment because of maternal, placental, or fetal aspects, lead to fetal adaptation
- Adaptations include the brain-sparing effect at the expense of other organ systems, and reduced production and sensitivity to the fetal insulin and ILGF-I with upregulation of the HPA axis
- Metabolic programming (epigenetic modification ie, those molecular mechanisms affecting gene expression patterns without causing alterations in DNA base sequence) at critical time window of fetal development ensures permanence
- Epigenetic changes are superadded with postnatal mismatched (normal or excessive nutrition) and suboptimal environment (sedentary life, less physical activity, and sedentary life habits), child's genetics & epigenetics: susceptibility to DoHaD

STRIDER TRIAL-Maternal sildenafil for severe FGR

EVERREST TRIAL - Maternal adenovirus gene therapy to increase expression of VEGF protein in the uterine arteries- to increase uterine artery blood flow and fetal growth. Awaited.

20 Growth Charts

What is growth chart?

Graphic representation of growth of reference population for clinical use

What are the Uses of growth charts?

- Diagnostic tool
- Educational tool
- Tool for action

Exponential growth occurs by six folds between 22 and 40 weeks

Rate of Intrauterine growth velocity decreases with increasing gestation

- **23 and 27 weeks - 21 g/kg/d (15 g/d)**
- 35 and 37 weeks -12 g/kg/d (33 g/d)
- Average growth velocity - 23 to 37 weeks 16 g/kg/d (25 g/d)

1. It is important to monitor the growth of infants to detect any deviation from normal.
2. Identification of babies at high risk of having poor neurodevelopmental outcome
   - Higher linear growth, weight gain, head growth associated with better neurodevelopmental outcome – including decreased incidence of cerebral palsy especially in ELBW
   - Rather than poor weight gain, slower head growth from birth to term was associated with worse neurocognitive outcomes in young adults born preterm with very low birthweights
   - Worst time to have poor head growth was after NICU discharge, but inferior head growth between admission to discharge was also associated with neurodevelopment impairment

Lubchenco's chart – 1st intrauterine growth chart to be widely used in neonates, also classified New-borns based on size at birth

Two common types of growth charts

- Growth references
- Growth standards

What do you understand by Growth Reference Chart?

- Statistical summary of anthropometry in a reference group of children, whose ***health status is not taken into consideration***
- Descriptive
- Show how children grow rather than how they should grow.

What are the two types of growth charts?

References growth chart	**Standards growth chart**
1. Descriptive tool	1. Prospective tools
2. How a fetal population *grew* at a specific location and period	2. How preterm infants should grow
3. Includes data from both low and high risk pregnancy	3. High risk pregnancy and maternal pathology are excluded
4. Fetal growth may be compromised due to maternal conditions	4. Sample of healthy neonates is taken with no growth restriction
5. Anthropometrics obtained from medical records (subject to error)	5. Standardised procedures and quality control measures to minimise error 6. (WHO child growth standards used same principle)

- Cross sectional data
- Easy to acquire large sample size

What do you mean by Growth standard charts?

- Statistical summary of anthropometry in a reference ***sample which is selected on health grounds***
- Prescriptive model – Represents healthy pattern of growth
- Shows how the child should grow
- Based on prospective and longitudinal monitoring of growth
- Difficult to acquire large sample size

Examples of Reference growth charts

1. Intrauterine growth charts
2. Post-natal growth charts
3. Fetal – Infant growth charts

Examples of Standard growth charts

1. WHO-MGRS charts
2. INTERGROWTH – 21st

Intrauterine Growth Curves

1. Assess growth status at birth, assign SGA, AGA, LGA
2. Monitor longitudinal growth of preterm
3. Assess EUGR at NICU discharge or term equivalent

Name some intrauterine charts are

1. Lubchenco (1966)
2. Usher and McLean (1969)
3. Brenner (1976)
4. Arbuckle (1993)
5. Alexander (1996)
6. Kramer (2001)

Discuss about Lubchenco charts

- Was most widely used
- 4700 New-borns b/w 26-42 weeks gestation
- Multi centric retrospective study
- Weight, Length & Head circumference
- First described SGA/AGA/LGA

Drawbacks of lubchenco charts

1. Single country (USA)
2. High altitude

Postnatal growth charts include

1. Dancis 1948
2. Infant Health and Development Program (IHDP) 1985
3. Shaffer 1987
4. Wright 1993
5. Berry 1997
6. Ehrenkranz 1999

Describe some features of Ehrenkranz chart (1999)

- Multicentric Prospective Longitudinal Cohort Study
- 12 centers in USA
- 1660 infants with BWt between 501 and 1500 g admitted within 24 h of age
- Longitudinal data on Wt, Lt, HC, MUAC were measured from birth until discharge, transfer, death, age 120 days, or a body weight of 2000 g
- Good sample size, n =1660
- Included if infants survived > 7 days and free of major anomalies
- 100 gms increments
- With and without major morbidity (CLD, severe IVH, NEC, or late onset sepsis).
- SGA vs AGA
- Not sex specific

Drawbacks of ehrenkranz chart

- Small sample size
- Population of a single country
- Only provides a single line trajectory and not major centiles

What are Fetal – Infant growth chart

- Constructed by merging two sets of reference data:
    1. Cross-sectional data of anthropometric measurement of preterm infants at
    2. Postnatal longitudinal anthropometric data of term infants birth
- Permit growth comparison with fetus first and then to term standards
- Advantage – assessment of catch up growth

Name some Fetal – Infant growth chart

- Babson and Benda charts 1967

- Fenton chart 2003
- Fenton charts 2013

Describe salient features of Fenton chart published in year 2003

- Updated the Babson–Benda charts
- Gestation – 22 to 50 weeks
- Canada
- Allows comparison of growth of a preterm infant with that of fetus initially starting as low as 22 weeks till 36 weeks and then later with term infants upto 50 weeks
- Wt, Lt, HC included
- Large sample size with large preterm population
- Data from multiple sources

DRAWBACKS of 2003 fenton chart

- Cross sectional data (predominantly)
- Not sex specific
- Change in wt. pattern not represented
- Do not show infant growth velocity
- Longitudinal growth influenced by medical and nutritional conditions
- Designed for plotting as completed gestation weeks
- Limitation in methodological quality and heterogeneity(affected its validity)

Features of Fenton chart published in 2013

- Revised in 2013
- Large preterm birth sample size(approx. 4 million infants)
- 1991 and 2007
- Developed countries (Germany, Italy, United States, Australia, Scotland & Canada

ADVANTAGE of fenton chart 2013

1. Data from recent population based surveys
2. Sex specific
3. Can be used to assign size for gestational age up to 36 weeks
4. The curves are equivalent to the WHO growth curves at 50 weeks of PMA
5. Enables to plot growth parameters of infants in between weeks and not as completed weeks

DRAWBACKS of fenton chart 2013

- Growth reference and not a growth standard
- Does not address the physiological postnatal loss of body water after birth.
- Different centers used variable methods for measurement of crown-heel length, making its reliability doubtful

Describe about INTERGROWTH – 21st growth chart

Intergrowth-21st Project was initiated by International Fetal and New-born Consortium

- Aim : to produce new prescriptive standards describing normal Fetal and New-born growth
- Data collected from 8 geographically different areas
- Countries included were China, India, Italy, Oman, Brazil, Kenya, UK and USA

Eight study sites: Pelotas, Brazil; Turin, Italy; Muscat, Oman; Oxford, UK; Seattle WA, USA; Shunyi County in Beijing, China; the central area of Nagpur, India; and the Parklands suburb of Nairobi, Kenya

Three graphs were developed based on various studies

1. Fetalgrowth longitudinal study (FGLS)
2. Postnatal growth of preterms: Preterm postnatal follow-up study (PPFS)
3. New-born size at birth : New-born cross-sectional study (NCSS)

(See Table on next page)

Salient features of FGLS

- Both LMP and USG combined over a time by a two stage process were used as a measure to ascertain gestation age
- Anthropometric data of fetus from 14 weeks gestational age to birth
- Fetal growth monitored in a healthy population

Features of PPFS

- Preterm New-born of more than 26 weeks and less than 37 weeks were followed post-delivery for evaluation of postnatal growth 201 eligible preterm New-borns from FGLS ,healthy or stable preterm
- All babies followed till 64 weeks PMA
- Standards for postnatal growth in preterm infants for weight, length and head circumference
- Can be used for assessment up to 64 weeks PMA

Intergrowth-21st size at birth charts	Intergrowth -21st size very preterm size at birth charts	Intergrowth-21st preterm postnatal growth standards
Prescriptive standards Cross sectional measures at birth	Descriptive references Cross sectional at birth with infants with some risk factor	Prescriptive standards Postnatal repeated longitudinal measures
Infant and maternal factor for fetal growth restriction excluded	Some Fetal growth restriction factors (except smoking and severe obesity)	Infant and maternal factor for fetal growth restriction excluded
n=1022	n=408	n=201
33-43wk	24-32wk	27-37wk

Features of NCSS

- 20,486 eligible women were enrolled between May 2009 and August 2013
- Weight, length and head circumference of all New-born infants whose mothers were enrolled in FGLS
- Centile curves for 3rd, 10th, 50th, 90th, and 97th were obtained according to gestational age and sex
- Prescriptive international anthropometric standards
- To assess New-born size from 33 to 43 weeks gestation were obtained from this study
- Prospective study
- Monitor child growth continuously from early prenatal life up to the age 5 years.
- Population based, multiethnic, multi-country and sex-specific

Across all the eight study sites, not only a uniform research method and same protocol was used but also accurate gestational age estimation was ensured by 1st trimester USG

Therefore, the standards are prescriptive and describe the optimum size in New-born infants without congenital abnormalities

- Despite a large sample size, there were relatively few early preterm births below 33 weeks for PPFS study
- In NCSS the lower limit of the curves was set at 33 weeks of gestation, because it was not possible to enroll preterm below this gestation age with very strict criteria

Comparison of Fenton chart with Intergrowth 21

The SGA rate was higher (12% vs. 15%, P=0.004) and the EUGR rate was lower (40.2% vs. 31.5 %, P< 0.001) with the INTERGROWTH-21st charts compared with the Fenton.

24% of the infants who were accepted as SGA according to the INTERGROWTH-21st standards were AGA according to the Fenton preterm growth charts

77% of the cases who had EUGR due to the Fenton standards were categorized as EUGR when evaluated using the INTERGROWTH-21st standards

Z SCORE

Indicates how far and in what direction the observed value deviates from a central value of the reference population (eg, mean or median)

Expressed in units of the population standard deviation (SD) o Values – negative, equal to zero, or positive

Negative Z score – observed value is below the central value of the population (E.g.: the 10th percentile corresponds to a z score of -1.28)

Positive Z score – observed value is above the central value (E.g. the 90th percentile corresponds to a z score of +1.28) Zero z score – observed value is equal to the mean of the reference population

Percentiles are more understandable and easier to use in clinical settings o Z scores allow to quantify the degree of "abnormal" growth

Z scores allow for quantification of the degree of their growth failure

GROW chart- Customised antenatal growth chart

GROW – Gestation Related Optimal Weight Customised growth chart

Adjusted for maternal Height Weight Ethnic origin Parity.

21 Neonatal Hypothermia

Thermo Neutral environment: The range of ambient temperature required for the infant (for each gestational age and weight) to keep a normal body temperature and a minimal basal metabolic rate. In practice, the core temperature of the infant at rest is between 36.5°C and 37 at the ambient temperature. 5°C and the core and mean skin temperatures are changing less than 0.2°C/hr and 0.3°C/hr, respectively

Cold stress: The infant senses heat loss as a stress and responds with increased heat production and peripheral vasoconstriction, with centralization of circulation, in an effort to maintain the core temperature

Hypothermia can be a sign of sepsis.

a. Mild hypothermia (cold stress): 36° to 36.4°C

b. Moderate hypothermia: 32° to 35.9°C

c. Severe hypothermia: Below 32°C

Effects of hypothermia

1. Hypothermia can lead to arrhythmias and death
2. Peripheral vasoconstriction: Acrocyanosis, pallor, and coldness to touch
3. Respiratory distress, apnea, and bradycardia
4. Depletion of caloric reserves and hypoglycemia, causing a shift to anaerobic metabolism and lactic acid production
5. Increased oxygen consumption and metabolic demands result in metabolic acidosis, a strong pulmonary vasoconstrictor inducing hypoxemia and central cyanosis
6. Norepinephrine release promotes pulmonary hypertension and pulmonary ventilation–perfusion mismatch
7. Decreased cardiac output, increased systemic vascular resistance, and decreased intestinal and cerebral blood flow
8. Decreased number, activation, and aggregation of platelets
9. Impaired neutrophil release and function
10. Poor weight gain with chronic hypothermia

Effects of hyperthermia or overheating

1. Peripheral vasodilatation: The skin is hot, the extremities are red, and the face is flushed.
2. Apnea, tachypnea.
3. Tachycardia and hypotension.
4. The infant assumes a spread-eagle posture.
5. Hyperactivity and irritability: The infant becomes restless and cries, then feeds poorly, with lethargy and hypotonia.
6. If hyperthermia is severe, shock, seizures, and coma may occur.
7. Hyperthermia is associated with adverse neuro-developmental outcome in infants with hypoxic ischemic encephalopathy

Effect of low admission temperatures -For each drop in 1oC in admission temperature (Laptook et al. Pediatrics; 2007)

- Mortality – increases by 28%
- Late onset sepsis – 11%

Mortality/morbidity Outcomes associated with low admission temperature

- Mortality
- Severe Neurological injury
- Severe ROP
- BPD
- Late onset sepsis
- Ventilation
- Severe NEC

Interventions to prevent hypothermia will lead to decrease in mortality and morbidities by18%– 42%.

What is thermos neutral zone of temperature?

That range of environmental temperature at which a baby can maintain normal body temperature with minimal oxygen consumption (and possibly minimal caloric expenditure

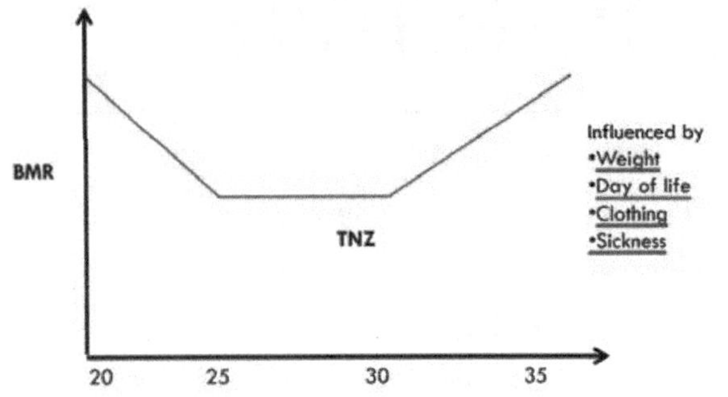

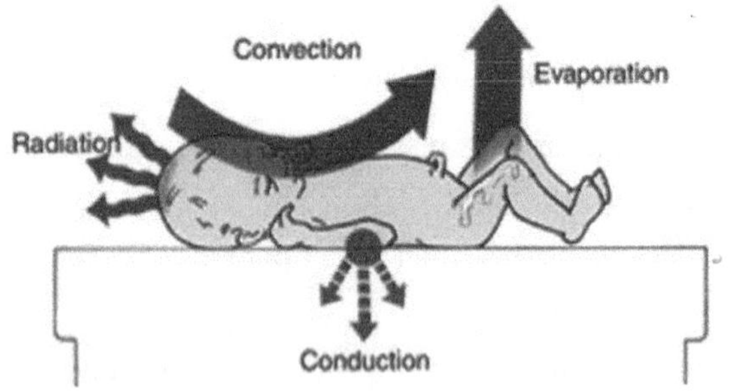

What are the 4 methods of heat loss in a neonate?

- Evaporation
- Convection
- Conduction
- Radiation

Polyethylene bags (20 cm × 50 cm) prevent evaporative heat loss in:

- Infants <32 weeks' gestation. Their diathermancy allows transmission of radiant heat to the infant.
- Immediately after delivery, open the bag under the Radiant warmer; wrap the wet infant's body from the shoulders down, and Dry only the head.
- Remove the wrap after the infant has been stable in the neonatal intensive care unit (NICU), in a humidified environment, for 1 hour.

Why neonates are at Risk factors for hypothermia

- Lesser brown fat tissue
- Larger surface area per unit kg of weight
- Skin Immaturity
- High trans epidermal water loss
- Low heat production per unit area
- Low resting metabolic rate
- Poor thermal insulation
- Less ability to change posture & No ability to adjust clothing
- Poor vasomotor control in immature infants
- Absent sweating in infants below 36 weeks gestation at birth
- Associated conditions further compromise the responses

What is Brown Fat?

- Brown fat constitutes 2% - 6% body weight in full term neonates. Contributes to 4-10% of fat tissue of body.
- Situated superficially between the scapulae and deep along the aorta, around the adrenals and kidneys.
- Highly vascularised Innervated by sympathetic nerves.
- Main source of non-shivering thermo genesis
- No detectable before 26-30 weeks of Gestation

Non-shivering thermogenesis is impaired in which conditions

- In all New-borns in the first 12 hrs
- Asphyxia
- Hypoxia

Evidence for preventing hypothermia in delivery room

- A Cochrane meta-analysis concluded that plastic wraps or bags were effective at reducing heat loss in infants of less than 28 weeks' gestational age, with a weighted mean difference for admission rectal temperature of 0.68°C (4 studies, n ¼ 223; 95% confidence interval 0.45–0.91).
- Studies show that the thermal mattress is effective and significantly associated with reductions in heat loss and admission hypothermia in VLBW infants.
- In a study of 115 VLBW infants, the addition of a thermal mattress to standard care (radiant warmer, hat, blankets) improved the admission temperature by 0.7°C.

Harmful effects of cold stress are

Hypoglycaemia, tachypnea and respiratory distress, increased peripheral vasoconstriction, decreased cardiac output, and metabolic acidosis.

Range of various thermometers

- Clinical thermometer reads from 35°C to 42°C (95 °F to 108 °F).
- Low reading thermometer reads up to 25°C (77°F)

Clinical features of hypothermia

Mild hypothermia (Cold stress): Restlessness, excessive cries, cold feet, acrocyanosis and poor feeding.

Moderate hypothermia – lethargy, refusal to feed, weak cry, decreased activity. Respiratory distress may be a feature.

Severe hypothermia – Respiratory depression (shallow and irregular respiration), edema, sclerema, Bleeding diathesis especially pulmonary hemorrhage and death

What is warm chain?

- Warm delivery room (28°C)
- Warm resuscitation.
- Immediate drying.
- Skin to skin contact between the baby and mother
- Breastfeeding
- Postponement of bathing and weighing.
- Adequate clothing and bedding
- Rooming in
- Warm transport.
- Training of healthcare providers

How to differentiate between fever and overheating in a neonate

Overheated infant	Febrile infant
1. High rectal temperature	High rectal temperature
2. Warm hands and feet	Cool hands and feet
3. Abdominal > hand skin temperature by < 2 C	Abdominal > hand skin temperature by > 3 C
4. Pink skin	Pale skin
5. Extended posture	Lethargic
6. healthy appear	Sick looking

22 Multiple Births

Types of twins it is of two types:

1. Dizygotic twins (80%), which results from fertilization of two ova leading to fraternal twin
2. Monozygotic twins (20%), which results from fertilization of one ova leading to identical twin.

Placenta consists of 2 parts: large fetal part derived from villous chorion and maternal part from decidua basalis.

Timing of formation of placental membranes

- Chorion: day 3 post fertilization
- Amnion: day 6-8 post fertilization

What is Hellin's rule for multiple gestations?

N (multiple gestations) $=1 \times 80^{(n-1)}$

- If frequency of twins in a population is 1/N, then-frequency of triplets will be $1/N^2$ and that of quadruplets $1/N^3$
- The rate of monozygotic twinning is constant

"The frequency of DZ twinning has a genetic tendency that is affected by the genotype of mother.

Parameter	25-30% (DCDA)	70-75 % (MCDA)	1-2% (MCMA)
Chorion	Two	One	One
Amnion	Two	Two	One
Time in days	**0-3**	**4-7**	**8-14**

Dichorionic-Diamniotic: early splitting at days 0-3

Monochorionic-Diamniotic: when splitting occurs at days 4-7

Monochorionic-Monoamniotic: when splitting occurs after day 7

Conjoined twins: late splitting after day 14

What are the two main factors accounts for the increase in multiple births?

- Fertility enhancing therapies (ARTs, IVF etc.)
- Older maternal age at childbearing (35-39yrs)

What is lambda or twin peak sign

Fused dichorionic placenta can be distinguished from true monochorionic placenta by internal dividing membrane or ridge at placental surface "LAMDA SIGN on scan.

The twin peak sign, also known as the lambda (λ) sign, is the triangular appearance of the chorion insinuating between the layers of the intertwine membrane and strongly suggests a dichorionic diamniotic twin pregnancy.

The T sign is really the absence of a twin peak sign (or lambda (λ) sign) and is used in ultrasound assessment of a multifetal pregnancy.

It refers to the lack of chorion extending between the layers of the intertwine membrane, denoting a monochorionic pregnancy. The intertwine membrane comes to an abrupt halt at the edge in a T configuration.

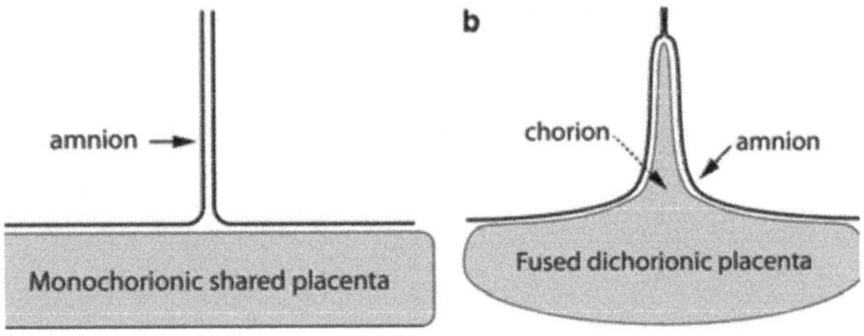

Dizygotic twin

• Identical or different sex
• Different genotype
• Same or different blood group
• Always dichorionic diamniotic (placenta can be one)

Monozygotic twin

• Identical sex
• Identical genotype
• Same blood group
• 70% monochorionic diamniotic, 30% dichorionic diamniotic, <1% monochorionic monoamniotic

- **Importance of zygosity**: monozygotic twins have genetic risk similar to singleton pregnancy; however dizygotic twins have double the risk.
- **Mean gestational age at birth** is 36, 33, and 29 and one-half weeks, for twin, triplets and quadruplets.
- Likelihood of birth weight < 1.5 kg is 8 and 33 times greater in twins and triplets or higher order multiples, compared with singletons.

What is discordance?

Intrapair difference in birth weight > 20% of the larger twins' weight.

- Mild discordance (<15%)
- Moderate discordance (15%-30%)
- Severe discordance (> 30%).

Significant risk (20-40%) of neurologic injury (multicystic encephalomalacia) in surviving co-twin as a result of associated severe hypotension or thromboembolic events upon death of the co-twin.

Congenital malformation

- MZ > DZ twins

STAGING SYSTEMS OF TTTS

A staging system proposed by fetal surgeon Dr. Ruben Quintero is commonly used to classify the severity of TTTS:

- Stage I: A small amount of amniotic fluid (oligohydramnios MVP <2 cm) is found around the donor twin and a large amount of amniotic fluid (polyhydramnios MVP > 8 cm) is found around the recipient twin.
- Stage II: In addition to the description above, the ultrasound is not able to identify the bladder in the donor twin.
- Stage III: In addition to the characteristics of Stages I and II, there is abnormal blood flow in the umbilical cords of the twins.
- Stage IV: In addition to all of the above findings, the recipient twin has swelling under the skin and appears to be experiencing heart failure (fetal hydrops).
- Stage V: In addition to all of the above findings, one of the twins has died. This can happen to either twin. The risk to either the donor or the recipient is roughly equal & is quite high in Stage II or higher TTTS.

Laser therapy is currently the optimal therapy for TTTS that develops before 26 weeks of gestation

Maternal Complications in twin gestation

- Hypertensive disorders of pregnancy
- Severe anemia
- Gestational diabetes
- Threatened and spontaneous abortions (vanishing twin)
- Hyperemesis
- Antepartum hemorrhage: abruption
- Preterm premature rupture of the membranes
- Operative delivery
- PPH : 3-4 fold increase
- Increased maternal mortality

Fetal and Neonatal Complications

- Prematurity and low birth weight
- Intrauterine growth restriction (IUGR)
- Fetal growth discordance
- Intrauterine fetal demise (IUFD) and Cord accidents
- Congenital malformations
- Conjoined twins
- Early vanishing twin
- Fetus papyraceus
- Twin to twin transfusion syndrome,
- Twin reversed arterial perfusion (TRAP).
- TAPS
- Monochorionic monoamniotic twins
- Conjoined twins

Intrauterine growth restriction (IUGR) in multiple pregnancy

- Till 28-30 weeks fetal growth is independent of number of fetuses

Causes of IUGR in twin pregnancy

- Overcrowding
- Limitation of placental perfusion,
- Anomalous umbilical cord insertion,
- Infection,
- Fetal anomalies,
- Maternal complications (e.g., maternal hypertension),
- Monochorionicity

What is Twin anemia polycythemia sequence?

Intertwin hemoglobin difference, without TOPS

Prenatal classification of TAPS severity:

- Stage 1– donor MCA-PSV >1.5 MoM and recipient <1.0
- Stage 2 – donor MCA-PSV >1.7 MoM and recipient <0.8
- Stage 3 – Stage 1 or 2 plus abnormal Doppler findings, such as absent or reversed end diastolic flow in umbilical artery, pulsatile flow in umbilical vein, increased PI or reversed flow in the ductus venosus
- Stage 4 – Hydrops of donor
- Stage 5 – Demise of one or both fetuses

Postnatal diagnosis OF TAPS

- Intertwin hemoglobin difference e"8.0 g/dL
- Intertwin reticulocyte ratio of >1.7 (reticulocyte count of the donor twin divided by the reticulocyte count of the recipient twin)

NORMAL PHYSIOLOGICAL VARIATIONS IN NEW-BORNS

What is the content of Meconium: Water (72-80%), desquamated cells from intestine and skin, GI mucin, lanugo, fatty material from vernix caseosa, amniotic fluid, intestinal secretions, blood group-specific glycoproteins, bile, enzymes including phospholipase A2.

What are the Characteristics of exclusively BF baby's stool:

- Golden-yellow in colour
- Curdy or paste-like in consistency
- Non-foul smelling

RISK FACTORS FOR HYPERBILIRUBINEMIA

J	Jaundice on day 1
A	Asian Race/ Male gender
U	Under 37 weeks (Prematurity)
N	Nursing difficulty (feeding issues)
D	Deficiency of enzymes (G6PD, PK)
I	Incompatible blood group (ABO, Rh)
C	Cephalohematoma –or any other bleed
E	Earlier sibling requiring phototherapy

What is pathological jaundice – presence of any of:

1. Jaundice in <24 hours of life
2. Rise in TSB > 5 mg/dL/day
3. TSB > 15 mg/dL
4. Lasting beyond 14 days of life
5. Clay/white-coloured stools and/or dark urine staining the clothes yellow
6. Direct bilirubin >2mg/dL at any time (or >15% of total, if total is >5 mg/dL

What is erythema toxicum neonatorum?

- Erythematous lesions with central yellow-white pustules
- On face, trunk, proximal extremities
- Seen in 30-70% of full-term New-borns
- Less frequent in preterms
- Most appear between days 2-3 of life
- Appearance as Flea bitten" appearance
- Etiology – Increased ground substance viscosity in neonatal skin with associated trauma can lead to eosinophilic inflammation within the skin.
- On HPE – Eosinophils in Wright-stained smear
- Asymptomatic. Waxes and wanes, and resolves spontaneously within the first week of life

Transient neonatal pustular melanosis

- More common in dark-skinned babies
- Less frequent in preterm
- 2-10 mm fragile, small pustules which rupture leaving collarette of fine scale and significant post-inflammatory hyperpigmentation which fades in weeks to months
- Can involve palms and soles
- If hyperpigmented macules are present at birth, the pustular phase presumably took place in utero
- HPE – Neutrophils in Wright-stained smear, no organisms
- D/d – Erythema toxicum, miliaria, infantile acropustulosis, eosinophilic pustular folliculitis

LANUGO

- Fine, soft, unpigmented hair
- Plays an important role in binding the vernix caseosa to the skin of fetuses

- Arises at about 3 months of gestation
- Hair growth starts around the scalp (around the eyebrows, nose and forehead) and proceeds in a cephalocaudal direction
- Shed at around 33-36 weeks of gestation, when it is subsequently incorporated into the amniotic fluid, eventually contributing to the composition of the meconium
- Ultimately replaced by villus (fine, thin hair) and terminal hair (thicker hair found on the scalp, axilla and genitalia)
- Often still present in 30% of neonates

CAPUT SUCCEDANEUM

- Swelling of the scalp secondary to pressure of the scalp and fetal head against the uterine and vaginal walls or cervix during labour and delivery.
- Results in accumulation of blood and serum in the tissue above the periosteum but below the skin
- Can cross suture lines: There can be abrasions of the skin overlying the area of caput that can develop a secondary infection
- Benign with infrequent complications: If the caput enlarges after birth or is very large at birth and a vacuum was used, consider an iatrogenic encephalocele

Cephalohematoma

- Represents a collection of blood underneath the periosteum
- Can occur in instrumented or non-instrumented deliveries
- Characterised by a swelling or mass on the cranium that does not cross the suture lines, and thus are usually unilateral
- Most prominent on the third day after birth. (Caput – most prominent after birth, and regress in around 24 hours)
- Involute over a course of several weeks Can form palpable nodules that resolve over a period of several months
- Monitor for development of hyperbilirubinemia
- Rare complications include secondary infections and osteomyelitis of the underlying skull

Subgaleal haemorrhage

- Represent bleeding (rupture of the emissary veins) that occurs in the large potential space beneath the epicranial aponeurosis and above the periosteum

  Can be large with potential loss of 40% or more of New-born's blood volume
- Bleeding is circumferential and thus extends downwards to the orbits, along the temporal and occipital regions and to the nape of the neck

  Each 1 cm increase in the OFC represents 30-40 m L of bleeding into the space
- Mortality rates are high due to shock (hemorrhagic) and coagulopathy (due to consumption of clotting factors)
- Highest risk period : 24-48 hours after birth
- Follow for hyperbilirubinemia

ESSENTIAL NEW-BORN CARE INTERVENTIONS CLEAN CHILDBIRTH AND CORD CARE

- Prevent New-born infection Thermal protection
- Prevent & manage New-born hypo/hyperthermia Early and exclusive breastfeeding
- Started within 1 hour after childbirth Initiation of breathing and resuscitation
- Early asphyxia identification and management

23 Nutrition and Lactation

Desired goals of nutrition in a preterm is

- Weight gain of 15- 20 g/kg/day till term gestation or once the infant reaches 2000-2500 g (based on intrauterine growth between 24 to 39 weeks GA gestation -fetal at a rate of approximately 15-20 g/kg/D.
- After term gestation a rate of 20-30 g/day is adequate.
- A growth rate of approxi-mately 1.0 cm/wk. is desirable for both length and head circumference

Calorie requirement of neonates

- Healthy term babies- **90-120 kcal/kg/D**.
- Preterms- **125 - 140 kcal/kg/D**
- Term neonates lose **5 to 10%** of BW- **first week** of life
- Preterms lose **10 to 20%** of BW- immature skin & kidneys, regain BW by **14-21 days**

	Average estimation (kcal/kg/day)
Energy expended	40-60
Resting metabolic rate	40-50
Activity	0-5
Thermoregulation	0-5
Synthesis	15
Energy stored	20-30
Energy excreted	15
Total	**90-120**

Associations with EUGR

- Lower Gestation age & birth weight.
- Male gender
- Need for assisted ventilation on day 1,
- History of NEC,
- Need for respiratory support at 28 days of age
- Exposure to steroids

TRANSITION		**INCIDENCE OF CEREBRALPALSY**
PRENATAL PERIOD	**POSTNATAL PERIOD**	
AGA	AGA	1%
AGA	SGA	20%
SGA	AGA	4%
SGA	SGA	5%

Indications for TPN

Indications	**When to start**
Preterm GA< 28 weeks/or <1kg	Day 1
Preterm GA < 32 weeks/or <1.5kg who are unable to achieve reasonable feeds	Day 3
Infants >32 weeks/or >1.5kg who are unlikely to achieve at least 50% enteral feeds	Day 5
Necrotizing enterocollitis	As soon as hemo-dynamically stable
Surgically correctable GIT anomalies i.e. gastroschisis, exomphalos etc	As soon as hemo-dynamically stable

Evidence based early nutritional practice for VLBW infants

- Starting GIR at 6mg/kg/min
- Increase GIR to about 10mg/kg/min by day 7 of age
- Main blood sugar 60-120 mg/dl
- Initiate amino acids at 3g/kg/day within hours of birth
- Increase to 4gm/kg/day by 0.5-1 g/kg/day steps
- Start lipid at 24 to 30 hrs of birth

- Start 0.5 to 1g/kg/day, advance to 3-3.5 gm/kg/day in steps of 0.5-1 g/kg/day

Aggressive Parenteral Nutrition (PN)

Recommendations include:

- Protein 1.5–2 g/kg/day grading to 3.5–4.4 g/kg/day
- Energy as tolerated to 120 kcal/kg/day (resting metabolic rate 40–60 kcal and 45–65 kcal for growth with variable additional requirements based on activity, thermogenesis)
- Glucose 4–6 mg/kg/min grading to 12 mg/kg/min;
- Fat 1–2 g/kg/day grading to 3–3.5 g/kg/day;
- Na 3.5 mmol/kg/day
- Calcium —-1.3–3 mmol/kg/day
- Phosphate — 1–2.3 mmol/kg/day
- Vitamin and mineral supplementation including vitamin A 700–1,500 IU/kg/day
- Vitamin D 40–160 IU/kg/day
- Selenium 2–4 μg/kg/day,
- Zn 400–500 μg/kg/day
- Iodine 1 μg/kg/day.
- Lipid should be started early as no harm has been demonstrated and no later than day 3 of PN

Minimal enteral nutrition (also referred to as **"gut priming" or "trophic feedings"**) may be described as the non-nutritive use of very small volumes of human milk or formula, for the intended purpose of preservation of gut maturation rather than nutrient delivery.

Advantages of Early Trophic Feeds (MEN) are

- promote intestinal maturation
- ↓time to reach full enteral feeds by facilitating feed tolerance.
- Improved levels of gut hormones
- Less feeding intolerance
- Earlier progression to full enteral feedings
- Improved weight gain
- Improved calcium and phosphorus retention
- Fewer days on PN

What is ADEPT TRIAL?

- Babies born preterm (up to 34+ 6 weeks of gestation)
- SGA (BW < below 10th centile)
- At <48 hours postnatal age
- Abnormal antenatal Doppler studies indicative of IUGR- *either*

  a) AEDF/REDF on at least 50% of the Doppler waveforms from umbilical artery on at least one occasion during pregnancy

  OR

  b) Cerebral redistribution, defined when both umbilical artery PI > 95th centile & MCA PI <5th centile for gestational age.

Two feeding regime was given DAY 2 (early group) VS DAY 6 (late group)

- Full, sustained, enteral feeding- achieved at an earlier age in the early group: median age- 18 days compared with 21 days.
- No evidence of difference in incidence of NEC: 18% in the early group and 15% in the late group
- All-stage NEC - 36 (18%) - early group and 30 (15%) -late group (relative risk [RR]: 1.20 [95% CI: 0.77–1.87; P = .42]).
- Early feeding resulted in - shorter duration of parenteral nutrition and high-dependency care, ↓ incidence of cholestatic jaundice, ↑ SD score for weight at discharge.
- The incidence of stages 2 and 3 NEC, which is of greater clinical importance, was 8% in both groups.
- Early group- ↑episode of "abdominal pathology": 59 (29%) vs 42 (21%; RR: 1.40 [95% CI: 1.00–1.98]), mainly d/t ↑dysmotility, meconium plug, & stage 1 NEC.

LACTATION

What are the stages of lactogenesis?

Stage I lactogenesis:

- Starts approximately midgestation or 12 weeks before parturition till first 2-3 days after birth.
- During pregnancy
- Gland developed to produce milk – but production limited by high estrogen and progesterone.
- Begins in mid-pregnancy (16 weeks)
- Detect lactose and a-lactalbumin levels
- Increase in lactose, proteins, immunoglobulin

Stage II lactogenesis:

Stage II starts at 2 to 3 days postpartum clinically when the secretion of milk is copious and biochemically when plasma Levels peak (paralleling the period when "the milk comes in"). 36-48 hours- 'Coming in' of milk

- Drop in progesterone levels a/w loss of placenta
- Maintenance of prolactin secretion
- First 4 days – 'Coming in' of milk (independent of infant suckling
- Sharp increase in citrate concentration (reliable marker
  a- Lactalbumin peaks in this stage.
  b- Prolactin surge precedes the onset of copious milk secretion by 2 days.

Secretory activation Mature milk – Day 10 onwards

- Most critical time in establishment of lactation
- Occurs at time of pregnancy to lactation transition
- Copious onset of milk secretion
- Also called lacto genesis stage II/ milk coming in
- Hormonal support – Prolactin, cortisol, thyroid and insulin
- Problems if unaddressed at this stage- Lactation failure
- Common causes – Childbirth stress, Problems with mechanics of suckling

What are the features of Colostrum in Human Milk?

- Provides 58-70 cal/100 ml.
- High in protein, electrolytes, sodium, potassium, chloride and vitamin A. Sodium, chloride, and magnesium are higher and levels of potassium and calcium are lower
- Low in fat and carbohydrate
- Produced in low quantities
- Produced in First few days postpartum
- Rich in immunologic components such as secretory immunoglobulin (Ig)A, lactoferrin, leukocytes, and developmental factors such as epidermal growth factor (EGF). Includes cytokines, antimicrobial peptides lactoferrin, lactalbumin,lysosomes, Ig's & growth factors
- Lactoferrin: Prebiotic & anti inflammatory actions
- EGF: Stimulates intestinal growth & repair
- Low concentrations of lactose
- Primary functions to be immunologic and trophic rather than nutritional.
- Oligosaccharides: Prevents microbial adhesion, Stimulates gut associated lymphoid tissues

What is Foremilk?

- Released first to satisfy the thirst of baby
- Higher in carbohydrate
- Lower in fat

What is Hindmilk

- Resembles cream, more calorie dense, helps in weight gain, so advised hind milk feeding
- Higher in fat
- Lower in carbohydrate
- Released after 10-20 minutes into the feeding

Cause of Delayed secretory activation

- Previous lactation experience
- Parity
- Cesarean section
- Diabetes (poor control), obesity, stress during parturition

Milk amount by fourth day – 600ml/day

Milk volume: By Day 10-14 after delivery:

Ideal: > 750 ml/day

"Borderline: 350-500 ml/day

Low: < 350 ml/day

Changes in milk content in First 72 hours:

- Fall in the sodium and chloride concentration in the milk and increase in lactose levels.
- Increase in concentration of serum immunoglobulin (IgA) and lactoferrin (max in first 48 hours)
- Oligosaccharide concentration high in early secretion – 2% on day 4

Lactogenic hormones:

Anterior pituitary – Prolactin, human growth hormone

Placenta- Human placental lactogen, human chorionic gonadotropin

Ejection hormone:

Oxytocin: From supra-optic and paraventricular nuclei of hypothalamus

Factors increasing prolactin secretion:

- Nursing
- Sleep
- Estrogen
- Metoclopramide

Factors decreasing prolactin secretion:

- Clomiphene citrate
- Dopamine

Oxytocin

- Released by: Nipple stimulation, Sensory – Visual, tactile, olfactory and auditory (touch, sound of baby)
- Receptors are located in canalicular system of breast, brain & uterus.
- Cause –Stimulation of myoepithelial cells forces milk out of alveoli to larger ducts and sinuses. (Neuro-endocrine)
- Oxytocin in Brain – Decreases stresses and improves interaction with infant.
- Multipara – More oxytocin release except in first 3-4 days.
- Spinal anesthesia has been associated with inhibition of oxytocin release after child birth\
- Significant increase in oxytocin occurs at 15 min after delivery when infant is placed in skin to skin contact.
- Levels return to baseline after 60 mins if infant does not suckle.
- Oxytocin release occurs both by infant suckling and mechanical dilatation of mammary ducts.

Feedback inhibitor of lactation

- Active whey protein
- Exerts reversible concentration dependent autocrine inhibition of milk secretion in lactating gland
- Affects secretion and not composition
- Probably presence of FIL regulates more of milk production as compared to alveolar distension.
- Alveolar distension causes interaction of lactocytes with basement membrane that inhibits prolactin receptors

Some Growth factors in breast milk

- **Heparin-binding EGF (HB-EGF)** is a member of the EGF family, and the primary growth factor responsible for damage resolution following hypoxia, ischemia-reperfusion injury, hemorrhagic shock/resuscitation injury, and necrotizing enterocolitis.
- EGF is highest in early milk and decreases over lactation.
- **VEGF** concentration is highest in colostrum in both preterm and term human milk, with preterm milk containing less VEGF than term milk.
- In retinopathy of prematurity (ROP), it is thought that pulmonary immaturity, supplemental oxygen, and negative regulation of VEGF lead to dysregulated vascularization of the retina suggesting a mechanism by which human milk may help reduce the burden of ROP.
- **Bile salt–stimulating lipase** (BSSL) also protects infants from viral infection, including Norwalk virus and HIV.
- **MUC1** blocks infection by HIV and rotavirus and both MUC1 and MUC4 block infection by Salmonella enterica serovar typhimurium and Norwalk virus

Flavor of foods in mother's diet influences taste of breast milk

Infants seem more interested in mother's milk if flavor is new

Exposure to a variety of flavors may contribute to infant's interest & acceptance of new flavors in solid foods

Breast feeding positions

1. Laid-back breastfeeding or reclined position
2. Cradle hold
3. Cross-cradle hold
4. Rugby ball hold
5. Side-lying position
6. Laid-back breastfeeding after a c- section
7. Upright breastfeeding or koala hold
8. Dangle feeding
9. Nursing in a sling
10. Double rugby ball hold
11. Dancer hand nursing. Position

Lipids in breast milk

Fat globule of milk contains a triglyceride core, inner membrane made up of phosphatidylethanolamine, phosphatidylserine and phosphatidylinositol.

Milk can be characterized as an emulsion of milk fat globules in an aqueous liquid. Milk fat globules with markedly variable sizes are formed in the mammary alveolar cells and contain a core of nonpolar lipids comprised primarily of triacylglycerol

Outer membrane is rich in phosphatidylcholine and sphingymyelin. Bioactive peptides cholesterol glycoprotein and cerebroside and gangliosdies are interspred in outer membrane.

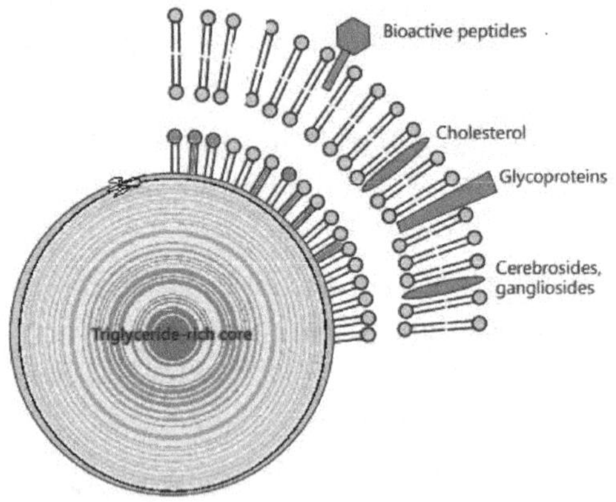

Human milk lipids provide a major portion of the energy supply to breastfed infants as well as essential vitamins, polyunsaturated fatty acids, complex lipids, and bioactive components

Phospholipids, plasmalogens, and sphingolipids including ceramides and gangliosides provide about 0.2– 1% of total milk lipids or about 100–400 mg/L. Gangliosides contribute some 10% of brain lipids, with high concentrations in the cerebral cortex. Total cholesterol content of 90–150 mg/L in human milk.

Triacylglycerol's contribute some 98–99% of human milk fat. The properties of milk triglycerides are very much influenced by their fatty acid composition. The saturated palmitic acid (C16:0) provides approximately 25% of all milk fatty acids and hence the major part of the total saturated fatty acid content.

The human milk contents of the mono-unsaturated fatty acid oleic acid (C18:1n-9) and of the essential PUFA linoleic acid (C18:2n-6) and α-linolenic acid (C18:3n-3) vary with the maternal dietary intake of these fatty acids.

Dietary DHA supply is a key determinant of milk DHA content. A balanced supply of both ARA and DHA appears to be relevant for the adequate incorporation of ARA and DHA into the growing brain.

The provision of DHA was shown to enhance the early development of visual pathways.

Fetal accretion of both DHA and ARA during pregnancy is facilitated by their active and preferential maternofetal placental transfer. Pregnant women's red blood cell levels of both DHA and ARA were positively associated with their children's IQ at school age. At birth, higher cord blood contents of both DHA and ARA predicted less later behavioural problems, emotional difficulties, hyperactivity, and attention deficit at the age of 10 years [55

Human milk lipids provide a major portion of the total energy intake in young infants, with a mean 44% of the energy supply. Among the macronutrients in milk, fat shows the most variable concentration. Milk fat content tends to increase with longer duration of breastfeeding and varies during the course of a day. Milk fat concentration increases with an increasing time interval to the preceding milk expression from the same breast, and it increases with maternal fat deposition in pregnancy indicated by the degree of gestational weight gain. Milk fat increases during the course of each breastfeeding meal, with markedly higher milk fat contents in hind milk (at the end of feeding) than in foremilk (at the beginning of the feed.

The increase of milk fat content during the meal is accompanied with a marked increase in the mean size of milk fat globule. Thereby, hind milk has a higher ratio of triglycerides in the core of the milk fat globule (providing energy) to the surface membranes (rich in phospholipids, complex lipids, and essential long-chain polyunsaturated fatty acids, LC-PUFA

The supply of long-chain polyunsaturated fatty acids in infancy is causally related to improving cognitive development and to reducing asthma risk at school age. Current evidence supports the provision of omega-3 docosahexaenoic acid along with omega-6 arachidonic acid with infant formula.

Cholesterol is an indispensable building block for all cell membranes and is incorporated in considerable amounts into myelin in the nervous system during the period of rapid brain growth, and it serves as the substrate for the synthesis of bile acids, lipoproteins, vitamin D, hormones, and oxysterols that modulate cholesterol, lipid, and glucose homeostasis.

Breast Pump

How to Manually Express Breast Milk - The Marmet Technique

All breast pumps consist of a few basic parts.

- **Breast Shield:** a cone-shaped cup that fits over the nipple & areola
- **Pump:** creates the gentle vacuum that expresses milk. The pump may be attached to the breast-shield or have plastic tubing to connect the pump to the breast-shield.
- **Milk Container:** a detachable container that fits below the breast-shield and collects milk as it is pumped. The container is typically a reusable bottle or disposable bag that can be used to store the milk or be attached to a nipple and used for feeding a baby.
- Manual pumps
- Battery-powered pumps
- Electric pumps
- Single-sided (can only pump one side at a time)
- Double-sided (option of pumping one or both breasts at once)

Electric pumps are generally more efficient than battery-operated or manual pumps.

What is nonnutritive sucking (NNS)?

Suck which is not for nutritional needs.

Appears between 28-33 weeks post-menstrual age

It is organized into alternating suck burst and pause periods.

- A mature NNS burst consists of
  - 6 to 12 suck cycles followed by pause periods to accommodate respiration.
  - Occurs at a pace of 2 suck cycles per second.
  - Involves minimal swallowing- allows sucking and respiration to function independently.

Immature suck pattern

- 3-5 sucks per burst
- A pause of equal duration often detaching from the breast

Transitional suck pattern

- 6-10 sucks per burst
- A pause of equal duration with occasional detaching
- An apneic episode can follow longer suck bursts

Mature suck pattern:

- 10-30 sucks per burst
- Brief pauses
- Suck/Swallow in 1:1 ratio

Disorganized sucking: Lack of rhythm of total sucking activity

Dysfunctional sucking: Interruption of feeding process by abnormal movements of tongue and jaw

Between 32 to 36 weeks, the most common pattern observed is apneic pauses in breathing (deglutition apnea [DA]) associated with pharyngeal swallows ("DA-swallow-DA")

If swallowing mechanism is not swift and efficient, duration of DA increases.

Such disruption to respiration (reduced tidal volume and minute ventilation) if prolonged can result in desaturations and bradycardia during oral feeding.

Healthy term infants: inhale-swallow- exhale

Some feeding assessment tools:

IBFAT – infant breastfeeding assessment tool – term – 6

Latch score – preterm Term – 5

NOMAS (neonatal oral motor assessment scale)-preterm/ term – 28

Preterm infant breastfeeding behavior (PIBBs) - preterm – 6

Systematic assesment of the infant at breast (SAIB) - term – 18

NOMAS consists of

- 28 items:
- 14 relate to movements of the jaw
- 14 relate to movements of the tongue
- 5 clusters

- Clinical tool that is used to diagnose sucking patterns in term and preterm infants' upto 48 weeks PMA.
- Best available instrument to distinguish a disorganised or dysfunctional sucking pattern from a normal or mature sucking pattern
- User-friendly and non-invasive assessment tool
- Performance on the NOMAS is predictive of developmental outcome at 24 months of age.

LATCH SCORING

Assessment	0	1	2	
LATCH	too sleepy/reluctant	repeated attempts to latch	good latch	**MAXIMUM SCORE – 10 SCORE LESS THAN 6 NEEDS INTERVENTION**
AUDIBLE SWALLOWING	none	few	good	
TYPE OF NIPPLE	inverted	flat	everted	
COMFORT	engorged	filling	soft	
HOLD	full assist	minimal assist	no assist	

PIOMI – Oral motor intrevention 8 steps

1. cheeck strech – 30 sec
2. lip roll – 30 sec –
3. lip curl/strecth
4. gum massage
5. lateral border of tongue/cheek – 15 sec
6. mid blade of tongue/palate
7. elicit a suck – 15 sec
8. support for non nutritive sucking – 2 min

EVIDENCE FOR OMS

An early oral stimulation program accelerates the transition to full oral feedings in preterm infants. This was associated with greater overall intake and rate of milk transfer observed in the experimental group when compared with the control group.

Feeding of Very Low Birth Weight Infants

- Cochrane review (four RCTs, 588 subjects) compared slow daily increments (15 to 20 mL/kg/day) versus fast daily increments of enteral feeding volume (30 to 35 mL/kg/day)
- Fast increment did not increase the risk of NEC (RR 0.97, 95% CI 0.54, 1.74), mortality (RR 1.41, 95% CI 0.81, 2.74), or interruption of feeds (RR 1.29 (95% CI 0.90, 1.85)
- Fast daily increment group regained birth weight and reached full feeds faster

Bolus vs continuous feeds

- Studies have failed to demonstrate differences between bolus and continuous feedings for VLBW infants.
- Systematic reviews comparing these methods have shown no differences in time to achieve full oral feedings, length of stay, NEC incidence, or postnatal growth rate
- However, in infants weighing less than 1,250 g, continuous feedings may improve weight gain and lead to earlier discharge.

Studies suggest that feedings every 2 hours improve feeding tolerance and reduce the time to achieve full volume.

CONTINOUS FEEDING

In an experimental study, continuous feeding resulted in (mean) 40% loss of fat, 33% of calcium, and 20% of phosphorus. Infusion via gravity resulted in 6%, 9%, and 7% losses, respectively.

Infusion by pump over 30 min resulted in intermediate losses. Fat adheres to the inner wall of the tubing, resulting in losses.

Most authors have started human milk fortification at 100 mL/kg/day and at a concentration of 1:50.

Fortification with a human milk-based fortifier at 100 mL/kg/day versus starting at 40 mL/kg/day, no difference in outcomes.

- < 28 weeks – iv fluid
- 28-31 weeks – og feed
- 32-34 weeks – paladai
- >34 weeks – breastfeeding

Feeding an ELBW neonate

- Preterm infants are at increased risk for nutritional compromise ***("Nutritional emergency")***
- **Limited nutrient accretion,**
- **Immature metabolic pathways,**
- **Increased nutrient demands**
- From 24 to 39 weeks GA gestation fetal growth increases at a rate of approximately 15-20 g/kg/D.
- Healthy term babies grow well with intake of 90-120 kcal/kg/D.

- Energy required by preterm infants is 125 - 140 kcal/kg/D

Energy needed for protein utilization of 1 gm amino acid: 30-40 kcal/kg/day

Advantage of early aggressive feeding regimen

- Poor early growth is associated with decreased neurodevelopmental and growth outcomes at 18 to 24 months' corrected age (CA), with early nutrition having an impact of 6 to 15 IQ points in various studies
- Children have growth parameter above 10th percentile at 18 months' CA if higher in-hospital growth rates are achieved, as well as lower incidences of cerebral palsy, neurodevelopmental impairment (including blindness and deafness), Bayley and Psychomotor Development Index scores less than 70, and rehospitalisation's.

Recommned daily enteral requiremnt of preterm infant

Fluid	140-200 ml/kg/day
Calorie	105-130 kcal/kg/day
Protein	3.4-4.5 g/kg/day
Carbohydrate	7-20 g/kg/day
Lipid	5-7 g/kg/day
Sodium	3-5 meq/kg/day
Potassium	2-3 meq/kg/day
Calcium	100-220 mg/kg/day
Phosphorus	70-140 mg/kg/day
Zinc	1-3 mg/kg/day
Vitamin A	1330-3300 iu/kg/day
Vitamin D	**800-100 iu**

Recommendation by NNF for feeding of LBW Clinical practice guidelines NNF 2020

1. Mother's own milk (MOM) is strongly recommended for feeding the low birth weight infant. Specific nutrient supplementation needs to be made in preterm very low birth weight infants.
2. If mother's own milk is not available, pasteurized donor human milk from human milk bank, should be used for feeding low birth weight infants.
3. If donor human milk is not available, formula milk is to be considered
4. Stable preterm very low birthweight infants may preferably be initiated on progressive enteral feeding from the first day of life.
5. Daily feed volumes are to be increased by 30-40 mL/kg in stable preterm very low birth weight infants with no signs of feed intolerance.
6. In the absence of other signs of feed intolerance in preterm LBW neonates, neither routine pre-feed abdominal circumference nor pre-feed gastric residue estimation is recommended for assessment of tolerance to enteral feeds
7. Preterm infants who cannot feed directly from the breast should be fed by cup, paladai or katori-spoon, rather than by bottle, to fasten the transition to direct breast feeding.
8. Preterm very low birth weight infants who do not accept cup, paladai or katori-spoon feeds should be fed by either nasogastric or orogastric route of tube feeding
9. Intra-gastric route of tube feeding is preferred over transpyloric route in preterm infants
10. Continuous feeding is not recommended as a routine strategy for feeding preterm low birth weight infants receiving intragastric tube feeding
11. Preterm low birth weight infants with birthweight >1250 grams and on cup, paladai or katori-spoon feeds or intragastric tube feeding may be given feeds fed every three hours.
12. Checking of position of feeding tube (NG/OG) after placement and before commencement of first feed is recommended in LBW infants. Of the available methods, abdominal x-ray seems to be the best method for checking the position of feeding tube.
13. Multi-nutrient fortification of breast milk can be initiated in preterm LBW infants with birthweight <1800 g and receiving enteral feeds of at least 50-80 mL/kg/day. For resource limited settings, fortification may be commenced only for those infants who fail to gain weight despite adequate breast milk feeding.
14. There is limited efficacy and safety data to recommend Human milk based fortifiers. In addition, there are ethical and cost concerns.
15. Routine supplementation of docosahexaenoic acid (DHA) / long chain polyunsaturated fatty acid (LC-PUFA) is NOT recommended in preterm LBW infants

What is early total enteral feeding?

Early Total Enteral Feeding- total enteral nutrition on day 1 (80 mL/kg) resulting in earlier achievement of full feeds in addition to other potential advantages.

- These neonates tolerate full oral nutrition sooner.
- Early feeding enhanced the maturation of small intestine motor activity.
- Early enteral feedings increase intestinal lactase activity
- Gastrointestinal barrier function is improved by early enteral feeding

GENERAL contraindications to early total enteral feeding

- Shock requiring inotropes
- Obvious abdominal distension/ blood/bilious vomit or aspirates
- Surgical conditions of GI tract
- Abnormal Antenatal Umbilical Artery Doppler flows (AREDF)

Possible Contraindication to ETEF

- Weight < 600 grams / Gestation ≤ 26 weeks
- Severe asphyxia
- Shock requiring inotropes
- Obvious abdominal distension/ blood/bilious vomit or aspirates
- Abnormal Antenatal Umbilical Artery Doppler flows (AREDF)
- Surgical conditions of GI tract

Indication of Fortification of feeds

- Indications: All preterm infants <1800 g (ESPGHAN) OR GA <32 weeks or BW <1500 g. Infants >1800 g-SGA or poor postnatal calorie intake & growth

What are the TYPES of fortification?

- Monocomponent / Multicomponent
- Bovine milk / Human milk based
- Solid/ Liquid

METHOD: Standardized / Individualized fortification method

Standard (STD) Fortification

- Used in most of the neonatal units.
- A fixed amount of fortifier is added to a fixed volume of mothers milk as per manufacturers' instructions
- Practically easy
- VLBW gets less protein with this method leading to suboptimal growth.

2. Individualized HM Fortification Methods

a. Adjustable (ADJ) Fortification

- Adequate protein intake is based on BUN monitoring
- Expected BUN is 10-16 mg/dl
- BUN < 10 mg/dl – add more protein
- Practically possible, more labor intensive than standard fortification.
- No need of expensive devices.
- Possible to Monitors protein intake of each infant.
- Prevents excessive or less protein intake.
- Proven to be effective in optimizing growth and protein intake with a RCT.

b. Targeted Fortification

- Macronutrient concentrations in mothers milk is analysed and based on the results milk is supplemented with extra protein and/or fat.
- All macronutrients can be supplemented.
- Bedside Human Milk analysers are required. Thus labor intensive. Not available easily
- Supplementation is done according to the recommendations, it does not include each individual infant's specific requirement which may vary among infants.

Human Milk Fortification

Component	ESPGHAN /kg/day	EBM 180ml/kg
Energy(Kcal)	110-135	120.6
Protein(g)	3.5-4.5	**1.98**
Fat(g)	4.8-6.6	6.3
Vit A(IU)	1320-3300	**86.4**
Vit D(IU)	800-1000	**14.4**
Calcium(mg)	120-140	**45.5**
Phosphorus(mg)	60-90	26.1
Iron(mg)	2-3	**0.16**

What is Individualized Fortification?

Adjusted fortification- Based on infant's ability to tolerate the protein

Targeted fortification -Based on protein content of mother's milk

What are the various types of fortifier available in market?

- Lactodex HMF
- Hijam HMF
- Similac HMF
- MMF

What is Mothers Milk Fortifier (MMF)?

- Made by Neolact, Australia
- 100% human donor milk
- 2:1 mothers milk: MMF
- Less reported complications like feed intolerance, NEC

The fortification methods in current use are:

1. Standard fortification,
2. Individualized fortification:
   - Adjustable fortification
   - Targeted fortification.

Adjustable fortification has been shown to improve protein intakes, somatic and head growth and seems to be a practical method to optimize HM fortification.

- Targeted fortification, being feasible and effective in some trials, needs to be improved.
- Human milk fortification can be started safely with multi-nutrient fortifiers when the milk volume reaches 50–80 ml/kg/d.
- Optimization of HM fortification is required. Individualized fortification (Adjustable or Targeted) is the recommended method for HM fortification.
- Targeted Fortification may need further research

HUMAN MILK FORTIFIER

- Sullivan et al evaluated an exclusively HM-based diet which consisted of mother's own milk or DHM and a HM–based fortifier, is associated with a lower rate of NEC than a diet of human milk and bovine milk-based products.
- The OptiMoM study in 2018, recently published by O'Connor et al, compared the efficacy of HM-based fortifier to bovine-based fortifier in the absence of formula. There was no difference in feeding tolerance, postnatal growth and morbidity, including NEC ≥ grade 2.

Disadvantages of human milk based fortifiers:

- Costly and supported by limited efficacy data
- Requires large amount of milk which can be infact used for feeding premature babies
- So Large studies needed to evaluate benefit risk ratio

Donkey milk fortifier: recently proposed as its composition is very close to human milk. Small RCT done by Coscia et al (2018) and Bernito et al (2019) studies has shown improved feed tolerance compared to bovine human milk fortifiers

Shortfalls with "Standard Fortification

- Actual protein intakes in preterm were consistently and significantly lower
- Assumed protein concentration by the manufacturers is 1.4-1.5 g/dl which only occurs during the first 2-3 weeks of lactation
- HM protein concentration decreases with the duration of lactation and drops to around 1g/dl by week 4 to 6

Multicomponent fortification vs control difference in parameters

- Weight gain – 2.33 gm/kg/day
- Weight gain per day – 4.74 gm/day
- Length gain -0.12 cm/week
- Head growth – 0.12 cm/week

Evidence for HMF VS BMF

- Six randomized controlled trials
- Lower risk of necrotizing enterocolitis (NEC; ≥ Stage II) (RR: 0.38; 95% CI: 0.15, 0.95; P= 0.04) and surgical NEC (RR: 0.13; 95% CI: 0.02, 0.67; P=0.02) in the HMF group;
- No significant difference in mortality (RR: 0.40; 95% CI: 0.14, 1.15; P=0.09,
- Lower weight gain in the HMF group
- No differences for length and head circumference
- No significant difference in late-onset sepsis

(See Table on next page)

Human Milk Oligosaccharides

HMOs are nondigestible glycan's that are produced in abundance in human milk with a high number of structures and striking diversity of structures among women

- HMOs are the third most abundant components of milk after lactose and lipids.
- HMOs are complex sugars present in free, unconjugated form in the milk aqueous phase.

Composition per sachet	Lactodex HMF (1gm)	HiJAM	Abbott simlac	Nestle Prenan FM 85	Neolac MMF
Calories(Kcal)	3.37	3.5	3.5	17	3.5
Protein (gm)	0.27	0.25	0.25	0.16	0.12
Vitamin D (mcg)	133	100	30		
Calcium (mg)	15.8	25	29.3	10.4	2.51
Phosphorus (mg)	7.9	12.5	16.8	7.2	1.77
Iron (mg)	0.3	0.36	0.08		
Zinc (mcg)	40	40	0.25		0.07

- *Neutral or fucosylated HMOs:* these HMOs contain fucose at the terminal position. Examples: 2'-fucosyllactose (2'-FL) and lactodifucopentose.
- *Neutral N-containing or non-fucosylated HMOs:* these HMOs contain N-acetyl glucosamine at the terminal end. Example: lacto-N-tetraose.
- *Acidic or sialylated HMOs:* these HMOs contain sialic acid at the terminal end. Example: 2'-sialyllactose.

Highest concentration of HMO in colostrum: 20-23 g/L

Mature milk HMO: 12- 14 g/L

Preterm milk HMO > Term milk HMO

Most abundant HMO – 2'- fucosyllactose

Highly variable in quantity and quality in lactating mother

- A proportion of 35-50% of fucosylated, 12-14% of sialylated, and 42-55% of non-fucosylated neutral HMOs has been reported in term breast milk.

Not significantly altered after donor milk pasteurization

- A **majority of HMOs reach the colon intact**
- In the colon, HMOs are either metabolized by an infant's gut bacteria and/or excreted intact in the feces, depending on infant age, maturity at birth.

Potential benefits of HMO

- Immune modulatory effects
- Anti-inflammatory effects
- Provides innate immunity – enhance barrier function
- Prebiotics effects – support beneficial bacteria
- Gut maturation, direct effect on enterocytes
- Ant adhesive
- Act as a decoy receptor for bacteria
- Support growth of bifidobacterium and bacteroides
- Decreases incidence of infectious diarrhea
- Decrease NEC severity
- Lower eczema
- Less respiratory infections
- Less food allergy
- Improved learning and memory
- Increases synaptic strength

What is Entero-mammary Axis?

- Human breast milk cells contain a limited number of viable bacteria but a range of bacterial DNA signatures, as also found in maternal peripheral blood mononuclear cells.
- Intestinally derived bacterial components are transported to the lactating breast within mononuclear cells.
- Colostral T cells - will respond by proliferation to enteric antigenic substances such as E. coli K-l
- T cells in colostrum are activated by enteric associated antigens rather than by systemic stimulation and probably derive from epithelial sites.
- A 28 weeker with klebsiella infection will not be able to mount a strong antibody response as we know that immunoglobulin production is robust only after 34 weeks. But if mother comes and does KMC she gets colonised with the same klebsiella and mounts a response and gives those klebsiella specific antibodies to her baby through breast milk.

Evidence on use of prebiotics Cochrane database (APRIL 2014 ON PROBIOTICS) -24 eligible trials

- NEC reduced the incidence of severe NEC (stage II or more) (typical relative risk (RR) 0.43, 95% confidence interval (CI) 0.33 to 0.56; 20 studies, 5529 infants)

- MORTALITY: Reduced mortality (typical RR 0.65, 95% CI 0.52 to 0.81; 17 studies, 5112 infants).
- SEPSIs no evidence of significant reduction of nosocomial sepsis (typical RR 0.91, 95% CI 0.80 to 1.03; 19 studies, 5338 infants).

Cochrane review on Probiotics database (2020).

- 56 trials, 10,812 infants
- The most commonly used preparations contained.
- Bifidobacterium spp., Lactobacillus spp., Saccharomyces spp., Streptococcus spp. alone or in combinations.
- NEC: RR 0.54, 95% CI 0.45 to 0.65 (54 trials, 10,604 infants number needed to treat for an additional beneficial outcome (NNTB) 33, 95% CI 25 to 50.
- Reduce mortality (RR 0.76, 95% CI 0.65 to 0.89; NNTB 50)
- Reduce late onset invasive infection NNTB 50.
- No effect on severe neurodevelopmental impairment

Cochrane review on Probiotics database (2023). Sahar sharif

60 trials with 11,156 infants

Very preterm or very low birth weight infants

1. Probiotics may reduce the risk of NEC (RR 0.54, low certainty (NNTB) was 33
2. Probiotics probably reduce mortality slightly (RR 0.77, the NNTB was 50
3. Probiotics probably have little or no effect on the risk of late onset invasive infection (RR 0.89,
4. Probiotics may have little or no effect on neurodevelopmental impairment

Extremely preterm or extremely low birth weight infants

1. Little or no effect on NEC and all cause mortality
2. Little or no effect on late onset invasive infection
3. No data for neurodevelopmental impairment in extremely preterm or ELBW infants.

Probiotics in Preterm infants (PiPS) trial

No evidence of benefit for the primary outcomes – sepsis and NEC stage > 2

The ProPrems trial (Susan et al)

- Daily administration of a probiotic combination (Bifidobacterium infantis, Streptococcus thermophilus, and Bifidobacterium lactis, containing 1 × 10(9)
- In infants born before 32 completed weeks' gestation weighing <1500 g.

Significantly reduced NEC of Bell stage 2 or more in very preterm infants, but not definite late-onset sepsis or mortality.

Zinc in Early Life (dose 1-2 mg/kg/day)

Zinc is functional for the activity of a number of proteins (i.e., enzymes, membrane proteins, gene-regulatory proteins, and hormonal receptors) involved in most major metabolic pathways [2]. Zinc interacts with proteins in different ways: (i) by promoting enzymatic processes; oxidoreductases, transferases, hydrolases, lyases, isomerases and ligases, all require zinc

Metallothioneins (MTs) are the most abundant cysteine-rich proteins containing zinc [5]. These proteins have an important antioxidant activity and stabilize cell membranes only in the presence of zinc [6]. Zinc is also required for the DNA binding proteins involved in the regulation of gene expression, zinc participates in cell division and growth, intestinal electrolyte absorption, neurotransmission, immune response, thymus activity, and vision

Maternal zinc deprivation increases the risk of fetal mortality, growth retardation and malformations, including neural tube defects

Most fetal zinc accretion occurs after the 24th week of gestation [40]. As gestation progresses, fetal zinc concentrations constantly increase. Zinc is stored in the fetal liver

In the last trimester, the mother transfers to the fetus up to 1.5 mg/Kg of zinc every day

Zinc Deficiency and Neonatal Complications

- Dermatitis
- Growth Retardation
- Necrotizing Enterocolitis
- Neurologic Damage
- Bronchopulmonary Dysplasia
- Infections
- Retinopathy of Prematurity

Zinc is the most abundant trace metal in the retina and may serve a critical function as antioxidant in this tissue

Donor Human Milk for Preterm Infants

Post pasteurization effect on donor human milk

Components	Percentage loss
IgA and secretory IgA concentrations	20-30 %
lactoferrin	(50%–75%)
lysozyme	(24%–74%)
IgG	(34%–76%)
interleukin-10, tumor necrosis factor-a) growth factors, and hormones (insulin-like growth factor 1, adiponectin, insulin, and leptin)	Significant loss
complete loss of lipase activity, IgM (concentrations) and white blood cells	Complete loss
oligosaccharides lactose, glucose long-chain polyunsaturated fatty acids, gangliosides vitamins A, D, E, B12, folic acid some cytokines (interleukin-2, 4, 5, 8, 13) (and some growth factors (EGF and TGF-b1),	are preserved

Lower versus Traditional Treatment Threshold for Neonatal Hypoglycemia HypoEXIT Study Group 2020

OBJECTIVE

- Management strategy that used a lower threshold (treatment administered at a glucose concentration of <36 mg per deciliter [2.0 mmol per liter]) would be non-inferior to a traditional threshold (treatment at a glucose concentration of <47 mg per deciliter [2.6 mmol per liter]) with respect to psychomotor development at 18 months, assessed with the Bayley Scales of Infant and Toddler Development.
- Cognitive and motor outcome scores were similar in the two groups
  – (mean scores [±SE], 102.9±0.7 [cognitive] and 104.6±0.7 [motor] in the lower-threshold group
  – 102.2±0.7 [cognitive] and 104.9±0.7 [motor] in the traditional-threshold group
- In otherwise healthy New-borns with asymptomatic moderate hypoglycemia, a lower glucose treatment threshold (36 mg per deciliter) was non-inferior to a traditional threshold (47 mg per deciliter) with regard to psychomotor development at 18 month

Infants were randomly assigned (1:1) to real-time CGM or standard care (with masked CGM for comparison) using a central web randomisation system, stratified by recruiting centre and gestational age (REACT TRIAL)

- Compared with infants in the standard care group, infants managed using CGM had more time in the 2·6–10 mmol/L glucose concentration target range (mean proportion of time 84% [SD 22] vs 94% [11]; adjusted mean difference 8·9% [95% CI 3·4–14·4]), equivalent to 13 h (95% CI 5–21).
- More infants in the standard care group were exposed to at least one episode of sensor glucose concentration of less than 2·6 mmol/L for more than 1 h than those in the intervention group (13 [15%] of 85 vs four [6%] of 70).
- There were no serious adverse events related to the use of the device or episodes of infection.
- Interpretation Real-time CGM can reduce exposure to prolonged or severe hyperglycaemia and hypoglycaemia.
- Further studies using CGM are required to determine optimal glucose targets, strategies to obtain them, and the potential effect on long-term health outcomes

Glucose Profiles in Healthy Term Infants in the First 5 Days: The Glucose in Well Babies (GLOW) Study

- Healthy, term, appropriately grown singletons had continuous glucose monitoring and repeated heel-prick plasma glucose measurements (4 in the first 24 hours then twice daily using the glucose oxidase method) from birth to 120 hours.
- Plasma glucose concentrations of 47 mg/dL (2.6 mmol/L) approximated the 10th percentile in the first 48 hours, and 39% of infants had ≥1 episode below this threshold.
- 39% healthy babies with no risk factors of hypoglycemia had at least one value <47 mg/dL
- Early term infants had lower mean glucose concentrations than those born at later gestational ages and were more likely to have episodes <47 mg/dL (<2.6 mmol/L) (19/32 [59%] vs 7/35 [20%]; relative risk, 3.0; 95% CI, 1.4-6.1; P = .001).

Conclusions: Healthy infants seem to complete their metabolic transition by day 4. Many have glucose concentrations below the accepted thresholds for treatment of hypoglycemia.

Evaluation of oral dextrose gel for prevention of neonatal hypoglycaemia (hpod): a multicenter, double-blind randomized controlled trail.

- To evaluate the relationship between the effects of oral dextrose gel on rate of NICU admissions and rate of hypoglycemia in different study sites.
- Population (p) : preterm babies (<37weeks gestation), infant of diabetic mother9any type), small (<2.5kg or <10th percentile), large babies (>4.5kg or >90th centile). Also satisfied all of the following >or equal to 35weeks, > or equal to 2.2kg,<1 hour old, no apparent indication for NICU admission, unlikely to require NICU admission for any other reason e.g: Respiratory distress syndrome
- Intervention(I): study group received single pre-packaged syringe of 40% dextrose gel and control group received identical-appearing 2% hydroxymethyl cellulose placebo gel
- Outcome(O): how many had hypoglycemia, NICU admission for hypoglycemia, hyperglycemia, exclusive breast feeding at discharge, formula feeding before discharge, formula feeding at 6weeks of age, maternal satisfaction with study participation
- The group of infants randomized to study group were given oral 40% dextrose gel with dose of 0.5 ml/kg (200 mg/kg) at 1 hour after birth
- However in this large multicentre randomized trail, dextrose gel prophylaxis did not reduce NICU admission

Stopping enteral feeds for prevention of transfusion-associated necrotising enterocolitis in preterm infants Cochrane Sys Review 2019

- Only one study involving 22 preterm infants was eligible for inclusion in the review.
- Randomised controlled trial evidence is insufficient to show whether stopping feeds has an effect on the incidence of subsequent NEC or death.
- Large, adequately powered RCTs are needed to address this issue.
- Conclusion: The overall body of evidence is not sufficient to promote a specific practice recommendation with respect to PRBC transfusions and preventing NEC.

Continuous nasogastric milk feeding versus intermittent bolus milk feeding for preterm infants less than 1500 grams Cochrane Database of Systematic Reviews 2021

- Babies receiving continuous feeding may reach full enteral feeding almost one day later than babies receiving intermittent feeding
- It is uncertain if continuous feeding has any effect on days to regain birth weight
- It is uncertain if continuous feeding has any effect on rate of gain in weight compared with intermittent feeding
- Continuous feeding may result in little to no difference in rate of gain in length compared with intermittent feeding
- Continuous feeding may result in little to no difference in rate of gain in head circumference compared with intermittent feeding
- It is uncertain if continuous feeding has any effect on the risk of NEC compared with intermittent feeding

Early or Delayed Enteral Feeding for Preterm Growth-Restricted Infants: A Randomized Trial Alison Leaf, Jon Dorling 2012 (ADEPT TRIAL)

- Infants with gestation below 35 weeks, birth weight below the 10th centile, and abnormal antenatal umbilical artery Doppler waveforms were randomly allocated to commence enteral feeds "early," on day 2 after birth, or "late," on day 6.
- Primary outcomes were time to achieve full enteral feeding sustained for 72 hours and NEC.
- Full, sustained, enteral feeding was achieved at an earlier age in the early group: median age was 18 days compared with 21 days (hazard ratio: 1.36 [95% confidence interval: 1.11–1.67]).
- There was no evidence of a difference in the incidence of NEC: 18% in the early group and 15% in the late group (relative risk: 1.2 [95% confidence interval: 0.77–1.87]).
- Early feeding resulted in shorter duration of parenteral nutrition and high-dependency care, lower incidence of cholestatic jaundice, and improved SD score for weight at discharge.
- CONCLUSIONS: Early introduction of enteral feeds

in growth-restricted preterm infants results in earlier achievement of full enteral feeding and does not appear to increase the risk of NEC.

Controlled Trial of Two Incremental Milk-Feeding Rates in Preterm Infants Jon Dorling, SIFT Investigators Group*

- Daily milk increments of 30 ml per kilogram of body weight (faster increment) or 18 ml per kilogram (slower increment) until reaching full feeding volumes.
- The primary outcome was survival without moderate or severe neurodevelopmental disability at 24 months.
- Secondary outcomes included components of the primary outcome, confirmed or suspected late-onset sepsis, necrotizing enterocolitis, and cerebral pals
- Survival without moderate or severe neurodevelopmental disability at 24 months occurred in 802 of 1224 infants (65.5%) assigned to the faster increment and 848 of 1246 (68.1%) assigned to the slower increment (adjusted risk ratio, 0.96; 95% confidence interval [CI], 0.92 to 1.01; P=0.16).
- Late onset sepsis occurred in 414 of 1389 infants (29.8%) in the faster-increment group and 434 of 1397 (31.1%) in the slower-increment group (adjusted risk ratio, 0.96; 95% CI, 0.86 to 1.07).
- Necrotizing enterocolitis occurred in 70 of 1394 infants (5.0%) in the faster-increment group and 78 of 1399 (5.6%) in the slower-increment group (adjusted risk ratio, 0.88; 95% CI, 0.68 to 1.16
- There was no significant difference in survival without moderate or severe neurodevelopmental disability at 24 months in very preterm or very-low-birth-weight infants with a strategy of advancing milk feeding volumes in daily increments of 30 ml per kilogram as compared with 18 ml per kilogram

Two-hourly versus Three-hourly Feeding in Very Low Birthweight Neonates: A Randomized Controlled Trial

- To study whether 3-hourly feeding is non-inferior to 2-hourly feeding with respect to time to reach full feeds VLBW neonates
- The primary outcome of time to achieve full enteral feed was comparable in the two feeding schedule groups (median 5 days IQR 4-6 days in both groups; p value 0.665).
- Among the secondary outcomes, there were no significant differences in incidence of hypoglycaemia (RR 0.86; 95% CI: 0.29-2.5) feed intolerance (RR 1.08: 95%CI: 0.5-2.3), necrotizing enterocolitis (RR 0.8; 95% CI: 0.22-2.3) in both the groups.
- Conclusion: Three hourly feeding does not increase the risk of hypoglycemia, NEC or feed intolerance.

Feeding infants below 29 weeks' gestation with abnormal antenatal Doppler: analysis from a randomised trial Stephen Kempley, 1 ADEPT sub group analysis

- To describe feeding and gastrointestinal outcomes in growth-restricted infants <29 weeks' gestation and to determine the rate of feed advancement which they tolerated
- Full feeds were achieved later in infants <29 weeks; median age 28 days {IQR 22–40} compared with 19 days {IQR 17–23} in infants ≥29 weeks (HR 0.35, 95% CI 0.3 to 0.5).
- The incidence of necrotising enterocolitis was also higher in this group; 32/83 (39%) compared to 32/312 (10%) in those ≥29 weeks (RR 3.7, 95% CI 2.4 to 5.7).
- Infants <29 weeks tolerated very little milk for the first 10 days of life and reached full feeds 9 days later than predicted from the trial regimen.
- Conclusions Growth-restricted infants born <29 weeks' gestation with abnormal antenatal Doppler failed to tolerate even the careful feeding regimen of ADEPT. A slower advancement of feeds may be required for these infant

Enteral lactoferrin supplementation for very preterm infants: a randomised placebo-controlled trial The ELFIN trial investigators group*

- Either enteral bovine lactoferrin (150 mg/kg per day; maximum 300 mg/day; lactoferrin group) or sucrose (same dose; control group) once daily until 34 weeks' postmenstrual age
- The primary outcome was microbiologically confirmed or clinically suspected late-onset infection (occurring >72 h after birth
- Interpretation Enteral supplementation with bovine lactoferrin does not reduce the risk of late-onset infection in very preterm infants. These data do not support its routine use to prevent late-onset infection and associated morbidity or mortality in very preterm infants.

Early fortification of human milk versus late fortification to promote growth in preterm infants

(Review) Thanigainathan S, Abiramalatha T

- We defined early fortification as fortification started at < 100 mL/kg/d enteral feed volume or < 7 days postnatal age, and late fortification as fortification started at ≥ 100 mL/kg/d feeds or ≥ 7 days postnatal age.
- Meta-analysis showed that early fortification may have little or no effect on growth outcomes including time to regain birth weight (MD -0.06 days, 95% CI -1.32 to 1.20 days), linear growth (MD 0.10 cm/week, 95% CI -0.03 to 0.22 cm/week), or head growth (MD -0.01 cm/week, 95% CI -0.07 to 0.06 cm/week) during the initial hospitalisation period.
- Early fortification may have little or no effect on the risk of NEC
- Early fortification may have little or no effect on incidence of surgical NEC, time to reach full enteral feeds, extrauterine growth restriction at discharge, proportion of infants with feed interruption episodes, duration of total parenteral nutrition (TPN), duration of central venous line usage, or incidence of invasive infection, all-cause mortality, and duration of hospital stay

Evidence is up-to-date as of August 2019

Fortification of breast milk with preterm formulae powder vs human milk fortifier in preterm neonates

- Open-label, parallel-group, non-inferiority randomized trial
- Neonates born at or before 34 weeks of gestation and having a b wt <1500 g
  – Receiving 100 mL/kg per day of enteral feeds and consuming at least 75% of feeds as EBM
- PTF arm g of PTF for every 25 ml EBM (Fe, Ca, P, MV, Vit D added separately
- HMF arm 1 sachet (1g) for 25 ml EBM (Vit D added separately
- At discharge, parents were advised to add fortification until the neonate reached a weight of 2 kg or until 40 weeks of PMA, whichever was later
- Primary outcome The rate of in-hospital wt gain measured as g/kg/d from the day of randomization to the day of discharge or 40 weeks' PMA, whichever was earlier
- There was no difference in the mean (SD) weight gain between the PTF and HMF groups (15.7 [3.9] vs 16.3 [4.0] g/kg/d; mean difference, -0.5 g/kg/d; 95% CI, -1.9 to 0.7).
- The lower bound of 95% CI did not cross the non-inferiority margin.
- The incidence of feed intolerance was lower in the PTF group (1.4 vs 6.8 per 1000 patient-days; incidence rate ratio 0.19; 95% CI, 0.04 to 0.95), and fewer neonates required withholding of fortification for 24 hours or more (5% vs 22%; risk ratio, 0.22; 95% CI, 0.07 to 0.75).
- The incidence of necrotizing enterocolitis stage II or more (0 vs 5%) and extrauterine growth restriction (73% vs 81%) was comparable between the groups.
- Conclusions and relevance: Fortification with preterm formula powder is not inferior to fortification with human milk fortifiers in preterm neonates. Given the possible reduction in feed intolerance and lower costs, preterm formula might be a better option for fortification, especially in resource-restricted settings.

Effect of Gastric Residual Evaluation on Enteral Intake in Extremely Preterm Infants: A Randomized Clinical Trial

- **Main outcomes and measures:** The primary outcome was weekly enteral nutrition intake in mL/kg for 6 weeks after birth.
- The no residual group had feedings that advanced more quickly compared with the residual group (mean weekly increase, 20.7 mL/kg/d vs 17.9 mL/kg/d; P = .02) and consumed more feedings at weeks 5 (137.2 [95% CI, 128.6-145.8]; P = .03) and 6 (141.6 [95% CI, 133.2-150.0]; P = .03).
- Among the secondary outcomes, the no residual group had higher mean estimated log weights (7.01 [95% CI, 6.99-7.02] vs 6.98 [95% CI, 6.97-7.00]; P = .03), had fewer episodes of abdominal distention (0.59 [95% CI, 0.34-1.01] vs 1.79 [95% CI, 1.27-2.53]; P = .001), and were discharged 8 days earlier (4.21 [95% CI, 4.14-4.28] vs 4.28 [95% CI, 4.19-4.36]; P = .01).
- Odds for necrotizing enterocolitis (0.058 [95% CI, 0.018-0.190] vs 0.026 [95% CI, 0.006-0.109]), death (0.004 [95% CI, 0.0003-0.046] vs 0.012 [95% CI, 0.001-0.131]), late-onset sepsis (0.970 [95% CI, 0.67-1.40] vs 1.38 [95% CI, 0.97-1.94]), and ventilator-associated pneumonia (0.084 [95% CI, 0.033-0.214] vs 0.056 [95% CI, 0.019-0.168]) were similar between groups.

- Conclusions and relevance: Among extremely preterm infants, the omission of gastric residual evaluation increased the delivery of enteral nutrition as well as improved weight gain and led to earlier hospital discharge; these results may translate into evidence-based practice.

Oral vitamin A supplementation in very low birth weight neonates: a randomized controlled trial Sriparna Basu

- Eligible infants were randomized to receive aqueous syrup of vitamin A (10,000 IU of retinol/dose; n = 98) or placebo (n = 98) on alternate days for 28 days.
- Primary outcome variable was composite incidence of all-cause mortality and/or oxygen requirement for 28 days.
- On intention-to-treat analysis, composite incidence of all-cause mortality and oxygen requirement for 28 days was significantly lower in vitamin A group (relative risk (95% confidence interval), 0.440 (0.229-0.844); $p < 0.05$, number needed to benefit, 7).

Requirement and duration of oxygen supplementation and non-invasive respiratory support, incidences of late-onset sepsis, patent ductus arteriosus, and duration of hospital stay were also significantly lower in vitamin A group.

- Postnatal intramuscular vitamin A supplementation improves the survival, respiratory outcome and other morbidities in very low birth weight neonates without major adverse effects.
- Limited studies on oral vitamin A supplementation did not document substantial benefits.
- Early postnatal alternate-day oral vitamin A supplementation at the dose of 10,000 IU/dose for 28 days improves the composite outcome of death and oxygen requirement in very low birth weight neonates with respiratory distress
- No major adverse effects were documented.

Early Human Milk Fortification in Infants Born Extremely Preterm: A Randomized Trial *Pediatrics* (2023) 152 (3): e2023061603

- Starting on feeding day 2, extremely preterm infants 28 weeks or younger fed maternal or donor milk were randomized to receive either a diet fortified with a human-based product (intervention group) or a standard, unfortified diet (control group).
- Addition of bovine-based fortifiers at approximately postnatal day 14 after full enteral nutrition has been established.
- The primary outcome was FFM fat free mass -for-age z score at 36 weeks of postmenstrual age (PMA).
- FFM-for-age *z* scores did not differ between groups. Length gain velocities from birth to 36 weeks PMA were higher in the intervention group. Declines in head circumference-for-age *z* score from birth to 36 weeks' PMA were less pronounced in the intervention group.

CONCLUSIONS

In infants born extremely preterm, human milk diets fortified soon after birth do not increase FFM accretion at 36 weeks' PMA, but they may increase length gain velocity and reduce declines in head circumference-for-age *z* scores from birth to 36 weeks' PMA

Role of probiotics VSL#3 in prevention of suspected sepsis in low birth weight infants in India: a randomised controlled trial

Interventions:

- Infants were randomised to receive probiotic (VSL#3, 10 billion colony-forming units (cfu)) or placebo for 30 days, and were followed up for 2 months.

Main outcome measure:

- Possible serious bacterial infection (PSBI) as per the Integrated Management of Neonatal Childhood Illnesses algorithm,
- Probiotics reduced median days of hospitalisation (6 days vs 3 days in probiotics) (p=0.018) but not the risk of hospitalisation (RR 0.66 (95% CI 0.42 to 1.04).
- The onset of PSBI in 10% of infants occurred on the 40th day in the probiotics arm versus the 25th day in the control arm (p=0.063).

Conclusions:

- Daily supplementation of LBW infants with probiotics VSL#3 (10 billion cfu) for 30 days led to a non-significant 21% reduction in risk of neonatal sepsis.
- A larger study with sufficient power and a more specific primary end point is warranted to confirm the preventive effect of VSL#3 on neonatal sepsis in LBW infants

Bifidobacterium breve BBG-001 in very preterm infants: a randomised controlled phase 3 trial e Probiotics in Preterm Infants Study 2016

Population

- 23 and 30 weeks' gestational age within 48 h of birth

Intervention

- Probiotic or placebo
- The probiotic intervention was B breve BBG-001 suspended in dilute elemental infant formula given enterally in a daily dose of 8·2 to 9·2 log10 CFU; the placebo was dilute infant formula alone.

Outcome

- The primary outcomes were necrotising enterocolitis (Bell stage 2 or 3), blood culture positive sepsis more than 72 h after birth; and death before discharge from hospital.
- Rates of the primary outcomes did not differ significantly between the probiotic and placebo groups.
- 61 infants (9%) in the probiotic group had necrotising enterocolitis compared with 66 (10%) in the placebo group
- (73 (11%) infants in the probiotics group had sepsis compared with 77 (12%) in the placebo group (0·97 (0·73–1·29); and 54 (8%) deaths occurred before discharge home in the probiotic group compared with 56 (9%) in the placebo group (0·93 [0·67–1·30]).
- No probiotic-associated adverse events were reported. Interpretation There is no evidence of benefit for this intervention in this population; this result does not support the routine use of B breve BBG-001 for prevention of necrotising enterocolitis and late-onset sepis in very preterm infants.

Probiotics for preventing NEC a network meta analysis 2021 nutrients

Exclusive HM fed infants For Single strain probiotics

- Bifidobacterium lactis - associated with reduced risk for NEC stage >= stage 2 both in exclusive and nonexclusive HM fed infants, (with relative effect size favoring infants fed exclusive Human milk).
- L. reuteri DSM17938 -reduced risk of stage 2 NEC in exclusively HM-fed preterm infants and with a reduced risk of NEC at any stage in non-exclusively HM-fed infants.

For multi-genus probiotics

- The authors found that combinations of one or more Lactobacillus spp. and one or more Bifidobacterium spp., Bifidobacterium lactis and Lactobacillus reuteri significantly reduced severe NEC in exclusively HM fed infants.

Non-Exclusive HM fed infants (Mixed Feeding)

For Single strain probiotic

- B. lactis Bb-12 OR B94 & L. Reuteri DSM17938 were associated with a reduced risk of any-stage NEC in non-exclusively HM-fed preterm infants. (mixed feeding)

For Multi-genus probiotics

- L.rhamnosus GG + L.paracasei + L.casei + L.acidophilus + Lactococcus lactis + B.bifidum + B.longum + B.infantis,
- B.longum R00175 + L.helveticus R0052 + L.rhamnosus R0011 + Sa.boulardii CNCM-I-1079 3. B.infantis ATCC15697 + L.acidophilus ATCC4356 • reported the best SUCRA values among the evaluated treatments in the multi-genus probiotic group with mixed feeding.

Characterisation and antimicrobial resistance of sepsis pathogens in neonates born in tertiary care centres in Delhi, India: a cohort study Investigators of the Delhi Neonatal Infection Study (DeNIS) collaboration

- The incidence of total sepsis was 14·3% (95% CI 13·8–14·9) and of culture-positive sepsis was 6·2% (5·8–6·6).
- Nearly two-thirds of total episodes occurred at or before 72 h of life (defined as early onset; 1351 [83%] of 1980).
- Two-thirds (645 [64%]) of 1005 isolates were Gram-negative including, Acinetobacter spp (22%), Klebsiella spp (17%), and Escherichia coli (14%).
- The pathogen mix in early-onset sepsis did not diff er from that of late-onset sepsis (i.e, after 72 h).
- High rates of multidrug resistance were observed in Acinetobacter spp (181/222, 82%), Klebsiella spp (91/169, 54%), and Escherichia coli (52/137, 38%) isolates.
- Meticillin resistance prevailed in 61% (85/140) of coagulase-negative staphylococci and 38% (43/114) of Staphylococcus aureus isolates

Early switching from intravenous to oral antibiotics in neonates with probable bacterial infection (RAIN TRIAL)

(P) In clinically well neonates born at or after 35 completed weeks' gestation with probable bacterial infection,

(I) is intravenous-to-oral antibiotic switch policy, at least as effective as,

(C) a full course of intravenous antibiotics,

(O) in reducing bacterial (re) infection within 28 days after finishing antimicrobial therapy (T)

- In the intervention group, intravenous antibiotics had been replaced by eight- hourly dosing regimen of 25/ 6.25 mg/kg of oral amoxicillin/ clavulanic acid, after 48 to 72 hours.
- In the control group, the full course of intravenous antibiotics had been accomplished.
- In both groups, neonates will be treated for a total of 7 days.
- The primary outcome of the cumulative reinfection rate at day 28 was reported in 1 of 252 neonates (<1%) in the amoxicillin–clavulanic acid group and 1 of 252 neonates (<1%) in the intravenous antibiotics group, between groups difference 0 [95% CI –1.9 to 1.9]; $p_{\text{non-inferiority}}$ <0.0001).
- Neonates in the in the amoxicillin–clavulanic acid group had significantly shorter duration of hospital stay [3.4 (3·0 to 4·1) vs. 6·8 (6·5 to 7·0), P = <0·0001] compared with than the intravenous antibiotics group.
- No statistically significant differences between both arms as regards adverse events either per intention-to -treat analysis (127 [50%] vs 113 [45%]; p=0·247) or per-protocol analysis (129 [52%] vs 82 [40%]; p= 0·074).
- The re-admission rates were similar between both groups.
- No statistically significant difference between both arms regarding the readmission rates and the quality of life assessment item

CONCLUSION:

The authors conclude that intravenous to- oral switch policy is not inferior to a full course of intravenous antibiotics completion in neonates with probable bacterial infection without increased the incidence of adverse events.

24 Total Parenteral Nutrition

Role of amino acids in Total Parenteral Nutrition (TPN)

Protein accretion rates in New-borns at 24-32 weeks GA is 3.3-4gm/kg/day.

- Dextrose 3.4 kcal/g
- Protein 4 kcal/g
- Fat -2 kcal/mL

Why preterms need protein in TPN?

- They have inefficient enzyme systems limiting the synthesis, transformation and degradation of essential amino acids (AA)
- Protein intake has direct co-relation with nitrogen retention
- Proteins are needed for improved cognitive function (head growth)
- Protein are needed for body growth thus prevent growth failure

Protein intake and its practical implications

- Maximum tolerated IV doses of Amino Acid is: 3.5g/kg/day
- Positive nitrogen balance achieved at 2.5gm/kg/day
- 30 non-protein calories per gm of Amino acid is needed for protein accretion
- Non-protein calorie: nitrogen ratio to be maintained between 150-250 (calorie protein ratio)
- For optimum protein accretion Non protein Energy Ratio (NER) or Calorie Nitrogen Ratio (CNR) should be between 150 and 250.
- **NER or CNR = Non-protein calories (CHO +Fats) / 0.16 × protein in gm**

Role of dextrose in TPN

- Chief energy source of brain
- Glucose intake should cover 60-70% of non-protein calories
- Starting GIR: 4-8 mg/kg/min on day 1 (45-150 mg %)
- Max GIR 12 (preterm) & 13 (term)
- When glucose is in excess, it undergoes lipogenesis, which leads to increased energy expenditure & increased CO_2 production exacerbating the lung disease.

Role of lipids in TPN

- Lipid is needed for proper cell metabolism
- It has important Role in brain development
- Lipid provides Essential fatty acids which are necessary for myelination
- Its usage decreases CO_2 production
- Hence, lipids should constitute 25-30% of non-protein calories and supplements of 0.1 gm/kg/day (term) to 0.25 gm/kg/day (preterm) of linoleic acid.

A Cochrane meta-analysis reported NO increase in sepsis, thrombocytopenia, NEC and increased duration of ventilation when lipids were introduced early (12 hrs) vs late (6 days)

What type of lipid is recommended for TPN?

- Latest recommendation: to use balanced composition of soybean oil (30%), MCT (30%), olive oil (25%) & fish oil (15%) plus tocopherol to counteract lipid peroxidation.
- Ideal ratio of w-6: w-3 fatty acids should be between 2 to 4 as it is most favourable for immune response and patient recovery
- Vitamins are added to lipid emulsion to increase stability & reduce peroxide formation

What Clinical Signs does a neonate shows in case of EFA Deficiency

Reduced growth rate • Flaky dry skin • Poor hair growth • Thrombocytopenia • Increased susceptibility to infections • Impaired wound healing.

Guidelines for using total parenteral nutrition

- Use central line for TPN if dextrose concentration is

> 12.5% or solution osmolarity > 900 mosm/l, if there is suggestion of prolonged TPN requirement.

- Single lumen central lines to be preferred
- Minimal handling with aseptic precautions
- PICC lines better as reduces number of lines needed and not associated with increased risk of sepsis
- Lipid is infused separately by syringe
- The two preparations can be infused thru same line by joining thru a 3 way connector
- Bacterial filter is used in line with AA, dextrose and electrolytes

What are the Complications of nutrition Over-correction?

- Excess CO2 production & increased minute ventilation
- Pulmonary edema and respiratory failure
- Hyperglycemia, which may lead to immuno-suppression, and increased infection rates
- Lipogenesis due to increased insulin production
- Generalized immunosuppression
- Hepatic complications: fatty liver, intrahepatic cholestasis, due to excess carbohydrate

Concentration of macronutrient in TPN

- Carb -50-60 %
- Lipid – 30-35 %
- Protein 10-15 %

Lipids contains three components in TPN

- Triglycerides (derived from soyabean, sunflower)
- Phospholipids for emulsification (from egg yolk)
- Glycerol to achieve isotonicity

What are the features of intralipid 20%?

- It's an Oil in water emulsion
- Contains Purified soyabean oil
- Purified egg phospholipid
- Has Osmolarity of 260 mosm/ l
- Energy content is 2 kcal / ml

What are the differences between 20 % Vs 10% Intralipids

- 1gm TG of 10% contains 120 mg phospholipid
- 1gm TG of 20% contains 60 mg phospholipid
- 10% intralipid infusion leads to - ↑ phospholipid , ↓ TG clearance
- The absorption of 20% lipid emulsion found to be better than 10% lipid Emulsions.
- Thus 20% intralipid is PREFERRED CHOICE

What is SMOF 20%?

- Contains: Soybean oil, Medium chain triglyceride, Olive oil and Fish oil
- A less marked increase of serum triglyceride concentration.

What is Omegaven 10%?

- Contain highly refined fish oil – 10gm
- Contains Eicosapentaenoic acid, Decosahexaenoic acid, α-Tocopherol.
- Glycerol: 2.5 g
- Purified egg phosphatide: 1.2 g
- Energy: 112 kcal/100ml
- pH: 7.5 to 8.7
- Osmolality: 308-376 mosm/kg

What's the Rationale for Providing Lipids Early in TPN?

- Good Energy substrate, iso-osmolar
- It's a Condensed energy source- prevents fluid overload
- Essential Fatty Acid (EFA) status in early infancy is low and is rapidly exacerbated with lipid free nutrition prevented by early lipid in TPN.
- Long Chain Polyunsaturated Fatty Acid (LCPUFA) derivatives from EFAs are important in brain and retinal development
- Lipids Prevent catabolism and protein sparing

How to give lipids?

- PN Lipid supplementation should start at 18-24 hr of life
- Maximum lipid dose ~ 3gm/kg/day
- Lipids should be given as continuous infusion over 18-24 hours
- Serum triglycerides should be monitored (< 200-250mg/dl)

Early Lipid Administration

NO differences in mortality, chronic lung disease or other morbidity in early versus late introduction of intravenous lipid.

Minerals in TPN

Phosphates

- 1mmol = 31mg of elemental P
- Available as organic and inorganic forms
- Inorganic forms available as dibasic or monobasic Na or K salts
- Availability in India still limited

Magnesium in TPN

- Given as 50% $MgSO_4$ solution
- I ml= 4mEq
- Dose is 0.2-0.3 ml/Kg/d

Vitamins in TPN

- All fat and water soluble vitamins needed
- No Pediatric MVI available
- Adult MVI 0.5ml/Kg should be added
- Recommended from Day 1 in preterms
- Vit K should be given weekly IM
- Extra Vit A may be beneficial to ELBW babies to prevent CLD

What are the Problems with vitamins infusion in TPN?

- Photo-degradation of vitamins A, D, E, B2, B6, B12, C, and folic acid
- AVOID exposure to light/phototherapy
- Cover with foil/use special tubing's
- Adsorption of vitamins A, D, and E occurs into the vinyl delivery bags and tubing
- Peroxide load from lipid peroxidation

Role of Trace Elements in TPN

- Present in <micrograms/L in serum
- Stores occur in last 12 weeks of gestation and last up to 3-6 months
- Zn, Cu, Cr, Se and Iron are most important
- Usually needed if TPN > 2 weeks
- Required for growth, skin and epithelial integrity

Complications associated with parenteral nutrition

- Sepsis, bacteremia, fungemia
- Fluid overload, dehydration
- Hyperglycemia, hypoglycemia
- Hypernatremia, hyponatremia
- Hyperkalaemia, hypokalaemia
- Hyperchloremia, hypochloremia
- Hyperphosphatemia, hypophosphatemia
- Hypercalcemia, hypocalcemia
- Hypermagnesemia, hypomagnesemia
- Bone demineralization Rickets, Osteoporosis
- Hepatobiliary dysfunction Cholestasis Cholelithiasis Steatosis
- Venous thrombosis
- Embolism Air embolism
- Extravasation of solution
- Catheter site infection
- Cardiac arrhythmia
- Deep vein or myocardial perforation
- Pneumothorax
- Hydrothorax Hemothorax
- Catheter dislodgement
- Vitamin or trace element deficiency
- Essential fatty acid deficiency Hyperlipidemia
- Fat overload syndrome Amino acid imbalance Hyperammonemia
- Acidosis

Implications in starting TPN in Resource Limited Settings

- TPN in term/late preterm: Starting TPN in these units will be a challenge due to understaffing, lack of training, and infrastructure for TPN prescription.
- TPN formulation (Standardized TPN): Availability and cost is a significant concern for widespread usage. In most developed countries, TPN is prepared and dispensed by trained central pharmacists. Manual mixing of various TPN constituents carries a risk of sepsis. There is an additional risk of errors in calculation or adding the right amount of TPN constituents with manual methods.
- Micronutrients: Availability of phosphate, trace elements, and multi-vitamin solution in appropriate customized doses for neonates is a concern.
- Venous access: Central line is preferred for delivery of TPN for long-term use. However, in most settings, maintenance of the central line and risk of sepsis are major limiting factors. Both guidelines allow peripheral line TPN for short-term use only.

- Infections: Due to overcrowding, understaffing, and lack of laminar flow, the risk of infection is higher with TPN usage. The risk of infection can be reduced by strict asepsis during preparation and Quality improvement approaches for central line-associated bloodstream infection reduction.
- Monitoring: Frequent monitoring can be a challenge, which can be overcome by using a standardized monitoring chart
- Cost: Cost of central lines, TPN constituents, and frequent monitoring is an additional co

Cochrane 2019 IV lipid in preterms

In preterm infants, meta-analysis found no evidence of a difference in the incidence of PNALD/cholestasis between fish oil based lipid infusion and all non-fish oil lipid low-quality evidence).

There was no evidence of a difference between fish oil lipid and all non-fish oil lipid for incidence of cholestasis; low-quality evidence).

There was no evidence of difference in subgroup meta-analyses of individual new lipids types in any comparison.

In preterm infants with surgical conditions or cholestasis, there was only one small study each reporting no evidence of a difference in incidence or resolution of cholestasis respectively with use of a pure Fish oil lipid versus soyabean based lipid

In preterm infants with PNALD/cholestasis (using any definition), the meta-analysis showed significantly less cholestasis with the use of fish oil-LE compared to Soyabean-LE (typical RR 0.54, 95% CI 0.32 to 0.91; typical RD –0.39, 95% CI –0.65 to –0.12; number needed to treat for an additional beneficial outcome (NNTB) 3, 95% CI 2 to 9; 2 studies; n = 40; very low-quality evidence). However, this outcome had a very low number of participants from two small studies with methodological differences, one of which was terminated early, increasing the uncertainty about effect estimates.

In the secondary outcomes for preterm infants, there was no difference between fish-oil lipid and non-fish oil lipid in meta-analysis for severe retinopathy of prematurity (ROP) (stage 3 or greater, or requiring surgery: typical RR 0.80, 95% CI 0.55 to 1.16; typical RD – 0.03, 95% CI –0.07 to 0.02; 7 studies; n = 731; very low-quality evidence). There were no differences in the LE types in pair-wise meta-analyses for death, bronchopulmonary dysplasia (BPD), ventilation duration, patent ductus arteriosus, sepsis, necrotising enterocolitis, intraventricular haemorrhage, periventricular leukomalacia, jaundice, hyperglycaemia, hypertriglyceridaemia, intra hepatocellular lipid content and conjugated bilirubin levels in any comparison.

25 Human Milk Banking

- Human milk is both **immunologically and nutritionally** ideal so called as -LIQUID GOLD
- According to NFHS what percentage of children under age 3 year were breastfed within 1 hr of birth - 41 %
- According to NFHS -5 what percentage of children under age 6 month are exclusively breastfed – 63.7 %

History of human milk banking

- First HMB in India established in 1989 by Dr. Armida Fernandez in Lokmanya Tilak Municipal Medical College and general hospital, Mumbai
- 2015 : IAP Guidelines
- 2017: National guidelines on lactation management in Public Health Centers.
- Currently there are more than **750 milk banks in 66 countries**
- In India there are approx. **100 HMBs**
- **Brazil** has the most comprehensive network of Human Milk Banks (HMBs), with 222 HMBs and 217 Collection Centres in Brazil

Which is the best milk for neonate according to WHO (best to worst)?

1. MOM
2. Donor fresh PT milk
3. Donated fresh term mature milk
4. PDHM
5. Preterm formula
6. Ordinary formula

Steps in human milk donation in bank

1. Screening of donor mothers
2. Milk collection
3. Processing of DHM –pre pasteurization – pooling – pasteurization
4. Testing of DHM
5. Storage of PDHM
6. Dispensing of PDHM

Which all mothers can donate their milk?

- Mothers whose babies are in the NICU
- Mothers in the postnatal wards and KMC wards
- Mothers of babies visiting well-baby follow-up clinics/ immunization sessions can be motivated to donate milk after ensuring they are in good health and complying with milk donation criteria.
- Lactating women among the staff of the hospital

What does SCREENING of donor mothers involves?

- Following screening blood tests are mandatory, if antenatal serological reports for them with in past 6 months are not available:
- a. HIV 1 or 2
- b. Hepatitis B
- c. Syphilis/VDRL
- d. Hepatitis C (optional)
- Antenatal serological tests conducted by a certified laboratory within the 6 months prior to donating milk will be considered and negative test results do not require confirmatory testing.
- If lifestyle or medical issues suggest an increased risk of donation, deferral or retesting is at the discretion of the pediatrician/neonatologist in-charge of the CLMC.

WHO CANNOT DONATE their milk?

- Receipt of a blood transfusion/blood product within past 12 months.
- Receipt of an organ or tissue transplant, within past 12 months.
- Permanent *tattoo*/ears or other body piercing with other than single-use instruments within the last 12 months.
- Daily use of alcohol

- Donors must not be users of tobacco or nicotine products including gum or e-cigarettes. These include casual and occasional smokers.
- Chronic Infection (HIV, active TB etc.) relevant to breastfeeding, a history of hepatitis B, hepatitis C (optional), or a history of leukemia or lymphoma or treatment of any other cancer within the last 3 years.
- A sexual partner in the past 12 months who is suffering from/at risk for HBV, HCV (optional), HIV and venereal diseases or one who has high risk behavior for contracting them

Who all can be given PDHM?

1. Premature and low birth weight babies: The largest group of recipients of donor human milk is preterm babies especially in the first few days, till their mothers are able to secrete adequate milk.
2. Sick preterm New-borns recovering from illnesses like necrotizing enterocolitis and GI surgeries
3. Severe IUGR.
4. New-borns not having access to her own mother's milk or when the mother has a contraindication to breastfeeding/expressing milk.
5. Babies of mothers with problems like eclampsia, PPH, febrile illnesses.
6. Babies admitted to the unit whose mothers are not available (due to physical absence or death).
7. Babies whose mothers have lactation failure.
8. Exceptional cases, with medical justification.
9. Multiple births (if needed).

LEVELS OF LACTATION MANAGEMENT CENTRES

CLMC – IN medical colleges with NICU and district hospitals (in phase 2) - complete milk bank

LMU – at district hospital /large sub district hospital with functional SNCU- only expression, storage and dispensing of milk

LSU- at all deliver points – skilled lactation support and counselling only.

Steps in manual expression of milk

1. Wash your hand well with soap and water
2. Place a clean container below your breast to collect milk
3. Massage the breast gently towards the nipple
4. Place your thumb and index finger opposite each other just outside the areola
5. Now press backwards towards your chest and gently squeeze to express milk
6. Repeat this at 5 different position around the areola
7. Express minimum 8 times/day or 100 minutes per 24 hours till baby starts to breastfeed.
8. Mothers should be encouraged to express milk from both the breasts completely each time to maintain the milk output

How milk is expressed by electric pump?

- Hospital-grade electric breast pumps are recommended for use in Lactation Management Centers (CLMCs and LMUs).
- Basic design-a funnel attachment, which fits over the nipple and areola, and work on a simple vacuum principle.
- Electric breast pumps are efficient and can be adapted to allow single or double pumping.
- Each mother should be provided sterilized tubing, funnel and milk container. There should be no sharing of breast pump tubing, funnel and milk containers among the donor mothers.
- Double pumping reduces time of expression by 10-15 minutes and also allows for higher prolactin reflex which results in higher amount in less time.
- Pause for 30-60 seconds when the milk slowsdown.
- Stop pumping after 20-40 minutes or when the milk stops flowing.
- Damaging of breast tissue should in no case be allowed by incorrect use of breast pump.

TYPE OF CONTAINER used for collection and storage of breast milk

- Containers of **polycarbonates, pyrexor polypropylene** are used across the world , **Food grade bisphenol A free hard plastic** -Nutrients and cells preserved - Reduce lactoferrin, lysozyme, S-IgA
- **Polythene bags** are fragile, prone to puncture and contamination and associated with a decrease in the IgA (60%), loss of vitamins, proteins and lipids
- In Indian setup, **stainless steel containers with tight fitting, screwed caps** are easily available, durable, easy to clean & autoclave- Cellular components are reduced

Important points to follow while storage and thawing of milk

- Mixing of raw milk to frozen milk of the same mother is not allowed due to hydrolysis of lipids because of sudden decrease in temperature of frozen milk.
- Shift the frozen DHM to a refrigerator overnight (not more than 24 hours) to allow milk to thaw slowly to 4°C.
- In case of an emergency, thawing can be done in a wide container of warm water (not to exceed 37°C) ensuring that water does not touch the lids of the containers and it does not fall over.
- Thawing should never be done in a microwave oven-destroy Immunoglobulin A and other antibacterial properties more than any other form of thawing.
- The content is gently agitated in order to uniformly distribute the constituents, as protein, water and fat of expressed milk freezes and thaws at different rate.
- ™The time and date of the thawing should be documented accurately.
- ™Thawed milk should never be refrozen.

PRE-PASTEURISATION TESTING OF DHM

- Before pasteurization, sample from each batch of pooled raw donor milk is to be tested for Staphylococcus aureus colony count. Milk would be discarded if colony count is more than 10^4 CFU.
- Other microbes are accepted irrespective of colony count.

PASTERUISATION of DHM

- Pasteurization eliminates bacteria while retaining the majority of the milk's beneficial components.
- This preserves Vitamin C content, prevents lipid peroxidation and inactivates CMV, HIV, and kills most pathogenic bacteria found in breast-milk.
- Pasteurisation should ideally be undertaken each day.
- However, the frequency of pasteurization will depend on the quantity of milk collected.

Two Methods of pasteurization used are:

- •Low temperature, long time (LTLT)
- •High temperature, short time (HTST)
- For CLMC - recommended to use a form of LTLT heat treatment also known as Holder Pasteurization method.
- Heating DHM to 62.5°C (+/–0.5°C) and holding at this temperature for 30 minutes.
- Following this, the temperature of the milk is then rapidly reduced to minimize heat damage to nutrients and provide a thermal shock to the organisms enhancing their destruction and preventing growth of spores.
- Milk temperature of 25°C to be attained within 10 minutes of the completion of holding period of 30 minutes and that a final temperature of 4°C be attained prior to transferring the pasteurized milk to a freezer.

Fully automated pasteuriser-Higher cost

Semi- automated pasteuriser- **SHAKER WATER BATH-**

a) Heat processing

Aliquots of milk are processed by submerging the containers in the well-agitated or shaking water bath preheated to a minimum of 62.5°C.

A control bottle containing the same amount of milk or water is also included for processing of every batch.

It should have temperature probe (data logger) in the control container to document the process of pasteurization throughout the process.

After the temperature of the monitored control bottle has reached 62.5°C the heat treatment continues for 30 minutes, maintaining the temperature and then ends immediately.

Fluctuation during the heating process may be seen for short periods of adjustment where heat may briefly fluctuate between 62.5°C and 64.5°C.

b) Rapid Cooling

- In this process cooling needs to be done immediately.
- Following heat processing, the milk is rapidly cooled to 4°C using either the processing equipment manufactured to cool milk or ice baths within 10 minute.
- If ice baths for cooling are used, water source must be of adequate sanitary quality and equipment creating ice must be maintained as per manufacturers' instructions.

The Effect of Holder Pasteurization on Nutrients and Biologically-Active Components in Donor Human Milk

	Donor Milk % activity
Living cells	0%
Secretory IgA	67
IgM	0%
IgG	70
Lactoferrin	27
Lysozyme	75%
Lipoprotein lipase	0%
Growth factors	60
Human milk oligosaccharides	100%
Gangliosides	100%
Free fatty Acids	100%

- Culture-negative pasteurized DHM kept at deep freezer –20°C can be preserved for 6 months.
- However, the milk may get rancid after 3 months due to lipolysis, but is still fit for consumption though it would have altered taste.
- Cooled or thawed pasteurized milk can be stored in the refrigerator at + 4°C, and should be used within 24 hours.
- Lid of any pasteurized DHM bottle should not be opened until the milk is dispensed for use.

Do not to transfer pasteurized milk in other containers as it has risk of contamination

- Prior to use, the DHM should be thawed preferably by transferring ™initially to refrigerator (at +4ÚC).
- It can be refrigerated for a maximum period of 24 hours.
- Before dispensing of DHM for use in the wards it should be brought to room temperature.
- ™Pasteurized frozen milk after bringing to room temperature should be used for feeding as soon as possible.
- DHM has to be consumed within two hrs preferably and latest by 4 hrs. Of storing at room temperature.
- The excess thawed DHM left after feeding the babies should be discarded immediately.

What is HACCP?

- It is an internationally recognized system used in the food industry to identify and reduce hazards during food processing.
- It stands for Hazard Analysis Critical Control Point
- Objectives: identify and prevent, eliminate, or reduce to acceptable levels any biological, chemical, or physical hazard that would be likely to occur in a food production or distribution environment.
- Milk bank uses this system as well to reduce hazards during food processing.

26 Polycythemia

Definition

Venous haematocrit > 65% or a Venous Hb > 22 gm/dL.

As viscosity increases, there may be impairment of tissue oxygenation and decreased glucose in plasma, leading to an increased risk of microthrombi formation.

Polycythemia is defined as venous hematocrit of at least 65%. The hyperviscosity syndrome is usually seen only in infants with venous hematocrit above 60%.Hyperviscosity is defined as a viscosity greater than 14.6 centipoise at a shear rate of 11.5 per second. The hematocrit peaks at around 2 hr of age and values upto 71% maybe normal at this age.

The relationship between hematocrit and viscosity is nearly linear below a hematocrit of 60%, but viscosity increases exponentially at a hematocrit of 70% or greater.

Incidence

- The incidence of polycythemia is 1% to 5% in term New-borns.
- About 15% of term SGA infants develop polycythemia as compared to 2% of term AGA infants.

Peripheral venous hematocrit sample is preferred to measure polycythemia. Arterial blood sample is not acceptable for hematocrit estimation as it would underestimate the hematocrit; capillary sample would overestimate the hematocrit by 5% to 15%.

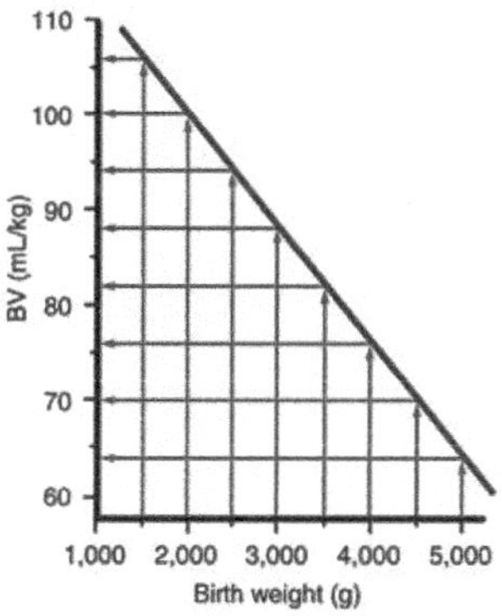

Blood volume in a polycythaemia neonate as per birth weight

There are three possible settings for polycythemia:

(i) Hypervolemia—placental transfusion;

(ii) Normovolemia placental insufficiency (fetal growth restriction [FGR])

(iii) Hypovolemia—dehydration

Partial exchange transfusion will likely treat symptoms, but has not been shown to affect the neurodevelopmental outcome.

Intravenous fluid supplementation does not decrease the need for partial exchange transfusion (for polycythemia). However, it may be considered in neonates with evidence of dehydration

A recent clinical trial that compared supplemental intravenous fluids with no supplementation in asymptomatic late preterm and term neonates with venous hematocrit between 65 and 75 did not find any evidence of clinical benefit with fluid supplementation.

Partial exchange transfusion: There seems to be no short- or long-term benefits of PET in polycythemia New-born infants who are asymptomatic or who have mild symptoms. PET may increase the risk of NEC. The developmental outcomes are reported to be variable.

Partial exchange transfusion should be performed with a crystalloid solution such as 0.9% saline. Usually, we take the blood from the peripheral artery and replace it with normal saline through a peripheral vein. Wherever possible, the umbilical vein should be avoided for pulling blood for PET due to the increased incidence of NEC when this vein is used.

Volume of exchange [mL]

$$= \frac{\text{(blood volume/kg} \times \text{weight in [kg]} \times \text{([observed hermatocrit] [desired hermatocrit])}}{\text{observed hermatocrit}}$$

The total volume exchanged is usually 15 to 20 mL/kg of body weight

Short term benefits of PET

- PET will lower hematocrit, decrease viscosity, and reverse many of the physiologic abnormalities associated with polycythemia hyperviscosity but has not been shown to significantly change the long-term outcome of these infants.
- Infants with polycythemia and hyperviscosity who have decreased cerebral blood flow velocity have been shown to have normal cerebral blood flow following PET.
- They also have improvement in systemic blood flow and oxygen transport
- There is no evidence for improvement in long-term neurologic outcome in infants with asymptomatic polycythemia/hyperviscosity.

27 Kangaroo Mother Care

History of Kangaroo Mother Care (KMC) - In 1978, Dr Edgar Rey Sanabria, Bogotá, Colombia. Instituto Maternal Infantil, Colombia, South America.

In 2003, WHO formally endorsed KMC and published KMC practice guidelines.

The WHO defines KMC with 4 components:

- Early, continuous, and prolonged skin-to-skin contact (SSC) between the New-born and mother,
- Exclusive breastfeeding,
- Early discharge from the health facility,
- Close follow-up at home

History of KMC in India

- 1995 – Few Paediatricians were trained in Kangaroo Mother care in India Mumbai, Ahmedabad, Rajasthan, Delhi, Chandigarh, Chennai, Lucknow, West Bengal
- 2001 — Kangaroo Mother Care in very low birth weight infants. Ramanathan K, et al. Indian J Pediatr. 2001
- 2004 – KMC Initiative – Network of five centers
- 2015 – 2KMC Foundation formed
- 2016 – KMC Guidelines by GOI
- KMC was introduced in India, in 1994 in BJ Medical College Hospital, Ahmedabad. This was followed by experiences in KEM Mumbai and at the All India Institute Medical Sciences (AIIMS).
- A KMC India Network comprising six institutions were started in 2003.

Innate behaviour of New-born immediately after birth

There is a sequence of nine innate behaviors described by Widstrom et al as birth cry, relaxation, awakening and opening the eyes, activity, a second resting phase, crawling towards the nipple, touching and licking the nipple, suckling at the breast and ûnally falling asleep

This 'sensitive period' predisposes or primes mothers and infants to develop a synchronous reciprocal interaction pattern, provided they are together and in intimate contact.

Who gave the theory of zero separation?

Nils Bergman -S chool of Child and Adolescent Health, and Department of Human Biology, University of Cape Town, Cape Town, South Africa

What is Zero Separation Policy?

Promotion of Zero Separation is based on the need for maternal sensory inputs that regulate the physiology of the New-born. There are harmful effects of dysregulation and subsequent epigenetic changes caused by separation.

Skin-to-skin contact is the antithesis to such separation; the mother's body is the biologically 'normal' place of care, supporting better outcomes both for normal healthy babies and for the smallest preterm infants

In the mother, there are needed neural processes that ensure enhanced reproductive fitness, including behavioural changes (e.g. bonding and protection) and improved lactation, which are supported by the practice of Zero Separation. When the infant is placed prone on the mother's abdomen or chest in direct ventral-to-ventral skin-to-skin contact"

Immediate skin-to-skin contact is done immediately after delivery, less than 10 minutes after birth

Early skin-to-skin contact was defined as beginning any time from delivery to 23 hours after birth.

Skin-to-skin contact should be uninterrupted for at least 60 minutes

What are the different types of KMC based on duration

- Short: 4 hours daily
- Extended: 5-8 hours daily
- Long: 9-12 hours daily
- Continuous: More than12 hours daily

KMC satisfies all five senses of the infant.

The infant feels the mother's warmth through skin-to-skin contact (touch), listens to her voice and heartbeat (hearing), sucks breast milk (taste) has eye contact with her (vision) and smells her odour (olfaction)

COMPONENTS OF KMC

- Kangaroo position: The kangaroo position consists of skin-to-skin contact (SSC) between the mother and the neonate in a vertical position, between the mother's breasts and under her clothes
- Kangaroo nutrition: Kangaroo nutrition is the delivery of nutrition to "kangarooed" neonates as soon as oral feeding is possible.
- Kangaroo discharge: Early home discharge in the kangaroo position from the neonatal unit is one of the key components of KMC
- Mothers at home require adequate support and follow-up; hence a follow-up program and access to emergency services must be ensured.

What is KMC POSITION?

- Upright positioning facing the mother's chest in between the breasts.
- Baby's chest and abdomen in skin -to-skin contact with mother.
- Head turned to one side in a slightly extended position.
- Avoid both forward flexion and hyperextension of the head.
- Frog positioning with hips flexed

Benefits of KMC

• Provides effective thermal control with a reduced risk of hypothermia.
• Facilitates physiological stability.
• Increases rate and duration of breastfeeding
• Reduces incidence of hypoglycemia
• Reduces incidence of apnea & sepsis
• Facilitates better weight gain thereby reduces hospital stay
• Improves follow up rates
• Alleviates pain in preterms
• Promotes lactation and facilitates the feeding interaction.
• Reduces stress, increases confidence, and provides deep satisfaction to parents with stronger bonding with the baby due to active involvement in care of the baby.
• Reduces health care cost as KMC saves money on equipment, medicines, artificial feeds, & prolonged hospital stay required during conventional care.
• KMC reduces mortality by 40%

Skin to skin care (SSC) and maternal oxytocin levels

SSC is a powerful vagal stimulant, through sensory stimuli such as touch, warmth, and odor, which among other effects releases maternal oxytocin. Oxytocin causes the skin temperature of the mother's breast to rise, providing warmth to the infant. In a study of infrared thermography of the whole body during the ûrst hour post birth found that SSC was as effective as radiant warmers in preventing heat loss in healthy full-term infants.

EEG and KMC

Preterm infants who received SSC experienced significantly greater EEG complexity of the right hemisphere, along with areas in the left and right parasagittal regions, when compared to preterm infants who did not receive KC. EEG complexity is correlated with advanced brain maturation.

Transcranial magnetic stimulation and KMC

The study applied TMS over the primary motor cortex of the brain of 39 adolescents who had been born preterm and found that the adolescents who had received KC as preterm infants had TMS outcomes that were more similar to adolescents who were born at full term relative to adolescents who were born preterm and did not receive KC (Schneider et al.)

Those who received KMC in New-born period had Decreased motor evoked potential (MEP) latency indicates improved primary motor cortex synchronization on TMS. Interhemispheric inhibition was longer, the latency was shorter indicating a faster transfer time between hemispheres, better control between the two hemispheres, and overall properly working interhemispheric pathways.

KMC and sleep

Study revealed that the preterm infants who received KMC experienced higher baseline respiratory sinus arrhythmia (RSA) more organized sleep-wake cycle. This suggests an increase in function of the autonomic nervous system compared to the preterm non-KMC group. At the term age assessment and ten year assessment, the baseline RSA and sleep organization continued to improve, suggesting that KMC has lasting effects of at least ten year on the function of the autonomic nervous system.

KMC AND CRYING

Preterm babies who received KMC were easily consolable after robust crying compared to those who did not receive KMC.

KMC AND BRAIN MATTER

KMC participants who weighed ≤1800 g (n = 264) at birth and had good-quality nuclear magnetic resonance (n = 195) had significantly larger cerebral volumes of total gray matter, cerebral cortex, and left caudate nucleus than control participants. Sensorial (visual and hearing) and motor (cerebral palsy) morbidity was comparable between the groups at 20 years, indicating that KMC did not protect children from these conditions.

Discharge criteria for KMC recipients

Generally the following criteria are accepted at most centres:

- Baby's general health is good and no evidence of infection
- Feeding well and receiving exclusively breast milk.
- Gaining weight (at least 15-20gm/kg/day for at least three consecutive days)
- Maintaining body temperature satisfactorily in room temperature.
- The mother and family members are confident to take care of the baby in KMC and are motivated to come for follow-up visits regularly

Post- discharge follows up for KMC recipients

- Follow up twice a week till weight gain is satisfactory: 15-20 gms/kg/day.
- Follow up subsequently weekly till 37-40 weeks of gestation or till the baby reaches 2.5-3 kg of weight.
- Follow up thereafter once in 2 weeks till 3 months of corrected age and later at an interval of 1-2 months during first year of life.
- Plan for more frequent visits if the baby is not growing well or his condition demands
- Assess growth, nutrition, neuromotor, neurodevelop-mental, neurosensory, neurophysiological status and provide early intervention therapy whenever indicated

Barriers for KMC - Lack of awareness, poor resources are cited as the major barrier for KMC.

What is ambulatory KMC?

The word ambulatory means to "walk around". Which is usually refers to the KMC, which is given after the infant has been discharged.

Their mother can give home (or ambulatory) KMC throughout the day while doing their household work (while walking, cooking, washing etc.) Ambulatory KMC can also given while attending clinic or visiting hospital.

KMC Cochrane review 2016

- Reduction in the risk of mortality (typical risk ratio (RR) 0.60, 95% confidence interval (CI) 0.39 to 0.93; seven trials, 1614 infants),
- Reduction in Nosocomial infection/sepsis (typical RR 0.42, 95% CI 0.24 to 0.73),
- Less Hypothermia (typical RR 0.23, 95% CI 0.10 to 0.55),
- Length of hospital stay (typical mean difference 2.4 days, 95% CI 0.7 to 4.1) at discharge or 40 - 41 weeks' postmenstrual age.
- At latest follow up, KMC was associated with a decreased risk of mortality (typical RR 0.68, 95% CI 0.48 to 0.96; nine trials, 1952 infants) and severe infection/sepsis (typical RR 0.57, 95% CI 0.40 to 0.80).

Twenty-year Follow-up of Kangaroo Mother Care Versus Traditional Care Charpak et al, 2017

- The effects of KMC at 1 year on IQ and home environment were still present 20 years later in the most fragile individuals.
- KMC parents were more protective and nurturing. It was reflected by reduced school absenteeism reduced hyperactivity, aggressiveness, externalization, and socio-deviant conduct of young adults.
- Neuroimaging showed larger volume of the left caudate nucleus in the KMC group.

Early intermittent KMC compared with late KMC significantly improved exclusive human milk feeding and direct breastfeeding, which continued post discharge in low -birthweight infants. Infants initiated on early KMC had less frequent apneas. Intermittent KMC with increased breastfeeding opportunities was found to be effective for improving weight gain in neonates who have delayed weight gain.

What are the various types of KMC?

- iKMC
- CiKMC
- eKMC

What is CiKMC?

Initiating kangaroo mother care at the community level is a promising strategy to increase coverage.

Pilot study in Haryana, India, babies weighing 1500–2250 g at home within 72 h of birth, if not already initiated in kangaroo mother care, irrespective of place of birth.

Mothers and infants in the intervention group were visited at home (days 1–3, 5, 7, 10, 14, 21, and 28) to support kangaroo mother care (i.e., skin-to-skin contact and exclusive breastfeeding)

The risk ratios for death were 28-day mortality 0·71, 95% CI 0·52– 0·97; p=0·032; 180-day mortality 0·76, 0·60–0·95; p=0·017.

What is i KMC – immediate KMC- kmc with 10 minutes of birth?

Up to 70% of neonatal deaths occur in LBW within the first 3 days after birth.

KMC is usually initiated 3-10 days after birth, which means that a large number of deaths among preterm/LBW babies have already occurred.

SDF- Supported Diagonal flexion in KMC

SDF positioning led to fewer disorganized gestures, negative vocalizations, and drowsiness, in favor of more deep sleep.

SDF led to more mother-infant eye-to-eye contact as well as maternal vocalizations, smiles, and caressing, although these differences did not reach significance.

What is KMC doula (Kangaroula)?

The definition of a doula is a person trained to advise, inform, and offer emotional and physical comfort to a mother before, during, and after the birth of her child.

The word doula comes from the Greek word doulç, the meaning of which translates to female helper or maidservant

A doula focuses on the mother's needs during labour and birth. A Kangaroula does this also, but primarily advocates for the baby during labour, birth and the first 1000 minutes of life.

The kangaroula has additional training in skin-to-skin contact (Kangaroo Mother Care),

Hence kangaroo + doula = kangaroula

Kangaroo mother care to reduce morbidity and mortality in low birth weight infants (COCHRANE)

21 studies, 3042 infants

19 studies evaluated KMC in LBW infants after stabilization, one evaluated KMC in LBW infants before stabilization, and one compared early-onset KMC with late-onset KMC in relatively stable LBW infants.

16 studies evaluated intermittent KMC, and five evaluated continuous KMC

KMC versus conventional neonatal care:

At discharge or 40-41 weeks' PMA, KMC was associated with

- Reduction in the risk of mortality (RR 0.60, 95% CI 0.39 to 0.92; eight trials, 1736 infants)
- Nosocomial infection/sepsis (RR 0.35, 95% CI 0.22 to 0.54; five trials, 1239 infants),
- Hypothermia (RR 0.28, 95% CI 0.16 to 0.49; nine trials, 989 infants; moderate-quality evidence).

At latest follow-up, KMC was associated with

- Decreased risk of mortality (RR 0.67, 95% CI 0.48 to 0.95; 12 trials, 2293 infants; moderate-quality evidence)
- Severe infection/sepsis (RR 0.50, 95% CI 0.36 to 0.69; eight trials, 1463 infants; moderate-quality evidence).
- Increase weight gain (MD 4.1 g/d, 95% CI 2.3 to 5.9; 11 trials, 1198 infants), length gain (MD 0.21 cm/week, 95% CI 0.03 to 0.38; three trials, 377 infants) and head circumference gain (MD 0.14 cm/week, 95% CI 0.06 to 0.22; four trials, 495 infants) at latest follow-up
- Increase in exclusive breastfeeding at discharge or 40 to 41 weeks' postmenstrual age (RR 1.16, 95% CI 1.07 to 1.25; six studies, 1453 mothers) and at one to three months' follow-up (RR 1.20, 95% CI 1.01 to 1.43; five studies, 600 mothers), any (exclusive or partial) breastfeeding at one to three months' follow-up (RR 1.17, 95% CI 1.05 to 1.31; nine studies, 1394 mothers)

No statistically significant differences were found between KMC infants and controls in Griffith quotients for psychomotor development at 12 months CA.

Immediate KMC and survival of LBW infants

POPULATION (P):

- All babies with B wt 1-1.8 kgs ll infants with wt between 1000 and 1799 gms regardless of gestational age, type of delivery, or singleton or twin status

INTERVENTION (I):

- Immediate initiation of KMC after birth COMPARISON
- Conventional KMC after stabilization

OUTCOME (O):

- Survival of neonates at 72 hrs and at 28 days

Primary objectives –

- To determine mortality rates in iKMC group in first 72 hrs
- To determine mortality rates in iKMC group at end on neonatal period
- Mother–NICUs – included mothers' beds and reclining chairs, were built or converted from existing NICUs

	Intervention	Control	P value
Death between enrolment and 28 days	12 %	15.7 %	0.001
Death between enrollment and 72 hrs	4.6 %	5.8 %	0.09

- NNT 27 (95% CI, 17 to 77
- NO significant differences between groups in the two pre-specified feeding outcome
- Being fully breast-fed by suckling at discharge being fed exclusively through breast-feeding at the end of the neonatal period
- Post-hoc analyses – intervention group had higher rates for initiating breast-feeding within 24 hours, putting the baby to the breast within 72 hours after birth, and reaching full breast-feeding within 7 days of birth

Effect on neonatal sepsis following immediate kangaroo mother care in a New-born intensive care unit: a post-hoc analysis of a multicentre, open-label, randomised controlled triaL

- Methods This is a post-hoc analysis of the previous iKMC trial, which was conducted in five level 2 New-born Intensive Care Units (NICUs) one each in Ghana, India, Malawi, Nigeria, and Tanzania, in neonates with birth weight 1 to
- The primary outcomes of this report were the incidence of neonatal sepsis in sub-groups, sepsis-related mortality and bacterial profile of isolates during hospital stay.
- Suspected sepsis was 14% lower in intervention group in sub-group of neonates with birth weight 1.0-<1.5 kg; RR 0.86 (CI 0.75, 0.99).
- Among neonates with birth weight 1.5-<1.8 kg, suspected sepsis was reduced by 24%; RR 0.76 (CI 0.62, 0.93).
- Suspected sepsis rates were lower in intervention group than in the control group across all sites.
- Sepsis related mortality was 37% less in intervention group than the control group; RR 0.63 (CI 0.47–0.85) which was statistically significant.
- The intervention group had fewer cases of Gram-negative isolates (n = 9) than Gram positive isolates (n = 16)
- Interpretation Immediate Kangaroo Mother care is an effective intervention to prevent neonatal sepsis and sepsis related mortality.

28 Developmentally Supportive Care

- 1880–83: Stephane Tarnier- Installed 1st incubator in Paris
- 1893: Pierre Budin - World first SCU for premature babies in Paris
- 1922: Julius Hess Incubator- 1st premature station in US in Chicago

What are the 5 components of DSC?

1. Pain protection- assessment and management
2. Protected sleep- cluster care, nesting/swaddling. KMC
3. Developmentally supportive activities of daily life – feeding, NNS, massage
4. Family centred care – KMC, education and participation collaboration with family.
5. Healing environment – noise, light, smell, positioning, KMC.

What is a normal intrauterine environment (maternal womb) is favourable for positive sensory inputs

The Intrauterine milieu is characterized by:

1. Generalized flexion and gentle, secure containment
2. Limited light and noise exposure
3. Normal sleep cycle preservation and development.
4. Unrestricted access to mother via somatosensory, chemosensory, and auditory pathways

"In 3rd trimester of fetal development and even in early infancy the brain is drastically changing with new brain cell production and migration, synaptic pruning and brain organization".

Third trimester of pregnancy is a most crucial period, during which the basic Foundation for the Neuromotor and Neurobehavioral systems is being laid in the growing fetus

What is Developmentally Supportive Care (DSC)?

Developmentally Supportive Care (DSC) practices are evidence based interventions that promote New-born brain and neurobehavioral development. They support autonomic stability, normal motor, sensory neurological development and promote behaviour state organization

The New-born brain can make both temporary and permanent changes to its synaptic neuronal connections, which are based upon sensory input from different environmental stimuli and experiences. **This adaptive capacity is known as neuroplasticity,** and can either be positive or negative.

Evolution of DSC Models

1. Coughlin et al, 2009 - proposed five developmental care core measures
   a. Protected sleep
   b. Pain and stress assessment and management
   c. Activities of daily living (positioning, feeding and skin care),
   d. Family-centred care
   e. The healing environment
2. The neonatal integrative developmental care model has seven neuroprotective core measures for family-centered developmental care. The Neonatal Integrative Developmental Care Model (Leslie Altimier, Raylene M. Phillips, 2013)
   a. The five neonatal core measures first introduced by Coughlin et al in year 2009 have been recategorized and expanded into seven distinct core measures of Neuroprotective neonatal care.
   b. Seven neuroprotective core measures for family centered developmental care of the premature neonate are depicted on petals of a lotus.
      i. The Healing Environment
      ii. Partnering with Families
      iii. Positioning & Handling
      iv. Safeguarding Sleep
      v. Minimizing Stress & Pain
      vi. Protecting Skin
      vii. Optimizing Nutrition and Feeding.

DSC is a continuous process and should be continued after discharge.

- It should start with birth of infant.
- It should be individualized rather than protocolized.
- DSC reduces stress and promotes growth.
- Providing a structured care environment which supports, encourages and guides the developmental organization of premature infant.

What is the sequence of development of Neonatal senses?

Tactile –Vestibular Gustatory –Olfactory -Visual /Auditory

Stimulation of early maturing senses should be done first.

Tactile –Vestibular stimulation in a neonate is done by?

Positioning :
– Nesting
– Swaddling
– Containment
– Facilitated tuck
– Massage

Gustatory – Olfactory stimulation

- Swaddling during breast feeding/ Katori Spoon feeding.

Babies >32 weeks -Differentiate, remember and habituate

Dos' • Mother's smell • EBM soaked gauze • KMC • NNS

Don'ts • Strong odours (perfumes, nail polishes) • Chemical disinfectants • cleaning agents

Vision-Auditory stimulation

Environmental and Behavioural modification to reduce Noise in Units.

The recommended sound level is 45 dB and not more than 60d**b**

- Attend alarms promptly.
- Adjust alarms to low noise.

NOISE IS HARMFUL →Increases stress →Disturbs sleep →Hearing loss, IVH, PVL

Visual stimulation

Last developing sense is Vision.

Bright light should be avoided, it leads to sleep deprivation.

Sleep enhances plasticity in the developing visual cortex.

Auditory stimulation

Mother singing in soft voice

Music therapy - Better sleep pattern • Improves vital signs • pacification

Retina –

- Critical retinal development – 24 weeks to 3 to 4 months of age
  - Random firing of retinal ganglion cells - This occurs during REM sleep
  - The fetus needs no outside light or visual stimulus - Safeguard sleep
  - Protect eye from direct light
  - Decrease excessive light levels whenever possible

After 38 to 40 weeks, the visual system is activated by the light and requires a variety of visual experiences

- Colour pathways become functional between 2-3 months corrected GA
- The visual stimulation for term infants should include light directed on to objects rather than the infants face.
- Mother face is the most important source of visual input

Nesting

- Aim for containment, rather than restraint.
- Flexible enough to allow spontaneous movement
- Firm enough to limit excessive activity

Touch

- When possible, hands should be able to move towards face/mouth for self-comfort
- Nurturing Touch activates parasympathetic nervous system.
- Procedural touch activates sympathetic nervous system.
- Parental touch should be allowed following a procedure.
- KMC during and after procedure is the best

What is developmentally supportive positioning of Newborn?

- Shoulders softly rounded forward
- Hands towards midline, able to touch face/mouth if possible for self-comforting
- Hips aligned and pelvis tucked

- Knees, ankles, feet aligned and softly flexed
- Neck neutral or slightly flexed, no hyperextension
- Head midline, or turned slightly right or left. Avoid turning more than 45° to either Side.

Pain

- Unpleasant sensory and emotional experience
- Associated with actual or potential tissue damage
- Infant born 25-42 weeks experience an average of 15 painful procedures daily
- Immature descending inhibitory pathway in preterm, Nociceptive pathways are active and functional as early as 25 weeks' GA
- Leads to impairment of brain development, sensory motor disintegration
- Altered neurodevelopment and stress response systems, can persist into childhood, psychological disorder

What is The Synactive Theory of Infant Development

Dr. Als H.

- The synactive theory: Theory on development of prematurely born infant
- Early Intervention program: Neonatal Individualized Development Care & assessment Program (NIDCAP)

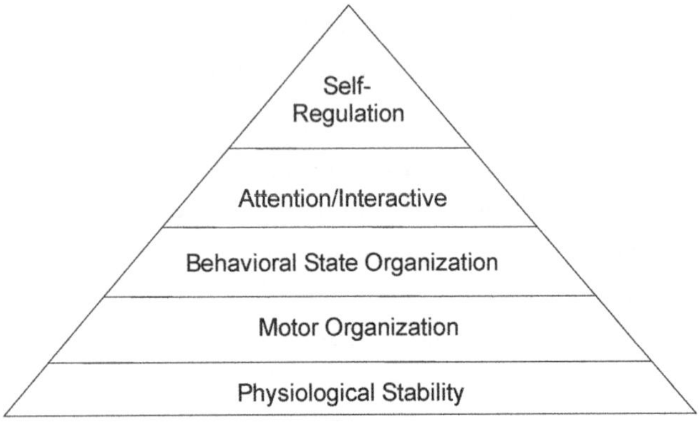

Lierarchical interaction and interdependency of five subsystems

Sound level in NICU and its equipment's

- In-utero, 40-60 db
- Usual noise levels in NICU, 50-80 db
- IV pump alarm 60-78 db
- Pulse ox alarm 86 db
- Tapping the finger on incubator 70-95 db
- Bubbling sound on ventilator 62-87 db
- Levels > 90 db for long time lead to hearing loss.

NICU Design:

- Location: Close proximity to labor suites
- 120 sq. ft per bed, excluding sinks & aisle
- Minimum 8 feet between the beds
- Nursing personnel: One nurse for 3 SC babies & 1 IC baby

Vision: Lighting Individual lighting should be at each baby

- All light should be indirect & not in direct line of baby's vision
- Special procedure focused controlled light
- Light levels not brighter than is necessary to complete the task Dimmer switch
- Working areas or Nurses' Charting areas with independent controls
- < 28 weeks: Dim light: < 10 lux (light level in candle lit room)
- > 28 weeks: Day light: 250-500 lux (Typical office)
- (Baby able to open eyes when awake & maintain sleep)
- Night light: < 10 lux

Octopus Therapy

This most innovative Idea originated at Aarhaus University Hospital in Denmark. The initiative appeared in Denmark in 2003 in the context of The Danish OCTO Project. In Denmark, there's an actual community—known as spruttegruppen—that's dedicated to crocheting octopuses for hospitals

Soft, curled Tentacles of the octopus mimic the umbilical cord and remind the babies of their time in utero and evoke the comfort and safety of the womb. Gripping the Tentacles is a similar experience as with the umbilical cord in utero along with chemosensory Stimulation.

29 Extrauterine Growth Restriction

What is the definition of Extrauterine Growth Restriction (EUGR)?

- EUGR is defined as a growth parameter value (weight/length/HC ≤10th percentile of intrauterine growth expectation based on the corrected gestational age(CGA) at the time of discharge or 36 weeks PMA or 40 weeks PMA (term-equivalent age)
- EUGR also defined as corrected weight-for-age Z-score ≤-2

Prevalence of EUGR in Indian population

- EUGR was 64.8% at discharge and 76.8% at term-KGMC, Lucknow[1]
- AIIMS data
  - EUGR (<10th percentile) at 40 weeks PMA in VLBW neonates
  - 73% (29/40) in PTF and 81% (42/52) in HMF group.

Factors independantly associated with EUGR are:

1. Male gender,
2. Need for assisted ventilation on Day 1 of life,
3. A history of NEC,
4. Need for respiratory support at 28 days of age, and
5. Exposure to steroids during the hospital course.
6. In addition, delayed initiation of feeding, delayed time to reach full feeding amount (100ml/kg/day) and delayed return to birth weight are also risk factors for EUGR

Growth and NDD in EUGR babies

- Infants with a suboptimal head size at the age of three months had a significantly lower median IQ than those with a normal head size
- Ehrenkranz *et al*, suggested that growth velocity during an ELBW infants NICU hospitalisation exerts a significant, and possibly independent, effect on neurodevelopmental and growth outcomes at 18 to 22 months corrected age.
- In addition to BW, in hospital growth velocity influenced likelihood of weight length and HC measurements below the 10th percentile at 18 to 22 months corrected age.

Nutritional strategies for prevention of eugr

1. Early aggressive nutrition:
   a. Initiate early parenteral (where indicated) and enteral nutrition
   b. Especially amino acid within hours of birth.
   c. Lipid emulsion within 24-30 hours of birth.
2. Growing care stage
3. Post discharge care

Growing stage care

1. Optimal increase in enteral feed
2. Fortification of human milk
3. Preterm infant formula
4. Fortification with preterm infant formula

30 Arterial Blood Gases (ABG) Analysis

Basics and some relevant points in ABG analysis

- Serum pH within the range of 7.35–7.45: Ideal environment for cellular metabolism
- Acid: Substance that yield free H+ in solution
- Base: Accepts H+ and in solution combines with an acid to neutralize it
- In the normal metabolic state, H+ are continuously produced and neutralized to maintain a steady pH balance.
- Rate of H+ production 2-3 times higher in neonates
  - Rapid growth rates
  - Increased acid production: Protein turnover, bone mineralization

How reliable is capillary blood gas analysis?

Arterialized capillary sampling - Fair estimates of pH, PCO2 & Not reliable for PO2 Not reliable when perfusion is poor.

Warm the heel to cause local vasodilatation. Warm water or steam towel.

Allen test- to ensure collateral blood supply by ulnar artery before puncturing radial artery.

How much heparin should be used for abg analysis - 0.05ml (1000 unit/ml) of heparin required. Objectively just coat the syringe.

How ABG sample should be transported- Ice (slush) container (allow immersion of the syringe barrel) - Will accurately reflect the condition at time of sampling for 2 hrs.

How heparin causes Sampling Errors in ABG analysis?

- Heparin is acidic and *lowers pH.*
- Dilution of electrolytes, HCO_3,PCO_2
- Na-heparin falsely elevates sodium
- Heparin binds cations (ca++, k+) causing hypocalcemia and hypokalemia.

How to reduce this heparin induced error?

- Use Pre-filled syringe
- Excess heparin should be expelled
- Use Lithium heparin is the current recommendation
- Sod heparin 1000U/ml instead of 5000 u/ml

How Air Bubbles affect ABG values?

- May falsely increase PO2 upto 150
- PaO2 -Greater than 100 mmHg will decrease -Less than 100 mmHg will increase
- PaCO2 will decrease.
- pH will follow PaCO2 change
- Expel bubbles by gently tapping the syringe, immediately after sampling and before mixing.
- Seal with cap immediately after taking sample.

Changes in ABG every 10 minutes in vitro

Parameter	37°C	4°C
PH	0.01	0.001
PCO2	0.1	0.01
PO2	0.1	0.01

MEASURED ABG PARAMETERS others are derived parameters

pH pCO2 and pO2

Provided by users

Hb FiO2 Temp

Normal Concentration of H+ : 40 nmol/L

Expressed as negative logarithm: 7.4

Chemical Buffer systems

Intracellular fluid (ICF)	Extracellular fluid (ECF)
•Phosphate Buffer System	Carbonic Acid–Bicarbonate Buffer
•Protein Buffer Systems·	Protein Buffer Systems·
•Hemoglobin buffer system·	•Hemoglobin buffer system·
•Amino acid buffers·	•Amino acid buffers·
•Plasma protein	•Plasma protein

Arterial Blood Gas		Capillary blood gas
pH	7.35-7.45	7.32-7.46
pCO_2	35-45 mm Hg	28.5-48.9 mm Hg
pO_2	50-70 mm Hg	30.2-60.3 mm Hg
HCO_3	20-24 meq/l	
BE	±5	

- Rule of thumb: compensation cannot overshoot 7.40
- Respiratory compensation is always FAST ...12-24 hrs
- Metabolic compensation is always SLOW...5 -7 days

Different types of compensations...defense mechanisms

1. By chemical Buffers..... Instantaneous...... HCO3, phosphates, proteins
2. Respiratory compensation ..... Hypo/hyper ventilation
3. By kidney.... Excreting H+ , retaining HCO3

WINTERS' FORMULA

- EXP.PCO, =1.5 × (ACTUAL HCO*f* {)+8 +/- 2 mmHg
- Quick rule of thumb : PCO, = last 2 digits of pH

Metabolic acidosis: Drop in pH is caused by the

- Accumulation of acid other than H2CO3 by the ECF(nonvolatile acids), resulting in loss of available HCO3", or
- Direct loss of HCO3" from body fluids

Measurement of anion gap gives a clue to differentiate metabolic Acidosis secondary to

- Loss of bicarbonate
- Accumulation of non-volatile acids

Anion gap (AG) = UA - UC

AG = Na – (Cl + HCO3)

NORMAL = 8 – 16 mEq/L

NORMAL ANION GAP ACIDOSIS suggests HCO3 loss or rapid dilution of ECF.

Chloride is proportionately increased in such conditions " GIT, Renal loss of HCO -3

(See Fig)

Increased anion gap suggest

- An addition of strong acid in the system as occurs in lactatemia, ketonemia, renal failure, excessive salt therapy (ringer lactate/acetate).

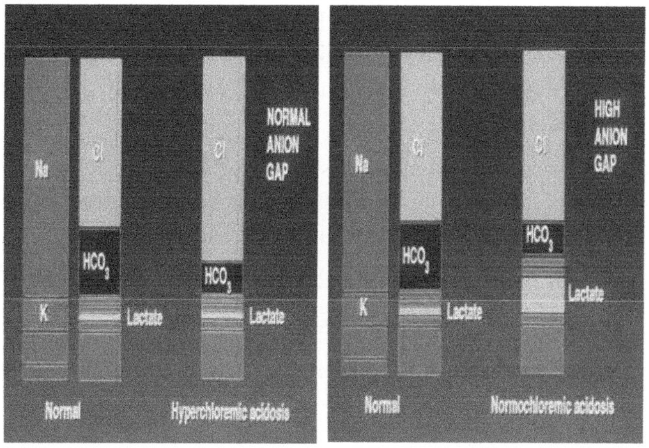

Anion gap is underestimated in hypoalbuminemia

Oxygen status of the baby can be assessed by

- Partial pressure of oxygen (pao_2)
- Alveolar arterial oxygen tension difference (AaDO2)- Normal AaDO2= 5-10mmHg Neonates, it can be as high as 25-35 mm Hg.(higher physiological dead space)- rough calculation AaDO2 = (7 × fio2)- paco2 – pa o2
- Oxygenation index (OI)
- Arterial to alveolar PO2 ratio- ratio does not change with varying inspired oxygen concentration.
- In healthy adult the ratio a/A O2 is more than 0.8.
- In infants with the severe RDS the a/A O2 ratio could fall to as low as 0.1 to 0.2.
- As baby recovers from RDS the a/A O2 improve gradually from low (0.1 to 0.3) to normal (0.7 to 0.9).
- A value of < 0.22 is indication for surfactant administration.

Oxygenation Index = MAP × FiO_2 / Postductal pO_2 × 100

- OI >25 – Indication for iNO.
- OI > 40 – Indication for ECMO.
- 40 – mortality risk > 80 – 90%
- 25–40 – Mortality risk 50 – 60%

Standard Bicarbonate Concentration (SBC)

NORMAL = 22–26 mEq/L

It is the concentration of the HCO3 - in the plasma which is equilibrated to bring the PCO2 to 40 mm of Hg at 37C i.e., it overcomes the changes in HCO3 - due to respiratory causes and reflects a non–respiratory acid–base change.

- If respiratory acidosis is present, HCO_3^- > SBC

(because this blood will have a PCO2 > 40 mm of Hg and therefore when equilibrated to 40 mmHg, some of the CO2 will leave the blood. Hence SBC will be lowered).

- If respiratory alkalosis is present HCO_3^- < SBC (because during equilibration to 40 mm some CO_2 gets absorbed and therefore SBC increases).
- SBC Low – Metabolic acidosis
- High – Metabolic alkalosis
- Respiratory acidosis if HCO_3^- > SBC
- Respiratory alkalosis if HCO_3^- < SBC
- When HCO_3^- = SBC then respiratory balance is present

The Base Deficit / Excess

- Assumption that all buffering of metabolic acids is by HCO3 and not other unmeasured ECF buffers is not totally correct.
- Buffer base (BB) : measure of the concentration of all the buffers present in either plasma or blood
- Total buffer base in a neonate is 48–49 mmol/L.
- Half of this is due to HCO -3
- 25% due to haemoglobin buffer.
- 25% due to protein, sulfate, phosphate buffers.
- A value of BE of +/-5 is considered normal.

Actual Base Excess (ABE)

- Refers to actual base above or below total buffer base (BB)
- The base excess allows an estimate how much base (if BE is negative) or acid (if BE is positive) is necessary to bring a liter of blood to pH 7.4
- Assesses all the extracellular buffers (in the blood sample) and is independent of pCO 2 (in vitro)
- BE is not independent of pCO2 *in vivo* (because blood contains Hb is a better buffer than the total ECF.)
- ABE does not distinguish compensation for a respiratory disorder from the presence of a primary metabolic disorder.
- So, the differences between in vitro and in vivo behaviour can be mostly eliminated If BE is calculated for a Hb -5g/dl instead of the actual Hb.

Standard Base Excess (SBE)

- Also called as BEecf and cBase (ECF)
- More reflective of in-vivo ECF conditions
- Calculated assuming Hb 5g%

SBE	ABE
In–vivo measurement	BE in the whole blood in vitro
BE–Equilibrated to PCO2, Temp, 5g/dl.	BE– Equilibrated to Hb-PCO2, Temp
Dependent on the equilibration of the interstitial or ECF compartment of the body and not only the blood with CO_2.	Buffering capacity is due to bicarbonate and hemoglobin

Consequences of metabolic alkalosis

- Decreased myocardial contractility, arrhythmias
- ↓ cerebral blood flow, confusion, neuromuscular excitability
- Hypoventilation: Pulmonary micro atelectasis, V/Q mismatch)

Consequences of respiratory acidosis

- Stimulation of ventilation (tachypnea), dyspnea
- ↑cerebral blood flow → ↑ICT
- Coma (arterial hypoxemia, ↑ICT, anaesthetic effect of ↑ PCO, > 100mmHg
- Tachycardia, bounding pulse
- Peripheral vasodilatation(warm, flushed, sweaty)

Consequences of respiratory alkalosis

- ↑neuromuscular irritability, altered sensorium
- CO & SBP ↑ (↑ SVR,HR), Arrythmias, ↓ myocardial contractility
- Hypokalemia, hypophosphatemia, ↓ Free serum calcium, Hyponatremia, hypochloremia

For an acute change in PCO2 of 10, the pH will change by 0.08

For a change in HCO3- of 10, the pH will change by 0.15

How Therapeutic hypothermia affects ABG values?

- Use uncorrected ABG values compared with the normal values
- A warmed ABG from a hypothermic patient will show a higher PaO2, higher PaCO2, and a lower pH than that actually present in the patient's blood in vivo.

31 Late Preterms

- Defined as 34 weeks 0 days to 36 weeks 6 days after last menstrual period
- Fastest growing population, accounts for > 70% of preterm population

Late preterm were earlier called Near term- misnomer, as this term gives a false security that these babies have features of term.

- May lead to false sense of security
- Less rigorous management & monitoring in the initial hours
- Early discharge - while still at risk

Term Late preterm: conveys they are still premature & still vulnerable

NICHD Workshop 2005 recommended the use of "Late Preterm" to describe infants born between 34 0/7 to 36 6/7 weeks, or 239—259 days counting from the first day of the LMP.

What is the incidence of RDS in late preterm?

- 33-34 weeks: 12%
- 35-36 weeks: 2%
- Term: 0.11%

Incidence of apnea in late preterm

Apnea: Incidence in Late preterm: 4 -7% Vs 1% in term.

Late preterms are more prone to hypothermia because of

- Decreased Brown adipose tissue & white adipose tissue
- Immature hypothalamic function
- Larger body surface area to body weight ratio
- Low concentration of hormones of brown fat metabolism – Prolactin, Norepinephrine, T3 and Cortisol

What significant events of brain development occur in final weeks of third trimester (which are missing in late preterm)

- Significant brain growth occurs in final weeks of 3rd trimester
- Critical phase of neuronal & glial maturation
- Brain weight: 60% to 80%, Cerebral volume: 53% of that of full-term infant is in a late preterm.
- Significantly less gyri and sulci & incomplete myelination.
- Relatively immature microstructural cerebral white matter than term
- Immaturity of laminar position & dendritic arborisation of neurons, as shown in Golgi drawings, in cerebral cortex of late preterm infant at 35 weeks GA is more compared with neurons at term.

32 Neonatal Pain

IASP (international association for the study of pain) definition of pain: An unpleasant sensory and emotional experience associated with actual or potential tissue damage.

1985: A landmark paper published by Anand *et al.* describing adverse physiological effects of the Liverpool method (pancuronium only, no anesthesia for PDA ligation) and improved outcomes with use of anesthesia for PDA ligation.

2004: The NEOPAIN trial (Neurologic Outcomes and Preemptive Analgesia In Neonates). Concluded that preemptive morphine infusion did not improve outcomes in ventilated neonates and did not relieve procedural pain – Anand *et al.*, 2004

Fast pain: Arises immediately without latency and is carried by A delta fibers. This is sharp and highly localized.

Slow pain: It arises slowly after 1 second and is carried by C fibers. It is dull diffuse and unpleasant pain.

Centers for pain sensation:

Subcortical centers- midline and interlaminar nucleus of the thalamus, periaqueductal grey matter and reticular formation.

Cortical centers- 3 areas in the cortex – SS1, SS2 and Cingulate gyrus (area 24)

NEONATAL PAIN SCALES

1. Neonatal facial coding system
2. Premature infant pain profile (PIPP AND PIPP-R)
3. Neonatal pain agitation and sedation scale (N- PASS)
4. Behavioral infant pain profile
5. CRIES - cry, requires O2, increased vital signs, expression, sleeplessness
6. COMFORT scale (calmness, movement, facial tension, rate and BP)

Which are the pain assessment tools in preterm?

2 scales have metric adjustments for prematurity.

- PIPP-R
- N-PASS

Only 1 scale takes sedation into account. N-PASS

PIPP-R:

- GA: 26-term
- Physiologic components: HR, SaO2
- Behavioural: alertness, brow bulge, eye squeeze, NL furrow.
- Type of pain: procedural, post op
- Metric: 0-21

N-PASS:

- GA: 0-100 days
- Physiological: HR, RR, BP, SaO2
- Behavioural: crying/ irritability, behaviour state, facial expression, tone
- Type: acute & prolonged pain, sedation
- Metric: Pain: 0 to 10
- Sedation: -10 to 0

(See Table on next page)

- Total score = sub-total score + GA score + BS score

Oral Sucrose

- Proposed hypothesis – endogenous opioid release by unknown mechanism.

Oral sucrose 24 % commonly used

- The recommended dosing for oral sucrose – 24 %
- For glucose – 20 to 30 %

EMLA cream- eutectic mixture of 2.5% lidocaine and 2.5% prilocaine.

- EMLA is recommended for use in venipuncture and circumcision.
- Not recommended for heel stick procedures

Neonatal pain responses may exacerbate impaired physiological conditions such hypoxia, hypercarbia, acidosis, hyperglycemia, dyssynchronous breathing, and pneumothorax. Following invasive operations, changes in intrathoracic pressure brought on by diaphragmatic splinting and vagal reactions triggered by pain trigger hypoxemic episodes and affect cerebral blood flow and oxygen delivery.

PIPP-R scale

Indicator	**0**	**+1**	**+2**	**+3**
Change in HR (bpm)	0-4	5-14	15-24	>24
Change in O2 saturation (%)	0-2	3-5	6-8	>8 or increase in O2
Brow bulge (sec)	None (<3)	Minimal (3-10)	Moderate (11-20)	Maximal (>20)
Eye squeeze (sec)	None (<3)	Minimal (3-10)	Moderate (11-20)	Maximal (>20)
Naso-labial furrow (sec)	None (<3)	Minimal (3-10)	Moderate (11-20)	Maximal (>20)
Gestational age (weeks+days)	> 36 weeks	32-35 weeks + 6 days	28 weeks -31 weeks 6 days	<28 weeks
Baseline behaviour state	Active and awake	Quiet and awake	Active and asleep	Quiet and asleep

Umbilical catheterization – Non-pharmacologic measures, IV acetaminophen (10 mg/kg), avoid sutures to the skin-Cord tissue is not innervated, but avoid injury to skin

Heel stick Use non-pharmacologic measures 1 mechanical lance, squeezing the heel is the most painful phase

Venipuncture Non-pharmacologic measures, use topical local anesthetic

IV cannulation Non-pharmacologic measures, use topical local anesthetics

Tracheal intubation (e.g., for mechanical ventilation) Give fentanyl (1 mcg/kg) or morphine (10–30 mcg/kg), with midazolam (50–100 mcg/kg), ketamine (1 mg/kg) use muscle relaxant only if experienced clinician, consider atropine

Morphine advantage

- Potent pain relief
- Better ventilator synchrony
- Sedation
- Hypnosis
- Muscle relaxation
- Inexpensive

Morphine Disadvantage

- Respiratory depression
- Arterial hypotension
- Constipation, nausea
- Urinary retention
- Central nervous system depression
- Tolerance, dependence
- Long-term outcomes not studied
- Prolonged ventilator use

Fentanyl advantage

- Fast acting
- Less hypotension

Disadvantage of fentanyl

- Respiratory depression
- Short half-life
- Quick tolerance and dependence
- Chest wall rigidity

Benzodiazepines advantage

- Better ventilator synchrony
- Antianxiety
- Sedation
- Hypnosis
- Muscle relaxation
- Amnesia
- Anticonvulsant

Benzodiazepines disadvantage

- No pain relief
- Arterial hypotension
- Respiratory depression
- Constipation, nausea
- Urinary retention
- Myoclonus
- Seizures
- Central nervous system depression
- Tolerance, dependence
- Alters bilirubin metabolism
- Propylene glycol and benzyl alcohol exposure

Long-term consequences of neonatal pain

Behavioral and neurologic studies suggest that preterm infants who experience numerous painful procedures and noxious stimuli are less responsive to painful stimuli at 18 months' corrected age.

33 Neonatal Palliative Care (NPC)

Palliative Care embraces physical, emotional, social and spiritual elements and focuses on the enhancement of quality of life for the baby and support for the family and also includes care through death and bereavement.

NPC considered under 5 broad categories

1. Antenatal/ postnatal diagnosis of a condition that is not compatible with long-term survival e.g. bilateral renal agenesis, anencephaly.
2. Antenatal/postnatal diagnosis of a condition, which carries a high risk of significant morbidity or death e.g. severe bilateral hydronephrosis and impaired renal function, severe spina bifida.
3. Babies born at the margins of viability where intensive care has been deemed inappropriate.
4. Postnatal conditions with a high likelihood of severe impairment of quality of life e.g. severe HIE, severe ICH
5. Postnatal conditions with baby experiencing 'unbearable suffering' e.g. severe NEC

Tissue donation in neonates

It may be possible for parents to donate baby's heart valves, cornea and hepatocytes for transplantation.

Post end of life care

- Assisting parents in
- Completing formalities at the earliest in order to reduce the stress in parents
- Certification and registering of death
- Funeral organization
- Communication and Follow-Up

34 Basics of Neonatal Jaundice

- Jaundice occurs in 60 % (Term) & 80% (Preterm)
- 15 % require intervention

Bilirubin formed from

- Destruction of circulating RBCs accounts for 75% of total bilirubin
- 25% of the remaining comes from:
  - Non-Hb heme protein (myoglobin, catalase) and free heme
  - Erythropoietic component from ineffective erythropoiesis from bone marrow

1g of Hb yields 35mg of bilirubin

Bilirubin is nonpolar hence insoluble at pH-7.4 Therefore must be conjugated

Enzymatically combined with a sugar glucuronic acid by uridine diphosphoglucuronic glucuronosyltransferase (UDPGT) producing monoglucuronide and diglucuronide.

UDPGT activity at birth is around 1% of adult & reaches adult levels by 6-14 weeks

Causes of neonatal jaundice

1. **Production -increased bilirubin production**
   - High Hb → More Hemolysis
   - Shorter life-span of RBCs (60-90days)
   - Incompatible blood groups – ABO/Rh
   - Enzyme deficiencies – G6PD/ PK
   - Collection of blood – bruising/cephalohematoma
2. **Transporation -↓ Capability of albumin in bilirubin transportation**
   - Less albumin in neonates
   - Drugs displace bilirubin from albumin
3. **Conjugation -The low capability of heptatocyte to conjugate bilirubin**
   - Less Y protein and ligandin
   - Immature hepatocytes
   - Reduced enzyme activity (UDP Glucuronyl transferase) – genetic/racial/familial traits
4. **Feeding issues/increased enterohepatic circulation**
   - Increased gut transit time
   - Less bacterial action
   - Increased entero-hepatic circulation
   - Dehydration

Mechanism of physiological hyperbilirubinemia

- Higher red blood cell volume
- Decreased red blood cell life
- Increased enterohepatic circulation
- Decreased membrane transport and ligandin in liver
- Decreased activity of UPGT

Physiological jaundice

- Appears after 24 hours, Rarely appears on day 1
- Maximum intensity by 4th-5th day in term & 7th day in preterm
- Rarely exceeds day 7 in term baby, day 14 in preterm baby
- TSB levels within normal centiles for age in hours based on normogram.
- Clinically not detectable after 14 days
- Disappears without any treatment.
- Rarely exceeds bilirubin >15mg/dl
- Rise of bilirubin is d" 5mg/day
- Has a cephalocaudal progression and never involves palms and soles

Pathological jaundice

- Appears within 24 hours of age
- Increase of bilirubin > 5 mg/dl/day or at a rate of >0.2mg/dl/hr
- Serum bilirubin >95 percentile for age in hours based on normogram.

- Jaundice persisting after 14 days in full-term babies.
- Stool clay/white colored and urine staining clothes yellow Direct bilirubin> 2 mg/dl or >20% of TSB.

Approach to a Jaundiced Neonate (questions to be asked)

- Gestational age- term or preterm?
- Is the Jaundice physiological?
- Does the baby have any risk factor?
- Is the baby sick?
- Are there signs of Bilirubin induced neurological dysfunction (BIND)?
- Does baby need phototherapy or exchange transfusion?
- Where does baby lie in nomogram (for prediction) at discharge?

The various photoisomers of bilirubin are Z-Z, Z-E, E-Z, E-E,E-Z and E-E.

The oxidative lysis of Hb results in Z-Z isomer of bilirubin

Bilirubin has been demonstrated to have antioxidant properties in physiological concentrations

Pattern of Physiological Jaundice?

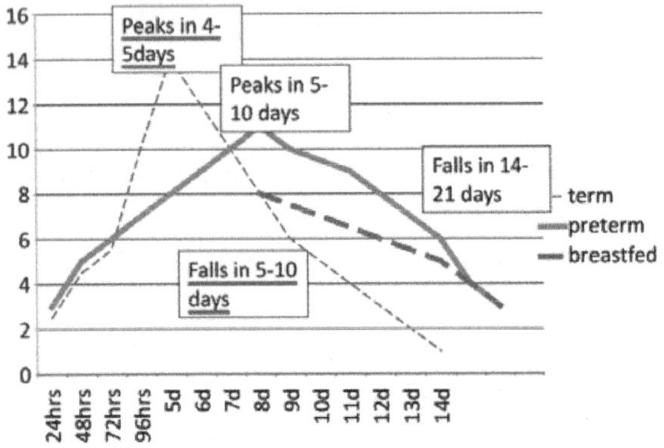

Identification of at risk New-borns for jaundice

Major risk factors

- Pre-discharge TSB or TcB level in high-risk zone
- Jaundice observed in first 24 h
- Blood group incompatibility, G6PD deficiency
- elevated ETCOc,
- Gestational age 35–36 wk
- Previous sibling received phototherapy
- Cephalohematoma or significant bruising
- Inadequate breastfeeding and East Asian race

Minor risk factors

- Pre-discharge TSB or TcB level in the high intermediate-risk zone
- Gestational age 37–38 wk
- Jaundice observed before discharge
- Previous sibling with jaundice
- Macrosomic infant of a diabetic mother
- Maternal age
- Male gender

Breast Milk Jaundice

- Benign unconjugated hyperbilirubinaemia is a common cause of prolonged jaundice in the otherwise healthy breastfed term infant
- Incidence has been reported at 36%
- In Isolated breast milk jaundice TSB rarely exceeds >12mg/dl
- Fatty acid and pregnanediol inhibit conjugation.
- Spontaneous resolution by 12weeks

Kramer's criteria for progession of jaundice

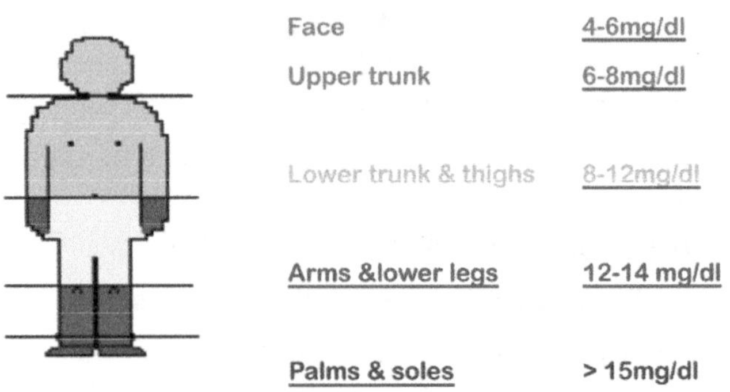

What is the reason for Cephalocaudal Progression of Jaundice?

- Conformational changes in bilirubin-albumin complex
- Bilirubin at proximal parts more loosely bound than distal parts
- Transcutaneous bilirubin, skin temperature and capillary refill time shows a similar cephalocaudal gradient
- New-born infants preferentially perfuse their head and proximal parts of their body in the first few days of life
- Leading to higher temperatures and increased bilirubin deposition at these sites

Transcutaneous bilirubinometer

- Minolta line (JM-101 and JM-102) Dräger JM-103 - two optical pathways
- Dräger JM-105 - barcode scanner, touch screen display, internal data storage, and use in preterm neonates
- BiliChek has – disposable tip – increased cost
- BiliMed - possibility to print out results and does not require touching the infant's skin. Lack sufûcient accuracy

What are the Advantages of TcB

- Study showed the mean difference between TcB and TSB values was -1.7micromol/l (suggesting accuracy of TcB),The correlation between TcB and TSB by is linear
- TcB seems to be a reliable screening method for hyperbilirubinemia in outpatient population
- TcB screening can increase the identification of New-borns needing phototherapy and significantly decrease the incidence of severe hyperbilirubinemia.
- Use of TcB Reduces the need for TSB measurements by roughly 40 %.

What are the Limitations of TcB

- Cannot be used when
  - < 35 weeks of gestation
  - < 24hrs of age
  - Child on phototherapy
- If Bilirubin is high (> 13- 14mg/dl), sensitivity of TcB decreases ØFor decision making, TSB values should be used

Automated Image Based Bilirubin (AIB)- AIB consists of cloud based off-line learning module and on-line prediction module. Skin image, by smart phone is uploaded to a specific cloud server. • provides an individualized and immediate predicted bilirubin index. • 82% sensitivity and 60% specificity.

Role of EtCOc in neonatal jaundice

- High ETCOc measurements (>3 ppm) correlated with known hemolytic conditions.
- AAP Guidelines recommend the use of ETCO testing in New-borns 35 weeks' gestation or more who:
  - are receiving phototherapy
  - have TSB rising rapidly
  - have TSB approaching transfusion levels
  - have jaundice unexplained by history and physical examination

Types of tubes for phototherapy

- Fluorescent Tubes - up to 11 $\mu W/cm^2/nm$ (1:1) up to 24 $\mu W/cm^2/nm$ (blue).
- Fluorescent lamps - Advantage-inexpensive but, light intensity, irradiance reduces with time change the lamps-after 1,000 to 2,000 hours
- Halogen Spotlights - >20 $\mu W/cm^2/nm$, Generate heat – dehydration, burns. Quartz halogen lamps- Produces heat
- Do not reduce in intensity with age but they are quite fragile especially when hot
- Fibreoptic systems - metal halide bulb – upto 35 $\mu W/cm^2/nm$, Insignificant heat – in contact with baby
- LED - gallium nitrate LEDs , much longer lifetime (20,000 hrs), Light emitting diodes Uses high intensity gallium nitrate • Produce less heat / placed closer • Low power consumption • Easily movable • Longer life(20,000hrs)

Use of filtered sunlight for phototherapy.

- Filtered sunlight - efficacious on 93% of treatment days as compared with 90% for conventional phototherapy.
- Filtered sunlight - higher mean level of irradiance (40 vs. 17 $\mu W/cm^2/nm$, P<0.001)
- Temperatures >38.0°C - 5% of the infants receiving filtered sunlight and in 1% of those receiving conventional phototherapy (P<0.001

The 2004 AAP guideline reserves the use of IVIG to direct Coombs-positive infants whose TSB continues to rise despite intensive phototherapy or whose TSB is within 2–3 mg/dL of the exchange level

Each gram of albumin binds 8.3 mg bilirubin

Phototherapy –

- LES (light emission spectrum) within Bilirubin absorption spectrum (400 to 520 nm)
- A Peak emission at 460±10 nm
- An irradiance level ≥ 30μW/cm2/ nm as measured by a specific irradiance meter
- An irradiance footprint that exposes at least one horizontal body surface or optimally entire circumferential (360) BSA

- Photooxidation – color less products
- Configurational isomerization – water soluble E, Z isomer.
- Structural isomerization - lumirubin

Factors modifying efficacy of phototherapy

- The spectral qualities -wavelength range and peak
- Intensity of light – spectral irradiance
- Exposed body surface area (BSA),
- Skin thickness and pigmentation
- The total bilirubin at clinical presentation, and duration of exposure.
- Line the bassinet with aluminium foil/white clothes (increases efficacy)

Baby factors affecting efficacy of phototherapy

- The thickness of skin (Maturity)
- The Initial Bilirubin level (at start)
- The rate of production of bilirubin (etiology)
- An enterohepatic circulation
- Hydration of the baby

What is Spectral Irradiance?

- Number of photons as directed to or received per square cm of the exposed body surface area.
- Measured as µW/cm2 /nm
- As measured for a wavelength spectrum, hence called "Spectral irradiance"
- Changes with-Distance and spot where measured

What is foot print (irradiance mapping)?

Distribution of irradiance levels within the footprint of the phototherapy light

Bronze baby syndrome

Dark grayish discoloration of the skin, impaired biliary excretion of bilirubin photoproducts that undergo polymerization

What are the Side effects of phototherapy?

- Increased insensible water loss
- Loose stools
- Skin rash
- Bronze baby syndrome
- Hyperthermia, retinal damage
- Seizures, thrombocytopenia
- Hypocalcemia
- Reopening of PDA

Blood for exchange transfusion

- Double volume exchange transfusion (Blood Volume = 70-90 ml/kg for term and 85-110 ml/kg for preterm infants)
- In cases of ABO incompatibility- Use O blood of same Rh type, ideal O cells suspended in AB plasma
- In cases of Rh isoimmunization- Emergency 0 -ve blood; Ideal 0 –ve suspended in AB plasma OR baby's blood group but Rh -ve
- In Other situations- Baby's blood group
- Have a known haematocrit of 0.5-0.6
- Negative for antigens determined by maternal antibodies
- Leukocyte depleted
- Irradiated and used within 24 hours of irradiation
- CMV negative
- As fresh as possible (ensure at least less than 5 days old)

Complication of exchange transfusion

- Cardiac Arrhythmias
- Apnoea
- Acid base instability
- Circulatory overload
- Hypocalemia/hypoglycaemia
- Embolism
- Infection
- Necrotising enterocolitis
- Thrombocytopenia
- Intraventricular haemorrhage

Role of IVIG in neonatal jaundice

- Used for a alloimmune neonatal thrombocytopenia, neonatal infections, Rh and ABO hemolytic disease etc.
- Acts by blocking Fc receptor sites of reticuloendothelial cells
- American Academy of Pediatrics, recommends high dose IVIG (0.5–1 g/kg) as an additional treatment of Rh and ABO hemolytic disease

Cochrane review (2018).

Nine studies with 658 infants, Term and preterm infants with Rh or ABO (or both) incompatibility were included. The applicability of the results is limited because of very low quality of evidence • Further studies are needed before the use of IVIg for the treatment of alloimmune HDN can be recommended.

Metalloporphyrins in neonatal jaundice - They cause competitive inhibition of rate-limiting enzyme in the bilirubin production.

35 Preterm Jaundice

Risk Factors for Neurotoxicity in neonatal jaundice

- Birth weight <1000 g (immature BBB)
- Apgar Score <3 at 5 min of age
- Arterial oxygen tension <40 mm Hg for >2 h
- Arterial pH <7.15 for >1 h
- Core temperature <35C for >4 h
- Serum albumin <2.5 g/dL
- Sepsis

Morris et al Aggressive vs. Conservative Phototherapy for Infants with Extremely Low Birth Weight N Engl J Med 2008;

Primary Outcome – Death or NDI at 18-22 months age

Results

- No difference in primary outcome
- Mild decrease in profound impairment / severe hearing loss
- Post-hoc – increased mortality in 500-650gm sub-group

Reason for decreasing incidence of kernicterus

- Prevention of Rh disease
- Early feeding & hydration
- Prevention or early treatment of neonatal sepsis
- Safe use of drugs
- Reduction of birth trauma
- Use of conservative phototherapy guidelines

Thresholds/Guidelines for treating preterm jaundice

- Maisels MJ & Bhutani VK – widely used in North America
- Stanford – Premie BiliRecs (27-34 weeks)
- NICE – UK based consensus guideline 2010

In preterm jaundice

- Use PMA for PT e.g. 29 0/7 week infant is 7 days, use 30 0/7 cut-off
- Discontinue PT if 1-2mg/dL (20-35mmol/L) below threshold

NICE Guidelines (2010)

•Consensus based

- Charts for phototherapy and exchange from 23 week onwards
- It incorporates day of life
- Does not take into account risk factors
- Phototherapy cut-off high after 48 hrs
- Exchange cut-off lower in first 48 hrs

Safety of irradiance 70-105 mW/cm2/nm not shown in studies ?Safety of irradiance 50-70 mW/cm2/nm not shown in studies for preterms

Monitoring of TSB on phototherapy

- TSB at 4-6 hourly intervals on phototherapy, if levels rising/not stable (after 3-4 hrs if critical hyperbil)
- TSB 6-12 hours, if levels are stable
- TSB 12-24 hours, if levels are falling

Cephalocaudal progression of jaundice can be explained by conformational changes of bilirubin albumin complexes.

- Although the initial binding of bilirubin to albumin is extremely rapid, final conformational changes may not occur for about 8 minutes.
- Thus, blood leaving the reticuloendothelial system and going to the proximal parts of the body contains bilirubin that is less tightly bound to albumin than that which subsequently reaches the distal parts of the body.
- Bilirubin that is less tightly bound is more likely to precipitate as bilirubin acid in phospholipid membranes in the skin and subcutaneous tissues, which is why the face appears jaundiced before the abdomen or the legs

Site for checking TcB

Because the forehead is exposed to ambient light, both in

the nursery and following discharge (while the sternum almost always is covered), measurements from the sternum might be a better choice)

Guidelines for optimising phototherapy – equipment factors

- Use special blue tubes or LED light source
- Using only white tube lights is less effective
- Monthly irradiance check with flux meter is a must – Ideal irradiance of at least 30 microW/cm2 /nm
- Keep the phototherapy unit as close as possible [up to 15 cms] ensuring that the neonate maintains normal temperature
- Align the phototherapy unit so that the neonate lies directly beneath the centre of the unit
- Increase the exposed body surface area of the infant under phototherapy – by placing another phototherapy unit beneath/ by the side of the neonate – reflecting material around the incubator or radiant warmer bed is optional
- Keep the diapers as short as possible
- Ensure adequate hydration- Continue breast feeding/ breast milk feeding
- No role of routine intravenous fluids or supplemental feeds, unless baby is clinically dehydrated
- May interrupt for feeding/ clinical care procedures provided total serum bilirubin is lower than exchange threshold
- Monitor urine output
- Cover the eye with opaque eye patches
- Monitor temperature every 2 hours
- Routine position changing is not recommended

Identification of jaundice in preterm neonates

- Visual assessment
- Transcutaneous bilirubin (TcB)
- Total serum bilirubin levels (TSB)

Examine the neonate in bright day light or white light. Examine blanched skin, sclerae and palate of the neonate. Assess frequently during every examination of the neonate, during the first week of life.

Visual assessment dose not reliably reflect severity of jaundice and hence, any jaundice on visual assessment in preterm neonates should be further evaluated using Tcb/ TSB

Rapidly rising TSB levels (>0.5 mg/dL/h), suggesting hemolysis

Bilirubin isomers

4Z,15Z-bilirubin - A structure of 4Z,15Z (unconjugated) bilirubin produced from normal heme catabolism

The 2 double bonds at positions 4 and 15 can have the groups attached to them either in the Z (zusammen, meaning same side) or E (entgegen, meaning opposite side) configurations When bilirubin absorbs a photon its electronic structure is altered, weakening the double bonds at positions 4 and 15, and allowing a twisting around one or the other of these bonds. This twisting can occur quickly, within picoseconds.

4Z, 15E-bilirubin cannot form a completely internally hydrogen-bonded structure as does bilirubin, and so it is more polar and water soluble than bilirubin. This property allows direct excretion of 4Z, 15E-bilirubin into the bile without conjugation

Lumirubin - Photoexcited bilirubin undergoes another kind of isomerization in which the double bonded carbon atoms on one end ring form new bonds with atoms in the adjacent ring-forming isomers, collectively called lumirubin. Lumirubin does not revert to bilirubin with light and is also thermally stable. Like the other isomers, lumirubin binds to albumin.

36 Bilirubin Induced Neurological Dysfunction

Bilirubin Induced Neurological Dysfunction (BIND) was defined as subtle neurodevelopmental disabilities without classical findings of kernicterus that, after careful evaluation and consideration, appear to be due to bilirubin neurotoxicity. These may include disturbances of sensory and sensorimotor integration, central auditory processing, coordination, and muscle tone.

Incidence of BIND

0.4 to 2.7 cases per 100,000 live births ($\geq$ 35 weeks) in developed countries

Incidence is 100 times higher in developing nations

Factors that contributes to higher incidence of BIND in developing nations

- Inadequate screening for neonatal jaundice
- Inability to measure total serum bilirubin levels
- High prevalence of medical conditions like G6PD deficiency, Rh isoimmunisation and sepsis
- Delay in referrals
- Long distances to be traveled to medical clinics
- Prolonged travel time to hospitals and poor transport facilities
- Challenge of implementing effective phototherapies
- Limited availability of blood and safe blood banking practices
- Lack of sensitivity to healthcare workers and parent
- Home deliveries
- Lack of parental and medical caretaker education with regard to the dangers of severe neonatal hyperbilirubinemia
- Application of home remedies, some of which may have hemolytic properties (e.g., menthol and henna)
- Absence of Rh isoimmunization prevention programs
- Inability to obtain serum or TcB testing
- Poor or erratic electricity supply
- Ineffective phototherapy equipment
- Inability to perform exchange transfusion

Neurotoxicity risk factors in preterm hyperbilirubinemia

1. Albumin levels < 2.5 g/dL
2. Blood pH < 7.15
3. Blood culture positive sepsis
4. Apnea and bradycardia requiring cardiorespiratory resuscitation (bagging and/or intubation) during the previous 24 hours
5. Hypotension requiring inotrope treatment during the previous 24 hours
6. Mechanical ventilation

What is ETCO?

1 mole heme produces 1 mole of bilirubin, during the process releases 1 mole of CO.

Which is detected by tracing gas analysis of CO in expired breath (ETCO)?

Bilirubin exists in plasma as bilirubin anion (monoanion/dianion) or bilirubin acid.

Anionic forms of bilirubin at physiological pH adds two + 2 H+ ions → formation of bilirubin diacid.

At physiological pH, free bilirubin is - 82% diacid, 16% monoanion, and 2% as dianion.

Pathophysiology of Bilirubin entry into brain

- Bilirubin production that saturates the normal buffering capacity of the blood/ tissue.
- Alterations in the bilirubin-binding capacity of albumin leads to higher unconjugated bilirubin in the circulation
- Increased CNS permeability to bilirubin secondary to disruption of the BBB

What are the Determinants of neuronal injury by bilirubin?

Concentration of unconjugated/free bilirubin-

- Free Bilirubin-bilirubin not bound to albumin is critical for neuronal damage

- No significant effect of the additional use of the bilirubin– albumin ratio compared with total serum bilirubin (TSB)

Concentration of serum albumin and its binding to bilirubin -

- Human albumin molecule binds 2 molecules of bilirubin
- First molecule more tightly bound than the second
- At a molar ratio of 1, each gram of human albumin binds 8.2 mg of bilirubin
- At albumin concentration of 3 g/dL, the first binding site- 25 mg of bilirubin per deciliter of serum/ plasma
- The second binding site - additional 25 mg/dL- total binding capacity of 50 mg/d
- Thus low albumin levels leads to higher free bilirubin levels.
- Bilirubin-binding capacity of albumin - ↓↓ in sick term and premature neonates.
- Serum albumin concentration is lower in these patients than in healthy, term counterparts.
- The bilirubin-binding capacity of albumin ↓ as pH drops below 7.4.
- Numerous agents compete with bilirubin for binding sites on albumin, to displace Bilirubin and ↑ the ratio of free to bound bilirubin in the serum
- FFA, ↑ in sepsis and hypoxemia- displace bilirubin.
- IV lipid emulsions- ↑ free fatty acids – displacement of bilirubin.
- Sulfisoxazole, other sulfa drugs, indomethacin, and salicylates displace bilirubin.
- Ampicillin— rapid injection– displace bilirubin
- Benzyl alcohol—preservative in various medications—competitively inhibit bilirubin binding

Neuronal susceptibility

- Damaged Blood brain barrier
- Acidosis increases the pH / H ions- ↑ the neurotoxicity of bilirubin
- Acidosis decreases - level of cellular binding, at the uptake of bilirubin, or both.
- Enhanced susceptibility of neurons to hypoxic-ischemic excitotoxic injured neuron
- Increased blood-brain transport of bilirubin due (hypercarbia, increased bilirubin acid, and impaired ATP dependent transporters
- Increased proportion of bilirubin as bilirubin acid (acidosis)

Bilirubin enters through –BBB and BCB (blood CSF barrier)

- ABCB 1transporter - transport bilirubin out of brain through blood brain border
- ABCC1 transporter – transport bilirubin out of brain through blood CSF barrier
- These transporters are up regulated in hyperbilirubinemia

Bilirubin transport across intact BBB

- Unbound free bilirubin: passive diffusion
- Increased cerebral blood flow in -hypercarbia and seizure

Bilirubin transport across disrupted BBB

- Hyperosmolar load (soda bicarbonate, 3% NS)
- hypercarbia with acidosis
- Asphyxia
- Acidosis
- Vaculitis (meningitis)
- Abrupt ↑in arterial /venous pressure

Hypoglycemia, metabolic aberrations, intracranial hemorrhage, infection, trauma, or exposure to toxic agents may ——additive effects on bilirubin toxicity to brain

Kernicterus mostly involves following areas of brain

- Globus pallidus,
- Sub-thalamic nuclei,
- Hippocampus,
- Oculomotor nuclei,
- Ventral cochlear nuclei and
- The Purkinje cells and dentate nuclei of the cerebellum

Bilirubin spares the cortex the striatum and thalamus.

The Hippocampus - most sensitive brain region, followed by the Inferior colliculus.

Auditory abnormalities in bilirubin toxicity

- Sensorineural hearing loss, High-frequency loss (bilateral)
- Auditory neuropathy spectrum disorder/auditory dyssynchrony - Defined as absent or abnormal BERA screening with normal tests of inner ear function. Tests of the mechanical integrity of the inner ear

(otoacoustic emissions) or of the outer hair cells of the inner ear (cochlear microphonics) are normal with absent BSAERs or abnormal brain stem latencies.

- May have little or no hearing loss but exhibit abnormal processing of sound
- Conduction in the large, heavily myelinated afferent auditory pathways is not synchronized.
- One of the earliest features of acute bilirubin encephalopathy
- It may be seen even in the absence of other clinical manifestations of bilirubin encephalopathy
- Functional effects include difficulties with sound localization and speech discrimination.
- Abnormal BSAERs may resolve. Central auditory processing disorder becomes apparent.
- Children with auditory neuropathy and hearing loss may respond favourably to cochlear implantation

Visual abnormalities in bilirubin toxicity

- Paralyses of upward gaze
- Horizontal gaze dysfunction and
- A blank stare or "scared appearance" caused by the combination of upward gaze paresis and facial dystonia.

Dental abnormalities

- Dental enamel hypoplasia of the deciduous (baby) teeth and,
- Green stained teeth

Extrapyramidal disturbances

- Dystonia,
- Athetosis,
- Chorea

BIND scoring interpretation (minimal score 0 maximum score 9)

The BIND score is a tool to objectify and facilitate a clinical diagnosis of acute bilirubin encephalopathy as well as to monitor the neonatal neurological exam in infants with progressive hyperbilirubinemia as a predecessor to encephalopathy.

The BIND score uses the mental state, muscle tone and cry pattern to categorize neonates into three levels of increasing abnormality (mild, moderate, severe).

The simplicity of the BIND scoring system, similar to the Apgar score, makes it an attractive tool for clinical diagnosis of ABE in resource limited locations that lack ready access to MRI) and ABR testing.

Score 1–3 -consistent with subtle signs of acute bilirubin encephalopathy in infants with hyperbilirubinemia.

Scores 4–6 — moderate acute bilirubin encephalopathy and are likely reversible with urgent and prompt bilirubin reduction strategies.

Scores 7–9 — advanced acute bilirubin encephalopathy; urgent, prompt, and individualized intervention are recommended to prevent further brain damage, minimize severity of sequelae, and possibly reverse acute damage.

El Houchi et al (32) studied the predictive ability of the BIND score and found that a BIND score of ≥ 4 had a specificity of 87% and sensitivity of 97% for predicting a poor neurologic outcome, and a specificity of 87% and sensitivity of 93% for predicting long-term hearing impairment.

What is modified-bind score?

The BIND score was modified for use primarily in low-resource settings often without ABRs and MRIs. The modified bilirubin-induced neurologic dysfunction scale (M-BIND). It is a 12-point score, incorporates eye abnormalities such as a divergent gaze, paralysis of upward gaze, anxious appearance and nystagmus, and serves to better discriminate degrees of BIND severity and to aid in distinguishing ABE from other common causes of neonatal morbidity and mortality such as tetanus still seen in low-resources settings.

In modified bind score gaze has been incorporated

- Normal gaze - 0
- Sun setting or paralysis of upward gaze – 3
- Maximum score is 12
- Score 1-4 indicative of mild ABE
- Score 5-6 indicative of moderate ABE
- Score > 7 indicative of severe/very severe ABE

Some factors responsible for the persistence of kernicterus spectrum disorder in developing countries

Low bilirubin kernicterus- Kernicterus at TSB level below commonly recommended exchange transfusion thresholds and that develop during the first year of age.

In year 2021 A New Hour Specific Serum Bilirubin Nomogram for Neonates >35 weeks of gestation was published

Last was Bhutani et al published hour specific bilirubin nomogram in 1999

Deficiency in old hour specific bilirubin monogram

- No data of bilirubin levels in first 0-12 hours of life was available
- A dip in bilirubin level was noted at 24 hours
- No subgroup analysis was done : sex, race, gestation-wise groups
- This nomogram was constructed from pre-hospital discharge total serum bilirubin (TSB) values of 2840 neonates who had negative direct anti-globulin tests.
- Small sample size
- Nomogram generated from New-borns who had one outpatient follow up TSB, obtaining the outpatient TSB was at the discretion of clinician, hence likely a biased sample

2021 updated nomogram by Bhutani et al

- Inclusion criteria • All births >35 weeks
- exclusion criteria
  - Neonates with a positive direct anti-globulin test.
  - Neonates with diagnosis of hemolytic disorders.(Hereditary spherocytosis, G6PD deficiency)
- Hour specific bilirubin nomogram from birth to 144 hrs of life was generated
- Subgroup analysis: for gestation, gender, race & ethnicity was also done
- 40th, 75th and 95th percentile of each epoch calculated

The main Results of the updated Bhutani nomogram

- Higher TSB values among late-preterm vs. term neonates
- No difference in TSB values between male and female neonates
- Neonates of black race have lower initial TSB values
- Neonates of Asian race have higher initial TSB values

Strengths of 2021 Bhutani nomogram

- Large sample size
- 0-12 hours
- No dip at 24 hours
- Higher 75th and 95th centiles Similar 40th centiles

Comparison of the two charts 1999 Bhutani chart

• Small sample size (2976)
• Follow up data included
• No subgroup analysis possible
• No data for 0-12 hours of life
• Trough at 24 hrs
• Lower 75th and 95th centiles between 60 and 144 hr of life
• Peak/plateau between 96 and 120 hours of life

2021 updated Bhutani chart

• Large sample size (3,97,395) Follow up not included
• Subgroup analysis done
• Hour specific TSB information for 1st 12 hrs period
• No trough at 24 hrs
• Higher 75th and 95th centiles between 60 and 144 hr of life
• Plateau around 144 hours of life

Similarities of old and new Bhutani charts

- 40th percentile values from the 1999 and new curves are similar.
- Estimate similar TSB values between 36 and 60 hours of life.
- The time at which 1st bilirubin value obtained was not random, biased by confounding factors.
- Absence of data regarding breastfeeding vs bottle feeding.
- Very small number of babies from whom follow up data was obtained.
- Not created from a cohort with proportions of races and ethnicities equal to global averages.

37 Ventilation Case

- **Case allotted**
- **Detailed Examination done**
- **Relevant history to be asked in presence of examiner**
- **Examination finding presentation**
- **Discussion on case**

History

In a DM exam at my center the usual process is that you will be given a one line history of the baby. You are supposed to do a detailed examination of the baby in the allotted time.

After finishing your examination the examiners will come and will ask you to ask relevant history about the case from the doctor managing the baby.

You have to ask specific and relevant questions based on your examination of the baby.

If you ask questions which are not relevant at this point you will be questioned for the purpose of that question.

When you are done with the relevant questions examiner with ask you to tell the examination findings. Usual pattern is the examiner asks what relevant history would you like to ask retrospectively.

Relevant questions to be asked which can vary case by case

1. What is the primary mode of ventilation (to get a basic idea what Q you have to focus in history)
2. At what time baby needed respiratory support
3. Maximum respiratory support needed by the baby
4. Did the baby cried immediately after birth

Now you can shift to ANC history

5. Primi/multi para / registered or unregistered pregnancy/ regular follow up
6. Maternal age (increasing maternal age —> risk of downs syndrome and other aneuploidies), age at marriage. Consanguinity (for genetic or metabolic disorders)- IF RELEVENT
7. Any leads to twins or bad obstetric history /previous abortions. Always ask about the other twin clinical status.
8. Any known significant medical history in mother / preconception medication if any
9. Product of spontaneous conception/assisted/IVF, if yes reason for the same
10. Any complications in first trimester- there is no history of any, fever, rash or Bleeding PV
11. Second trimester - calcium and iron supplementation and had 2 doses of tetanus toxoid.
12. Anomaly scan findings
13. Any Doppler changes or any other abnormality in ANC scans. Ultrasound- fetal well being • Doppler indices of umbilical and MCA vessels
14. Mother blood group/father blood group - HIV ELISA, Hep B, VDRL, were reported as normal. TORCH profile
15. Antenatal steroid – dose / duration/ type/ repeat dose
16. Magnesium suphate for neuro protection
17. Iv antibiotics – if any /indication of antibiotics in mother /uti/pprom
18. Any h/o aph, pih, dm, leaking pv, any signs of chorioamnionitis /bleeding pv/ precipitous labor/spont onset of labor/ Doppler changes leading to preterm delivery, no h/o of gestational hypertension/ gestational diabetes, BPV/LPV or h/o of decreased fetal movements, excess or decreased amniotic fluid.
19. Intrapartum monitoring details. Amniotic fluid was clear and fetal well-being was monitored by CTG and intermittent fetal heart auscultation.
20. Duration/ complication of labour/indication for LSCS
21. CIAB/DNCIAB – Apgar score/extended Apgar score
22. Cord abg and its interpretation
23. Placenta examination – if available
24. Details of Resuscitation required and for how long

25. Time of onset of spontaneous effort

Now go to the onset of presenting complains (O/D/P)

26. RD at what minute of life – what support was given
27. Maximum support required/ maximum oxygen requirement
28. Surfactant dose type and indication and at what hrs of life, technique of surfactant administration
29. Reason for escalating the respiratory support
    a. frequent episodes of apnea
    b. increasing RD
    c. CPAP/NIMV failure based on ABG
    d. Poor respiratory efforts
    e. Severe shock requiring multiple inotrope
    f. Apnea requiring B&M ventilation
    g. Poor sensorium
    h. Pulmonary HGH
    i. Post surgery
    j. Etubation failures
    k. look for causes for prolonged respiratory support
30. Maximum support required and at which hr of life
31. First abg, abg at the time of deterioration and abg after intervention
32. X-ray first and later X-rays
33. Any usg lung findings if done
34. Relevant blood investigation at this point

SHOCK (IF ANY)

35. HOW shock was detected and at which hr of life
36. Hr/bp/pi/pp/2decho at the time of shock
37. What intervention done for shock bolus/inotrope
38. Dose of inotrope and number of inotrope required
39. Hr/pp/bp/pi /2decho after intervention for shock – abg pre and post intervention
40. Etiology of shock – asphyxia, prematurity, hypovolemia, bleeding (ivh, pul hgh, gi bleed), HSPDA, sepsis. Anemia, severe APH,
41. When was shock under controlled

HSPDA

42. Pda parameter at 24 /12 h or life
43. What treatment given
44. Current PDA status
45. Any gi bleed/aki/pulmonary hgh

Sepsis parameters

46. Sepsis screen- cbc, tlc, anc, it ratio, crp, and micro esr. X-ray chest, blood cs, maternal hvs – if leaking PV. Procal if done. Lp if done
47. Ask relevant history related to nutrition – when was the feed started / any feed intolerance/
48. Current status of TPN
49. Ask about KMC and developmentally supportive care
50. All screen should be covered pda screen/ivh screen/ sepsis screen/ aki screen/electrolyte screen/ hypoglycaemia screen/hypocalcemia screen/ jaundice screen/ stooling and urine output/

You **should be able to summarize your case after history taking with a probable reason for**

Prematurity

Shock

Respiratory distress

Current respiratory staus

Current feeding status

EXAMINATION But 1st hand washing

Environment - Start from outside to inside (vice versa), less important to more important like

Baby is being nursed in open care system with set temperature of 36.5C and measured 36.6C and heater output of 10%. Placement of probe • Condition of skin underneath the probE

There are 5 infusions includes dextrose, TPN, dopamine, adrenaline and milrinone with total of 8.7 ml/hr that comes to 90 ml/kg/day. Infusion pumps – types of pumps? • Medications going? • Fluid rate? • Amino acids (10%) – how much g/kg • Lipids (20%) – dose? Covered? • Inotropes – rate, dose?

Baby in under phototherapy.

ET tube fixed at 7 cm, secured well with no soakage.

NG tube 6F fixed at 17cm. Orogastric tube • Fixed at —— • Left open or feed in the tube or aspirate.

Baby has a PICC inserted at rt saphaneous vein. Pulse oximeter and temperature probes are attached to the baby.

UVC UAC PICC line Fixed at Blood in the circuit? Peripheral

lines- Redness, color change around lines

Being ventilated in TCPL AC mode with pressures of 16/5 @ 40 Bpm no significant distress noted FiO2 of 35%, humidification chamber is reading temperature of 37C , with adequate water level, with minimal condensation noted in the expiration limb. Long press power button on humidifier shows temperature of plate and end of heater wire. Flow sensors if attached

Ventilator settings • Set parameters • Measured parameters • Tidal volume delivered? • Respiratory efforts • Graphics – leak, air trapping, compliance, secretions, efforts • Synchronisation

If on CPAP, Interface – nature, appropriateness Cap Settings Bubbling, Nasal injury

She is being continuously monitored by HR and pulse oximeter, with no alarms activated currently. Pulse oximeter with saturation of 95% with probe placed in right hand, limits of 90- 96. Heart rate is 144 with limits of 120-180. There was no episode of desaturation or bradycardia during the examination.

VITALS

1. PULSE / HEART RATE- Rate, volume, regularity, all peripheral pulses palpable
2. Respiratory rate and pattern / SAS OR DS SCORE
3. Color, CFT, PI
4. Blood pressure ± SBP, DBP, MBP, PP and Centiles.
5. Temperature ± set, measured and axillary temperature

Saturation ± reading with fio2.ANY Pre and post ductal difference. PVI if available

Anthropometry

Weight – birth and todays

Head

Length

Chest

Abdomen cir

Ponderal index if FGR

Penile length if dsd

Gestational age assessment

Use modified ballard scoing system- if stable to tolerate the examination

Otherwise use – parkins score

General Examination (head to toe)

- GENERAL EXAMINATION- looks for things relevant for your case
- Head – shape/size/ anterior fontanel- size, level, pulsatality/ PF/ SUTURES – separated or overriding or fused. Soft tissue swelling, discoloration, opening or lack of continuity of skin over scalp, face and neck
- Any birth injury to skull- caput/cephal/subgaleal HGH.
- Eyes – slant, cataract, subconjunctival hemorrhage, periorbital edema
- Facial dysmorphism, malformations, Symmetry, size, shape and relationship of all individual components of face • Observe facial tone and strength at rest and crying/ yawning
- Neck - Any neck mass (Cystic hygroma, Brachial cleft cyst, Thyroglossal duct cyst) • Mobility (Decreased- Torticollis d/t trauma to SCM or developmental abnormality) • Excessive skin (Turner's) • Palpate clavicle bilaterally- Fractures/ partial or complete absenc
- Ear - EARS- Position, size and appearance. • Normal position- Helix intersected by a horizontal line drawn from outer canthus of eye perpendicular to vertical axis of head. Examine preauricular and postauricular area • Examine tragus, attachment of ear lobe, and external auditory meatus: patency and size
- Skin - jaundice, pallor, cyanosis, sclerema, polycythemia, injury, odema, neurocutaneous markers, Redundancy of skin esp in face, neck and over abdomen, Any lesions • Take scrapings of scaling lesions if any • Pustular lesions- Aspirate and make stains
- Umbilicus- 2 A 1 vein, staning, surrounding redness, discharge, cord fall on which day, cord size .
- Back – any pit, sinus, tuft of hair
- Genitalia as per GA.

SYSTEMIC EXAMINATION

RESPIRATORY

- INSPECTION • Shape and size of chest • Symmetry and any sternal prominence • Count the RR for one whole minute • Respiratory pattern and chest movements-Retractions/ Protrusions of any soft tissue adjacent to the bony rib cage • Work of breathing- Nasal flarings/ retractions/ head bobbing

- Description includes interface, mode and settings on ventilator.
- On these settings baby is well synchronized with the ventilator and has adequate chest rise minimal retractionX, OR
- The baby is comfortable on CPAP, with respiratory rate of 48 pm and has minimal intercostal retraction with SAS of 2. The saturation is 95 % in the right upper limb On auscultation air entry is equal on both sides
- Baby's spontaneous resp rate is 45 and maintaining a saturation of 95 % on right upper limb. On auscultation the air entry is equal on both sides and there are no added sounds.

CVS

- Describe vitals, precordial examination, perfusion, inotrope support/ any other medications
- Palpate anterior chest for impulses • Locate the point of maximal impulse activity(PMI)
- The baby is pink with HR is 145/min with peripheral pulses palpable, regular rhythmic and normal volume. The femoral pulses are palpable b/l. The CFT is <3 sec.
- The BP is in right upper limb 46/32 is at 50th centile as per the ZUBRO chart .
- No visible precordial impulse. Heart sounds are normal, no murmer.
- Auscultate for the first and second heart sounds and murmur with a warmed stethoscope while the baby lies quietly. • All areas of the precordium, the back and axillary areas. • Heart sounds are best heard along the left sternal border. • S1 is best heard at the apex and S2 is best heard at the left upper sternal border. • Murmurs-Intensity, quality, location, time of occurrence in the cardiac cycle, and the area of transmission.
- Baby is receiving following inotropes currently .

ABDOMINAL SYSTEM

- Inspect abdomen for contour and size, bilateral symmetry, umbilical cord location and anatomy
- Palpate for muscle mass and tone in abdominal wall, location and size of viscera, tenderness
- Auscultate bowel sounds. If sounds are infrequent-listen for atleast 5 mins before diagnosing absent BS
- Transillumination in cases of suspected pneumoperitoneum

CENTRAL NERVOUS SYSTEM

1. Higher mental functions
2. Cranial nerves
3. Motor function
4. Reflexes (deep tendon, superficial, neonatal)
5. Sensory examination
6. Behavioural assessment

Volpe staging - Levels of alertness

- Habituation
- Latency
- Consolability
- Stereotypical movement

State of consciousness

Prechtl

1. NREM sleep
2. REM sleep
3. Awake quiet
4. Awake active

Brazelton

1. Deep sleep
2. Light sleep
3. Drowsy
4. Awake alert
5. Awake active
6. Crying

1. Cranial nerves
2. Motor function
   a. -Tone
   b. -Power
3. Reflexes (deep tendon, superficial, neonatal)
4. Sensory examination

Not possible to do all in a venti case

Do minimum what is need with disturbing the baby much.

Posture of baby

Examination of head if not done earlier

- CN 1: Response to strong odour – sucking movements,

grimace, change in activity level,

- Transient change in heart rate. (Breast crawl)
- CN 2: (Optical blink reflex /Dazzle reflex) – Blinking on exposure to a light source seen after
- 32 weeks GA.
- CN 3: Pupillary reflex – not reliably present until after 35 weeks. • CN 3,4,6: Position and movement of eyes
- CN 5: Rooting reflex, Sucking reflex, corneal reflex – sterile thread of cotton
- CN 7: Facial movement – absence of depressor anguli oris or facial palsy, Glabellar tap
- CN 8: Hearing response – Change in sucking rate, startle/arousal response Acoustic blink reflex (Cochleo-palpebral reflex)
- CN 9, 10, 12: Rooting, Sucking & Swallowing
- CN 11: Horizontal movements of head

MOTOR FUNCTION

- Quantity, quality and symmetry of movements
- Posture

Tone: Passive tone – Resistance to passive extension of muscles Active tone – Active contraction of muscles

APPENDICULAR SKELETON (PASSIVE TONE) – done only when baby is stable for the procedure otherwise don't do it.

- Scarf sign
- Arm recoil
- Square window
- Adductor angle
- Popliteal angle
- Heel to ear
- Dorsiflexion of foot

APPENDICULAR SKELETON (ACTIVE TONE)

- Palmar grasp
- Pull to sit
- Axillary suspension
- Plantar grasp
- Magnet reflex
- Crossed extensor reflex

FINAL DIAGNSOSIS

PLAN FOR MANAGEMENT

What will you do for ventilation?

Whats your plan for feeding

What will you plan for inotropes?

What counselling will you do to parents?

Developmentally supportive care.

Relevant theory

New Ballard score important points

- 2 score for eyelid tightly fused
- -1 score for eyelid loosely fused
- -2 plantar surface < 40 mm (heel to toe length)
- -1 plantar surface 40- 50mm
- 5 – popliteal angle
- 5 – for skin

Weight as per GA

- 24 weeks – 600 gms
- 25 weeks – 750 gms
- 26 weeks – 850 gms
- 27wks – 1000 gms

Antenatal Steroids

Dexa/ Beta – Synthetic (resistant to inactivation)

Benefits

- Inducing surfactant synthesizing enzymes
- Inducing genes for production of surfactant proteins
- Improving quality of surfactant produced
- Mature non surfactant producing tissues of lung – septa become longer, thinner & less cellular with larger air spaces and ↑ no of alveolar divisions
- Anti-oxidant enzyme activity and reduced oxidative stress

Max benefit: 2-4 days after administration, no longer than 7 days

- Smaller but useful benefit <24hrs
- Greatest benefit – 30-34wks

Dexamethasone sodium phosphate and betamethasone acetate + phosphate are two safe corticosteroid to be used in ANC period

Acetate salt of betamethasone is not available in India only phosphate salt is available .acetate is long acting salt.

Betamethasone is more costly and less stable than dexamethasone at high temperature.

Dose:

- Betamethasone 12mg IM × 2 doses Q24H
- Dexamethasone 6mg IM × 4 doses Q 12H
- Repeated courses
- Maternal hyperglycemia, infections
- Fetal HPA suppression
- ↓ HC, ↓Wt, ↓ht – at time of discharge

A single repeated dose of antenatal betamethasone given for imminent preterm birth at least one week after standard betamethasone treatment, however, was not shown to influence Neurodevelopment outcome and had no significant effect on growth at 2yrs of age

Daily weight checks on infants in incubators and warmers should be done using the in-bed scale.

To protect the infant's FRC, NCPAP-using infants should be weighed while the NCPAP is in use.

Shock is a pathological state in which tissue oxygen delivery is inadequate to meet the demand

Hypovolemic shock – low PRELOAD

Cardiogenic shock - PUMP FAILURE

Distributive shock AFTERLOAD

Signs of shock

- Prolonged CRT (>3-4 seconds)
- Poor peripheral pulses
- Arterial lactate > 2
- Significant metabolic ocidosis (base deficit > 8)
- Oliguria/anuria

Recommended room temperature for neonatal care units - 22-26°C (AAP/ACOG 2007)

Delivery Room

Recommended DR air temperature: NRP 8th edition – 23-25°C.

Place infant < 32 weeks and/or < 1250 grams in a pre-warmed convertible incubator.

Place infants between 32 and 35 weeks and > 1250 grams in a pre-warmed standard incubator.

Place infants > 35 weeks and/or 1700 grams on a pre-warmed radiant warmer or open crib.

Lung development Time period Development	Defects
Embryonic Wks 3-6 Proximal airways	TEF, pulmonary agenesis, pulm sequestration
Pseudoglandular Wks 6-16 Lower conduction airways	CDH, Lobar Agenesis
Canalicular Wks 16-26 Gas exchanging acini Terminal sac	
Wks 26-36 Refinement of acini Alveolar	
Wks 36- 3yrs Alveolar proliferation & development	

D/D of cystic.lung lesion

- CPAM
- CDH
- Pulmonary sequestration
- Bronchogenic cyst

Anatomy of Neonatal Airway

- Narrow nares
- Short neck
- Large tongue
- High glottis
- Large, floppy epiglottis
- Narrow cricoid ring
- Cylindrical rib cage
- Horizontal cartilaginous soft pliable ribs
- Horizontal angle of insertion of diaphragm
- Short length of bronchial tree

38 Basics Respiratory

What is Respiratory Distress? In a quiet & resting baby, any of the 2:

- Respiratory Rate > 60/min (tachypnea)
- Retractions
- Cyanosis, Desaturations
- Expiratory grunting or inspiratory stridor

What are the constituents of surfactant?

Major constituents of surfactant are • dipalmitoyl phosphatidylcholine (lecithin) • phosphatidylglycerol, • apoproteins (surfactant proteins SP-A, -B, -C, -D), • cholesterol

Saturated phospahtidyl choline – 50 %

Unsaturated phosphatidylcholine -20 %

Neutral lipids – 8 %

Phasphatidylglycerol – 8 %

Other phospholipids – 8%

SP A- 5 % - innate defense and regulator protein

SP B 2 % - surface activity and lamellar body formation

SPC 1 % - surface activity

SP D 1 % - innate defense

Role of surfactant proteins

- SP-A and SP-D play a central role in the protection of the lungs against respiratory infection
- SP-A & D also play a role in the metabolism of surfactant and its recycling
- SP-B more efficient in reducing surface tension
- SP C stabilises the alveolar surfactant film by enhancing the adsorption rate of phospholipids

Surfactant production begins at

- Begins at 24-28 weeks of gestation, and gradually increases until full term

Factors that affect normal functioning of surfactant

- Asphyxia, hypoxia, hypotension, hypothermia
- Hypoxia - ischemia and reperfusion injury - inhibits surfactant function
- Asphyxia - hypoxemia and academia - inhibits surfactant synthesis
- Cold - ↓ surfactant function
- Acidemia – impaired surfactant synthesis

How Maternal DM affect surfactant production in fetus

Fetal high Insulin levels secondary to maternal hyperglycemia –

- delays maturation of Type II alveolar cells
    - ↓proportion of saturated Phosphatidylcholine in surfactant
- ↓ SP-A in amniotic fluid

Name some Tests for surfactant estimation

1. LS ratio: Thin layer chromatography • >2 – very low risk of RDS; >3.5 in IDM • Contaminants – blood, meconium
2. TDx-FLM II measures surfactant albumin ratio. • Clinically significant RDS < 55 mg/g• Contaminants – blood, meconium
3. Lamellar body counts in amniotic fluid – ↑ with advancing GA • <50,000 lamellar bodies/microlitre – Risk of RDS
4. Appearance of Phosphatidyl glycerol • NOT affected by blood, meconium• Appears late, low sensitivity, high false negative
5. Foam Stability Index • Formation of stable foam when fluid mixed with ethanol in test tube • Contaminants – blood, meconium

Content of endogenous surfactant

- Endogenous surfactant pool is major determinant of compliance of lung
- Term New-born : 100 mg/kg
- Very preterm with severe RDS: <5 mg/kg
- Preterm have 5% of amount of surfactant in term

Effects of Surfactant on pulmonary tissue and circulation and radiography

Pulmonary effects

- Increase FRC
- Slow and variable increase in lung compliance
- Decrease in pulmonary ventilation perfusion mismatch
- Improve oxygenation
- Decrease in mechanical ventilation support

Pulmonary circulation

- Decrease in pulmonary artery pressure or increase pulmonary artery flow
- Increase ductal flow velocity from systemic to pulmonary circuit

Radiographic changes

- Decrease in signs of RDS
- Clearing of lung can be uniform, patchy or asymmetric or disproportionate improvement on right lung

Effect of antenatal corticosteroid on lung

- It accelerate morphologic development of lung development
- It increases in transcription of responsive genes after - 1-2 hrs of exposure
- Accumulation of new proteins in - 12-24 hrs
- Optimal response occurs in 48 hrs and persistent for at least 7 days
- Reduction in RDS diminish 7-10 days after ANS completion- repeat the course

Which surfactants are Synthetic surfactants without proteins?

- Exosurf consists of 85% DPPC, 9% hexadecanol, and 6% tyloxapol (a spreading agent).
- ALEC (pumactant), (not manufactured) 7:3 mixture of DPPC and phosphatidylglycerol

Which surfactants are Protein-Containing Synthetic Surfactants?

- Lucinactant (Surfaxin)- which contains a mimic of SP-B called sinapultide or KL4 peptide. Lusupultide (Venticute) contains SP-C analogues, recombinant SP-C.

Advantage of Early surfactant

Significant decrease in

- Pneumothorax
- PIE
- Neonatal mortality
- Chronic lung disease

Benefit of surfactant therapy

- Decreased incidence / severity of RDS
- Increased survival from RDS
- Decreased need for oxygen
- Decreased ventilatory support
- Decreased pneumothorax / PIE
- Decreased incidence & severity of (CLD or death)

Surfactant

Major constituents of surfactant are • dipalmitoyl phosphatidylcholine (lecithin) • phosphatidylglycerol, • apoproteins (surfactant proteins SP-A, -B, -C, -D), • cholesterol

- **Beractant (survanta)** (1ml=25 mg) – bovine lung mince extract (4ml/kg) (100mg/kg)
- **Poractant (curosurf)** (1 ml= 76 mg) – porcine lung mince (2.5 ml/kg) (200 mg/kg)
- **Infasurf (calfactant)** – calf lung lavage
- **Neosurf** – 1 ml= 27 mg 5 ml/kg (135 mg/kg)

Complications of surfactant therapy

- Transient bradycardia and occasional tachycardia with or without fall in saturation
- Plugging of ET tube – slower rate of administration
- Reflex of surfactant – needs proper synchronization with the inspiration of baby and ventilator
- Pulmonary hgh – sudden fall in pulmonary artery pressure
- Fall in CBF
- Fall in systemic blood pressure

Causes of non responsiveness to surfactant therapy

- Improper ventilatory technique
- Severe RDS
- Pulmonary odema
- Fluid overload
- Air leak syndrome
- Extreme prematurity
- Associated pneumonia/hypoplasia

Risk of RDS as per GA

24 weeks—>80 % • 28 weeks—70 % • 32 weeks—25 % • 36 weeks—5 %

Which infection appears same as RDS radiologically

- Signs and radiographic findings of group B Streptococcus (GBS) sepsis/pneumonia are indistinguishable from RDS

Genetic causes of RDS

Genetic mutations in surfactant protein B and ABCA3 can result in an RDS picture in the immediate New-born period.

Recommendation of European Consensus Guidelines on the Management of Respiratory Distress Syndrome – 2019 Update

1. Mothers at high risk of preterm birth <28–30 weeks' gestation should be transferred to perinatal centres with experience in management of RDS
2. Single course of prenatal corticosteroids to all women at risk of preterm delivery from when pregnancy is considered potentially viable until 34 weeks' gestation ideally at least 24 h before birth.
3. A single repeat course of steroids may be given in threatened preterm birth before 32 weeks' gestation if the first course was administered at least 1–2 weeks earlier
4. $MgSO_4$ should be administered to women in imminent labour before 32 weeks' gestation
5. In women with symptoms of preterm labour, cervical length and fibronectin measurements should be considered to prevent unnecessary use of tocolytic drugs and/or antenatal steroids
6. Clinicians should consider short-term use of tocolytic drugs in very preterm pregnancies to allow completion of a course of corticosteroids and/or in utero transfer to a perinatal centre.
7. Delay clamping the umbilical cord for at least 60 s to promote placento-fetal transfusion
8. In spontaneously breathing babies, stabilise with CPAP of at least 6 cm H_2O via mask or nasal prongs
9. Do not use SI as there is no long-term benefit
10. Gentle positive pressure lung inflations with 20–25 cm H_2O peak inspiratory pressure (PIP) should be used for persistently apnoeic or bradycardic infants.
11. Oxygen for resuscitation should be controlled using a blender. Use an initial FiO_2 of 0.30 for babies 100/min) should be achieved within 5 min
12. Intubation should be reserved for babies not responding to positive pressure ventilation via face mask or nasal prongs
13. Babies who require intubation for stabilisation should be given surfactant
14. Plastic bags or occlusive wrapping under radiant warmers should be used during stabilisation in the delivery suite for babies <28 weeks' gestation to reduce the risk of hypothermia
15. Babies with RDS should be given an animal-derived surfactant preparation
16. A policy of early rescue surfactant should be standard but there are occasions when surfactant should be given in the delivery suite, such as when intubation is needed for stabilisation
17. Babies with RDS should be given rescue surfactant early in the course of the disease.
18. A suggested protocol would be to treat babies who are worsening when FiO_2 >0.30 on CPAP pressure of at least 6 cm H_2O.
19. Poractant alfa at an initial dose of 200 mg/kg is better than 100 mg/kg of poractant alfa or 100 mg/kg of beractant for rescue therapy (A1).
20. LISA is the preferred mode of surfactant administration for spontaneously breathing babies on CPAP, provided that clinicians are experienced with this technique.
21. A second and occasionally a third dose of surfactant should be given if there is ongoing evidence of RDS such as persistent high oxygen requirement and other problems have been excluded
22. CPAP should be started from birth in all babies at risk of RDS, such as those <30 weeks' gestation who do not need intubation for stabilisation.
23. 2 The system delivering CPAP is of little importance; however, the interface should be short binasal prongs or mask with a starting pressure of about 6–8 cm H_2O.
24. Positive end-expiratory pressure (PEEP) can then be individualised depending on clinical condition, oxygenation and perfusion.
25. CPAP with early rescue surfactant is considered optimal management for babies with RDS.
26. Synchronised NIPPV, if delivered through a ventilator rather than BIPAP device, can reduce extubation failure

but may not confer long-term advantages such as reduction in BPD.

27. During weaning, HFNC can be used as an alternative to CPAP for some babies with the advantage of less nasal trauma.
28. After stabilisation, MV should be used in babies with RDS when other methods of respiratory support have failed.
29. Duration of MV should be minimised
30. The primary choice of ventilation mode is at discretion of clinical team; however, if conventional MV is used, targeted tidal volume ventilation should be employed.
31. When weaning from MV, it is reasonable to tolerate a modest degree of hypercarbia provided the pH remains above 7.22.
32. Caffeine should be used to facilitate weaning from MV.
33. Early caffeine should be considered for babies at high risk of needing MV such as those on non-invasive respiratory support.
34. A short tapering course of low dose or very low dexamethasone should be considered to facilitate extubation in babies who remain on MV after 1–2 weeks.
35. Inhaled budesonide can be considered for infants at very high risk of BPD.
36. Opioids should be used selectively when indicated by clinical judgment and evaluation of pain indicators.
37. The routine use of morphine or midazolam infusions in ventilated preterm infants is not recommended.
38. Core temperature should be maintained between 36.5 and 37.5°C at all times.
39. Most babies should be started on intravenous fluids of 70–80 mL/kg/day in a humidified incubator, although some very immature babies may need more.
40. Fluids must be tailored individually according to serum sodium levels, urine output and weight loss.
41. Parenteral nutrition should be started from birth.
42. Amino acids 1–2 g/kg/day should be started from day one and quickly built up to 2.5–3.5 g/kg/day.
43. Lipids should be started from day one and built up to a maximum of 4.0 g/kg/day if tolerated.
44. Enteral feeding with mother's milk should be started from the first day if the baby is haemodynamically stable
45. Treatment of hypotension is recommended when it is confirmed by evidence of poor tissue perfusion such as oliguria, acidosis and poor capillary return rather than purely on numerical values.
46. If a decision is made to attempt therapeutic closure of the PDA then indomethacin, ibuprofen or paracetamol can be used.
47. Haemoglobin (Hb) concentration should be maintained within acceptable limits. Hb thresholds for infants with severe cardiopulmonary disease are 12 g/dL (HCT 36%), 11 g/ dL (HCT 30%) for those who are oxygen dependent and 7 g/ dL (HCT 25%) for stable infants beyond 2 weeks of age.
48. Surfactant can be used for RDS complicated by congenital pneumonia.
49. Surfactant therapy can be used to improve oxygenation following pulmonary haemorrhage.
50. Use of iNO in preterm babies should be used with caution and limited to those in clinical studies or as a therapeutic trial when there is severe documented pulmonary hypertension.

Evidence of Antenatal MgSO4

1. Reduction in Cerebral Palsy by 32%. NNT 63.
2. Reduction in Germinal Matrix dysfunction by 39%
3. No sig. difference in Mortality and other neurological abnormalities.

Evidence for Use of heat loss preventing bags for maintain temp of preterms

1. Improved core body temperature by 0.58 deg Celsius
2. 33% Fewer neonates with hypothermia on admission. Or two hours after birth (NNT 4)
3. RR for hyperthermia 3.91 NNH-25
4. Risk of temp outside normothermic range reduced by 25%, NNTH 5

Evidence for sustained lung Inflation

1. Sustained Inflation has no significant impact on death and BPD
2. Sustained inflations had no effect and may even increase mortality in very preterm infants

Evidence for early use of caffeine (< 2 days)

- Less adverse neurodevelopmental outcome
- Lower BPD, PDA and severe neurological injury.
- Early caffeine therapy is associated with better

neurodevelopmental outcomes compared with late caffeine therapy in preterm infants born at <29 weeks' gestation.

Non RDS indication of surfactant

- MAS
- Pulmonary HGH
- Pneumonia

Techniques of Less invasive surfactant delivery

- Via thin catheter
- Aerosolized administration
- Pharyngeal surfactant administration
- LMA guided surfactant administration

LISA

- It allows combining surfactant delivery with spontaneous breathing.
- Allows maintained laryngeal function.
- Potential to improve patient comfort by avoiding mechanical ventilation.
- Improves outcomes when compared with mechanical ventilation, other modes of non-invasive ventilation or short-time intubation and surfactant instillation (INSURE).
- Recommended in recent surfactant guidelines on the basis of individual studies and metaanalyses.
- Needs further research in order to optimize patient comfort

Less invasive surfactant therapy

Three technique of LISA used in RCTs

Catheter size for LISA external diameter 1.33–1.7 mm.

Cologne method-

- 4-Fr feeding tube
- Inserted 1.5 cm below the vocal cords
- Under direct laryngoscopy with the aid of Magill forceps
- After premedication with atropine.

In the Take Care method

- 5-Fr feeding tube without Magill forceps
- Premedication was used.

In the minimally invasive surfactant therapy (MIST)

- 16-gauge vascular catheter (Angiocath)
- Without premedication was used

COLOGNE method	5 F feeding tube
Hobart method	16 G angiocath
Take care method	5 F feeding tube
Sonsure	4 F feeding tube
Karolinska method	5 F
Ecalmist	17 G vascular catheter

What is Cologne method of surfactant administration?

Thin catheter is placed into the trachea with aid of a Magill forceps under direct laryngoscopy for surfactant administration.

Hobart method of surfactant administration?

Uses a more rigid vascular catheter instead of a soft catheter for surfactant administration.

Introduced into the trachea without the use of a Magill forceps

Coughing, choking, desaturation, bradycardia, and surfactant reflux are some of the unfavourable effects of inserting a narrow catheter.

Success rate of catheter placement on first attempt -72% to 95%.

LISA vs INSURE/ OR OTHER METHODS

Metaanalyses of 14 studies in which LISA was compared with endotracheal administration of surfactant as a control demonstrated

1. A significant decrease in risk of the composite outcome of death or BPD at 36 weeks' postmenstrual age (PMA) (risk ratio [RR], 0.59; [NNTB], 9;
2. Decrease in the need for intubation within 72 hours (RR, 0.63; NNTB 8
3. Decrease severe intraventricular hemorrhage (RR, 0.63; NNTB, 22 ;),
4. Decrease death during first hospitalization (RR, 0.63; NNTB, 20;
5. decrease BPD among survivors (RR, 0.57; NNTB, 13;
6. There was no significant difference in risk of air leak requiring drainage.

TCA vs insure

- No change in mortality
- Decrease in BPD in TCA.
- The point estimate suggests that for every 25 infants treated with TCA there will be one less case of BPD

- 26% decrease in BPD/death in TCA
- Decrease in pneumothorax in TCA
- 26% decrease in need of MV in TCA

History of surfactant?

- 1959: Avery and Mead - HMD is due to deficiency of surfactant
- 1963: Patrick Bouvier Kennedy, the son of President John F Kennedy; born at 34-35 weeks; died due to HMD
- 1964- First synthetic surfactant trial
- 1980- Fujiwara- First human trial with natural surfactant
- Insure invented by Henrik Verder in 1989
- Late 1990. MIST
- MIST/LISA popularized in late 2000
- Surfactant administration with the use of a thin catheter, first described by Verder et al in 1992, has been the most studied less invasive technique

CALMEST approach - Catheter and Laryngeal Mask Endotracheal Surfactant Therapy

Recommendation for management of RDS as per European guidelines

- Babies with RDS should be given an animal-derived surfactant preparation.
- A policy of early rescue surfactant should be standard, but there are occasions when surfactant should be given in the delivery suite, such as when intubation is needed for stabilization.
- Babies with RDS should be given rescue surfactant early in the course of the disease. A suggested protocol would be to treat babies who are worsening when $FiO_2 > 0.30$ on CPAP pressure of at least 6 cm H_2O
- Poractant alfa at an initial dose of 200 mg/kg is better than 100 mg/kg of poractant alfa or 100 mg/kg of beractant for rescue therapy
- LISA is the preferred mode of surfactant administration for spontaneously breathing babies on CPAP, provided that clinicians are experienced with this technique.
- A second and occasionally a third dose of surfactant should be given if there is ongoing evidence of RDS such as persistent high oxygen requirement and other problems are ruled out.

MAS and surfactant

- Meconium contains cholesterol, FFA, bile salts, bilirubin and proteolytic enzymes which inhibits surface-tension lowering properties of surfactant.
- It alters surfactant morphology, changing the loosely stacked layers to spherical lamellar and folded linear structures
- Decrease levels of SP-A & SP-B

Evidence for Use of Exogenous surfactant in MAS

- Four trials (326 infants)
- No statistically significant effect on mortality
- Risk of requiring ECMO was significantly reduced in two trials

Role of surfactant in CDH

No statistically significant difference in duration of ECMO, duration of intubation and mechanical ventilation, or rates of BPD between those patients who received at least one dose of surfactant while on ECMO, and those who did not.

Evidence for Prophylactic vs rescue surfactant (Cochrane)

- No effect on neonatal mortality
- CLD more in prophylactic group
- No difference in pneumothorax

Evidence for Early vs delayed surfactant (Cochrane)

- Early group – 16 % less mortality
- No change in BPD
- 31 % reduction in pneumothorax in early group
- No difference in pulmonary hgh
- 17 % Reduction in CLD/Death combined outcome in early group

Animal vs protein free synthetic surfactant

- 11 % Reduction in mortality
- No significant difference in BPD
- 35 % Reduction in Pneumothorax
- 38 % increase in NEC
- No significant difference in grade III or IV IVH

Protein containing synthetic surfactant vs animal derived surfactant

- Protein containing synthetic surfactant group compared to animal derived surfactant extract group did not dhow significant different risks of:

- Mortality at 36 weeks
- Chronic lung disease at 36 weeks
- Combined outcome of mortality or chronic lung disease at 36 weeks
- Decrease risk of NEC was noted in infants who received protein containing synthetic surfactants compared to animal derived surfactant extract

Bovine vs porcine surfactant

- 44% increase in mortality in bovine group
- 30% increase in BPD/death in bovine group
- 57% increase in repeat dose in bovine group
- No difference in air leak

1. Difference in these outcomes was limited to studies using a higher initial dose of porcine minced lung surfactant extract
2. It is uncertain whether the observed differences are from differences in dose or from source of extraction (porcine vs. bovine) as lack of dose-equivalent comparison groups with appropriate sample size

Multiple vs single dose of surfactant

- 30% decrease in pneumothorax with multiple
- No change in pulmonary haemorrghae
- No significant on PDA
- No effect on IVH
- No significant on BPD
- 41% decrease in mortality

Early surfactant rapid extubation to CPAP vs selective surfactant and MV

- 33% less need of mechanical ventilation in early surfactant f/b CPAP
- 49% decrease in BPD in early surfactant f/b CPAP
- 43% less need of repeat surfactant in early surfactant f/b CPAP
- 48% decrease in air leaks in early surfactant f/b CPAP

"Absolute humidity" (AH) is defined as the amount of water vapor (in milligrams) per gas volume (in liters) at a given temperature.

"Relative humidity" (RH) is the actual water vapor content of the gas volume (in milligrams) relative to the water vapor content (in milligrams) of this same gas volume at saturation at the same temperature.

A gas holds 44 mg of water per litre at 37° C and 100% relative humidity.

The point where the gases are at 37 C and 100% RH is known as isothermic saturation boundary and usually is located just below the carina.

Harms of inadequate conditioning?

a. Increases water and heat loss, inflammation of airway epithelium leading to damage to airway.
b. Damage to mucociliary transport system (at 30% RH), which reduces clearance of secretions, increase airway blockage by mucus plugs, atelectasis.
c. Impairs action of surfactant

In non-invasive, the airway set point is lower (34C) as nose and upper airway of the baby add to the temperature and humidity of inspired gases and achieve core body temperature (37C)

Signs of inadequate conditioning?

1. Minimal consumption of humidifier water
2. Excess condensation in inspiratory limb (rainout) – VAP, Auto cycling
3. No condensate in expiratory limb
4. Lack of beading condensate on inner walls of humidification chamber

Third generation synthetic surfactant with SP-B and SP-C mimics -**CHF-5633**

Apneic Spell (AAP definition)

Cessation of breathing for 20 seconds or longer or a shorter pause accompanied by:

- Bradycardia (<100 beats per minute) OR
- Hypoxemia (detected clinically by cyanosis or by oxygen saturation monitoring: SpO2 <80%), OR
- Hypotonia, or pallor

REM sleep and Apnea

- Rapid eye movement (REM) sleep is marked by irregularity of tidal volume and respiratory frequency.
- REM sleep predominates in preterm infants and apneic spells occur more frequently in this state than in quiet sleep.

- Mechanism - loss of upper airway muscle tone, leading to pharyngeal collapse
- Preterm infants have a blunted ventilatory response to elevated CO2.
- Preterm infants have a biphasic response to hypoxia with transient hyperventilation, followed by hypoventilation and sometimes apnea
- GER does not prolong or worsen concurrent apnea
- Hyperbilirubinemia - Unconjugated bilirubin crosses the blood-brain barrier and causes brainstem dysfunction
- Results in decreased respiratory drive in response to either hypercapnia or hypoxia

Use of Nasal Continuous Positive Airway Pressure in apnea -

Splints upper airway with positive pressure and decreases the risk of pharyngeal or laryngeal obstruction.

CPAP also increases functional residual capacity (FRC) At a higher FRC, time from cessation of breathing to hypoxemia and bradycardia is prolonged.

Features of caffeine

- Clear colorless sterile, preservative free, single use only, storage <30 C, discarded if colored or with particulate matter
- Dose equivalent: 20 mg = 10 mg base
- Peak plasma levels after loading dose: 6-10mg/l and mean time to reach peak concentration is 30 mins to 2 hours
- Preparation 1ml= 20 mg caffeine citrate (10 mg base) compatible with dextrose solutions (D5, D10)
- Half life: 40-230 hours (prolonged in hepatic disorders esp-cholestatic jaundice)
- Bioavailability is almost 100% even after oral administration but not fully examined in preterm neonates

Respiratory Effects of Xanthine Therapy

- Increases minute ventilation
- Improves CO2 sensitivity
- Decreases hypoxic depression of breathing
- Promotes bronchodilation
- Enhances diaphragmatic activity

IN TOTAL MOLECULAR MECHANISM AND ITS EFFECT OF CAFFEINE AT BRAIN, LUNG AND HEART

MECHANISM IN BRAIN	EFFECT
1. Caffeine Increases respiratory neural output by antagonising the adenosinergic inhibition on inspiratory neurons in the brainstem. 2. Proposed based on animal studies Enhanced CO2 responsiveness and decreased hypoxic depression of breathing by action on A1 receptor and peripheral chemoreceptor 3. Neuroprotective anti-inflammatory effect against periventricular white matter injury and hypoxic insults by blocking adenosine action. 4. Increase in myelination, promotion of oligodendroglial maturation and process arborisation in hypoxia-exposed white matter 5. Anti-apoptotic effect possibly by blocking TNF-α	1. Enhanced cerebral cortical activity 2. Reduced incidence of death or clinical disability, cerebral palsy and cognitive delay at 18-21 months of corrected age compared to placebo. 3. No difference in death or severe impairment (motor impairment, behavioural problems, poor general health, deafness and blindness) at 5 years compared to placebo. 4. Improved motor function at 5 and 11 years. 5. No difference in the combined rates of functional impairment, academic performance and behavioural problems at 11 years compared to placebo 6. Improved fine motor coordination, visuomotor integration, visual perception, visuospatial organisation at 11 years

MECHANISM IN LUNG	EFFECT
1. Improvement in diaphragmatic contractility and function 30 min after loading dose in ELBW infants 2. Inhibition of pulmonary inflammation induced by hyperoxia by decreased proinflammatory cytokine expression (animal models] 3. Induction of surfactant protein B transcription through a cAMP-dependent pathway 4. Diuretic effect, probably by removal of excess fluids from the lungs and the facilitation of breathing	1. Reduction in ventilatory support and IPPV 2. Reduction in oxygen treatment at 36 weeks PMA 3. Lower rates of BPD at 36 weeks PMA 4. Improved minute ventilation and tidal volumes 5. [12] Reduced incidence of apnoea 6. Reduced extubation failure 7. Improved lung function at 11 years

MECHNISM AT HEART	EFFECT
1. Increased left ventricular stroke volume with inotropic effect accompanied by pressor effect	1. Reduced need for PDA treatment 2. Reduced need for surgical closure of PDA 3. Reduced rate of vasopressor requirement

Indications for Caffeine Therapy

- For treatment of infants who have documented apneic spells that are frequent, prolonged, or associated with bradycardia and/or oxygen desaturation
- For treatment of infants who have apneic spells that require intervention with bag and mask ventilation, or multiple episodes of tactile stimulation
- As prophylactic therapy given to all extreme preterm neonates to reduce the need for intubation and mechanical ventilation
- To facilitate extubation in extreme preterm neonates who are intubated

Loading dose of 20 mg/kg of caffeine citrate (10 mg/kg caffeine base) orally or intravenously

Maintenance doses of 5 to 10 mg/kg in one daily dose, beginning 24 hours after the loading dose

High loading dose and cerebellar injury on MRI in preterm infants has been observed

Insufficient safety data to routinely advocate higher doses of caffeine than the standard doses

Caffeine serum levels of 5 to 20 µg/mL are considered therapeutic

Toxic levels: > 40-50 micrograms/ml. Clinical monitoring: if HR>180bpm consider withholding

Toxic levels can produce:

- Tachycardia
- Cardiac dysrhythmias
- Feed intolerance
- Reduced weight gain
- Seizures (rare)

Caffeine for Apnea of Prematurity (CAP) Trial (2005)

- Randomly assigned 2006 infants with birth weights between 500 g and 1250 g to caffeine or placebo in the first 10 postnatal days to prevent or treat apnea or to facilitate extubation.
- Dosing - loading dose of 20 mg/kg followed by maintenance of 5 mg/kg per day, which could be increased to 10 mg/kg per day for persistent apnea.
- Caffeine-treated infants had a shorter duration of mechanical ventilation, lower incidence of bronchopulmonary dysplasia, and improved neurodevelopmental outcome at 18 months.
- Follow-up study – In survivors at 18 to 21 months corrected age, infants in the caffeine group had a lower incidence of cerebral palsy and cognitive delay. At five-year follow-up, the difference between groups for these outcomes was not statistically significant.
- Long-term neurodevelopment follow-up - caffeine therapy was associated with a reduced risk of motor impairment and improved visuomotor, visuoperceptual, and visuospatial abilities at 11 years of age.
- Use of caffeine was found to be safe with no adverse effect on general intelligence, attention, academic performance and behavior at 11-year follow-up.
- Early caffeine therapy within the first 3 days of life - beneficial in reducing BPD, PDA and duration of mechanical ventilation in preterm infants less than 32 weeks' gestational age.

Dobson et al, 2014:

Retrospective analysis of 29000 VLBW infants from Pediatrix Medical Group found that early initiation of caffeine therapy (within 3 d of life)- associated with a lower incidence of BPD, less treatment of PDA, and a shorter duration of mechanical ventilation

Early caffeine preferred

- Definite benefit in BPD (consistent)
- Decrease risk of PDA ,PDA requiring surgery
- Decrease risk of ROP and brain injury in retrospective studies

Hering- Breuer reflex

- Expansion of lung reflexively inhibits inspiration and promotes expiration and that deflation of lungs promotes inspiration and inhibits expiration.
- Factors increasing the strength of this reflex is- Premature birth, prone position , active sleep and respiratory distress syndrome

Ventilator associated pneumonia

Imaging evidence: Two or more serial chest radiographs with new/ progressive and persistent infiltrate, cavitation, consolidation, or pneumatoceles for patients with underlying pulmonary or cardiac disease (respiratory distress syndrome, bronchopulmonary dysplasia, pulmonary edema) or one chest radiograph with the aforementioned abnormalities for patients without underlying pulmonary or cardiac disease

AND

Worsening gas exchange

AND

- **At least three of the following:**

(1) temperature instability,

(2) white blood cell count less than 4000/µL or greater than 15,000/µL with 10% or more bands,

(3) new-onset purulent sputum, change in character of sputum, increased respiratory secretions, or increased suctioning requirements,

(4) physical examination findings consistent with increased work of breathing or apnea, (5) wheezing, rales, or rhonchi,

(5) cough,

(6) bradycardia (<100 bpm), or tachycardia (>170 bpm)

Ventilator-Associated Pneumonia

- Pneumonia (as defined above) AND
- Patient on ventilator for more than 2 days AND
- Ventilator in place on day of or day before VAP diagnosis

Key practices that may help reduce the risk of VAP include

1. Timely removal of tracheal tubes from patients,
2. Minimizing aspiration of pathogenic bacteria by elevating the head of the bed by 30 to 45 degrees, and performing oral hygiene with sterile water.
3. There is no clear evidence of the superiority of closed versus open suctioning systems in minimizing VAP risk.
4. Use of hand hygiene and gloves prior to management of ventilation equipment,
5. Developing standard practices for suctioning while minimizing contamination,
6. Optimizing non-invasive ventilation strategies whenever feasible
7. Oropharyngeal administration of human milk has been used to reduce VAP in infants <1.5 kg
8. Using sterile water in humidification systems, periodic drainage of condensate from breathing circuits
9. Extubating as soon as possible
10. Changing the ventilator circuit only when visibly contaminated
11. Avoiding saline instillation with ETT suctioning
12. Suctioning the ETT only when needed

Risk factors for VAP

- Length of stay in NICU (OR 23.45)
- Reintubation (OR 9.18)
- Enteral feeding (OR 5.59)
- Mechanical ventilation (OR 4.04)
- Transfusion (OR 3.32)
- Low birth weight (OR 3.16)
- Premature infants (OR 2.66)
- Parenteral nutrition (OR 2.30)
- Bronchopulmonary dysplasia (OR 2.21)
- Tracheal intubation (OR 1.12).

Closed vs open suction – No significant difference in rates of VAP – Easier to use, Faster, Better tolerated. CDC recommendations – do not endorse one system over the other – no recommendations addressing the frequency at which closed suctioning systems should be changed

CDC - Breathing circuits do not need routine changing unless they become visibly soiled or malfunction

VAP Bundle

Care bundles are groupings of usually 3 to 5 evidence-based practices specific to a disease process that individually improve care but, when applied together, may result in substantially greater improvement

Compliance (CL)

- The relationship between a given change in volume & pressure reqd to produce that change
- CL = σV/ σP
- Inverse of elastic recoil
- FTNB: 1 hr – 3.5 ml/cm of H_2O
- 24 hr – 4.5 ml/cm of H_2O8 days – 6 ml/cm of H_2O
- Adults: 200 ml/cm of H_2O

Upper inflation point

Pressure beyond which further increase would not result in

increase in tidal volume but would result in over distension of alveoli and risk of air leaks

Lower inflation point

Below this pressure the alveoli start collapsing and result in atelectasis and collapse Work of breathing increases

Time Constant (Kt)

- Kt is a measure of how quickly pressure in the proximal airways (or venti tubings) can be equilibrated in the alveoli
- Kt = CL × R
- One Kt is time taken to discharge 63% of Vt thru airways
- Three Kt equal to 95% of Vt discharge
- Normal neonatal 1Kt = 0.15 sec

Normal & Abnormal values

	CL (L/cm of H2O)	R (cm H2O/ L/se c)	Kt (Sec)
Normal	0.005	20	0.10
RDS	0.001	20	0.02
MAS	0.003	100	0.3

RDS = low compliance = short time constant

BPD = ▲resistance = long time constant

MAS = ▲resistance = long time constant

Short Time constant = alveolus needs short time for expiration (so u can have short Te and longer Ti)

- Long time constant= need longer Te, or it will lead to air trapping

Indications for CPAP - In 1971, Gregory- used CPAP in preterm infants with RDS

- Respiratory distress syndrome (RDS) (No role for free flow oxygen therapy)
- Apnea of prematurity (especially obstructive apnea)
- Post-extubation in preterm VLBW infants
- Transient tachypnea of New-born (TTNB)/delayed adaptation
- Others Pneumonia Meconium aspiration/ other aspiration syndromes Pulmonary edema/pulmonary hemorrhage Laryngomalacia/ tracheomalacia/ bronchomalacia

CPAP Failure

- Rising FiO2 requirement to > 60%
- CPAP pressure of >8-10 cm
- Frequent apneas on appropriate CPAP
- Absolute ABG criteria of respiratory failure

Contraindications to CPAP

- Progressive respiratory failure with PaCO2 levels >60 mmHg and/or inability to maintain oxygenation (PaO2 <50 mmHg)
- Certain congenital malformations of the airway (choanal atresia, tracheo esophageal fistula, congenital diaphragmatic hernia, etc.)
- Severe cardiovascular instability (hypotension) ? Poor respiratory drive (frequent apnea and bradycardia) that is not improved by CPAP

Nasal Masks vs Nasal Prongs as interface

- Nasal mask CPAP reduced the rate of intubation, reduced the need for surfactant and reduced the rate of BPD (RR, 0.47; 95% CI, 0.23–0.95) compared with nasal prong CPAP.
- Longer CPAP duration with nasal mask CPAP

NIPPV vs. nasal CPAP Primary therapy

- Less NIMV Failure
- Less intubation and mechanical ventilation
- No significant difference in BPD

NIPPV vs. nasal CPAP Postextubation

- Less NIMV Failure
- Less intubation and mechanical ventilation
- No significant difference in BPD

sNIPPV consistently showed lowest rates for ETT/MV and BPD vs. all other modes

Dominant REM sleep – irregular TV and respiratory effort – more chances of apnea especially in preterm

Rates not an efficient way of controlling CO2

In neonatal ventilation, Ti constant most of the time, So Increasing rates gives more breaths in one minute and allows better oxygenation if Ti is kept constant but it decrease the expiratory time.

CO2 elimination is determined by

- Tidal volume
- Expiratory time and rates

CO2 elimination is determined by

1. Recruit maximal number of alveoli

2. Minimize alveolar dead space
3. No collapse / over-distension
4. Minimize external dead space
5. Tidal volume
6. Reduce resistance & obstruction of airways
7. Expiratory time and rates

High CO2 causes - IVH

Low CO2 causes – PVL

Low CO2 indicates volutrauma

Bronchopulmonary Dysplasia

Lung Compliance – reduced

Airway resistance increased – markedly

Time constant – Increased

Pneumonia

- Pathophysiology is nearly similar to RDS • Initial ventilator settings similar to RDS
- Lung Compliance – Reduced
- FRC– Reduced
- Time constant – Short

Meconium Aspiration Syndrome

- Airway Resistance -⇧
- Time Constant -⇧
- FRC -⇧
- Compliance - N to⇩
- PIP – To achieve TV- 4-6 ml/kg. Usually 15-25 • Adequate PEEP – 4-5 cm of H2O • Te – Adequate to prevent air trapping (0.71.0 s)
- Rates- Relatively rapid 50-60 /min • FiO2 – 10% higher than required on hood

Apnea of Prematurity (AOP)

PIP – Minimal PIP- 7-15 cm of H2O suffices • PEEP –4-5 cm of H2O • Ti – 0.3-0.4 • Rates- Slow rates, 20 /min • FiO2 – <0.25 is generally sufficient

Pulmonary Hemorrhage

Marked alveolar hemorrhage ↓↓ lung compliance & gas exchange

- PIP – High PIP req. to achieve TV, usually 20-30 cm of H2O
- Moderate to High PEEP – 6-7 cm of H2O • Ti – 0.3-0.5 • Rates- 40-60/min • FiO2 – To maintain SpO2 92-95%
- AaDO2 > 250 – indicates need for assistant ventilation
- AaDO2 > 400 indicates shunt
- AaDO2 > 600 need for ECMO
- a/A ratio: < 0.8 indicates hypoxia < 0.3 indicates severe resp. compromize

Oxygenation index:

- 15 indicates severe resp. compromize
- OI > 25 – iNO
- OI> 40 – ECMO
- 40: mortality risk 80%

New BPD

- Saccular or immature air spaces with no new alveolarization
- Minimal or no airway pathology
- Minimal inflammatory infiltrate
- Dysmorphic pulmonary angiogenesis

Old BPD

- Alveolar injury, rupture and fibrosis
- Airway- hyperplasia of smooth muscles and metaplasia of epithelium
- Marked inflammatory infiltrate
- Vascular smooth muscle hypertrophy in pulmonary vessels

Disease	Compliance ml/cmH2O	Resistance cmH2O/ml/s	Time constant	Resistive work gm–cm/ kg
Term	4 – 6	20 - 40	0.25	20 – 30
Preterm / VLBW	2 – 2.5	20 – 40	0.1	↑
RDS	< 1	20 - 40	0.02	30 – 40
MAS	3	100	0.30	↑↑
BPD	< 1	> 150	↑	> 40

Non ventilatory strategies to minimize VILI

- Adequate sedation and pain control
- Proper fluid and electrolyte management
- Haemodynamic monitoring
- Prevention and aggressive treatment of sepsis
- Early diagnosis and treatment of HSPDA
- Nutrition

How to monitor adequacy of mechanical breaths

- Movt of chest – adequate
- Disappearance of retraction
- Adequate air entry
- Normal saturation
- ETCO2 monitoring
- ABG values
- Pulmonary graphics

Causes of acute deterioration (within minutes)

- Displaced tube
- Obstruction
- Pneumothorax
- Equipment failure
- Large IVH

Causes of gradual deterioration in a stable neonate

- Increase in primary pathology
- Infection
- Anemia
- Hypotension
- PDA
- Dyselectrolytemia
- Hypoglycaemia
- Progression to BPD

JENSEN classification of BPD 2019 Neonatal Research Network Definition

Highest mode of respiratory support administered at 36 weeks "PMA"

1. Grade 1 -Nasal cannula with flow ≤2 L/minute
2. Grade 2- Nasal cannula >2 L/minute, nCPAP NIPPV
3. Grade 3 Invasive mechanical ventilation

Delivery room interventions for Prevention of BPD

1. Use of CPAP/establishment of FRC
2. Avoid large tidal volume during resuscitation
3. T-piece most accurate and consistent for tidal volume delivery
4. Avoiding invasive ventilation
5. Blended air/oxygen should be available.
6. FIO_2 adjustments up or down should be guided by pulse oximetry

Initial tidal volume

1. Preterm RDS <700 g 5.5-6 mL/kg
2. Preterm RDS 700-1249 g 4.5-5 mL/kg
3. Term, late preterm, normal lungs 4-4.5 ml/kg
4. Term MAS with classic CXR 5.5-6 mL/kg
5. Term CDH 4-4.5 mL/kg
6. Preterm evolving BPD, 3 weeks old 5.5-6.5 mL/kg
7. Established severe BPD 7-12 mL/kg.

Evidence based Benefits of Volume-Targeted Ventilation (recent SRMA)

- Death at BPD at 36 weeks – RR 0.75
- BPD at 36 weeks PMA – RR 0.73 NNB - 8
- Grade 3-4 IVH – RR 0.53 NNB 11
- PVL ± severe IVH -RR 0.53 NNB 11
- Pneumothorax RR 0.52 NNB - 20
- Hypocapnia RR 0.49 NNB - 3
- Days of MV -1.35 DAYS

Risk Factors for Extubation Failure in Neonates

- Low gestational age (<26 weeks)
- Extremely low birth weight (<1000 g)
- Intraventricular hemorrhage (grade III and/or IV)
- Hemodynamically unstable patent ductus arteriosus
- Lack of caffeine administration pre-extubation
- Sedation (narcotics or benzodiazepines)
- Neurologic or neuromuscular disorder
- Airway abnormalities
- Hemodynamic instability
- Sepsis and necrotizing enterocolitis

Interventions to reduce BPD

1. Antenatal Steroids – indirect effect

2. Oxygen administration -Titrate supplemental oxygen to obtain preductal oxygen saturation as per Dawson chart. Maintain oxygen saturations 91-95%.
3. Surfactant – indirect effect- Use insure/LISA technique to administer surfactant
4. DR CPAP with early rescue surfactant through INSURE technique- NNTB -8
5. Consider volume targeted ventilation strategies: TV 4-6 mL/kg
6. If using pressure control mode then
   a. Use short inspiratory times (0.3-0.4 s)
   b. rapid rates (40-60 per min)
   c. low PIP on pressure control settings (14-20 cm H2O),
   d. moderate PEEP (4-6 cm H2O)
   e. PaO2: 40-60 mm Hg;
   f. PaCO2 :45-55 mm Hg
7. Early trial to NIPPV/SNIPPV if tolerating weaning to minimal settings on invasive ventilation
8. Intratracheal administration of budesonide and surfactant – more evidence needed
9. Fluid Restriction – trend towards lower BPD. Restrictive fluid intake may decrease BPD in first week of life
10. Caffeine – good evidence NNTB – 10
11. Low dose hydrocortisone in first week Low dose hydrocortisone (total dose 8.5 mg over 10 days) is associated with increased BPD free survival. Increased risk of late onset sepsis in infants <26 weeks. Increased risk of SIP in infants who receive indomethacin
12. Aggressive Nutrition and MOM – good evidence. Exclusive human milk feeding reduces the risk for BPD
13. Vitamin A- single RCT showing benefit. Improves BPD free survival with reported NNT 14-15. Dose: 5000 IU given intramuscularly 3 times a week for 4 weeks
14. Diuretics – if there is evidence of pulmonary odema. May improve respiratory mechanics and facilitate weaning of support.
15. Azithromycin – in some cases
16. Inhaled steroid – not very effective may improve symptoms in some
17. Decrease sepsis – supportive
18. Post Natal Steroids – good evidence. Low dose dexamethasone (0.89 mg/kg over 10 days) facilitates extubation but does not reduce BPD.
19. High dose dexamethasone (0.5 mg/kg-1 mg/kg) reduces BPD but may increase the risk of NDI and CP
20. Those who remain intubated at 3-4 weeks postnatal age maximum benefit for steroid
21. Blood gas targets: pH 7.25-7.35; PaO2 50-70 mm Hg; PCO2 50-60 mm Hg in evolving BPD

DART Dexamethasone a Randomized Trial

- 70 infants, <28wks, <1000, ventilation, >7days
- Dexamethasone over 10 days 0.83/kg cumulative Dose
- Less severe BPD, more extubations
- Long term 2yrs outcome - Death or cerebral palsy (23% vs 37%) but death or abnormal ND is similar (46% vs.43%)

DART dosing

1. 0.075 mg/kg/dose every 12 hours (6 doses)
2. 0.05 mg/kg/dose every 12 hours (6 doses)
3. 0.025 mg/kg/dose every 12 hours (4 doses)
4. 0.01 mg/kg/dose every 12 hours (4 doses)

Cumulative dose = 0.89 mg/kg

Attempt to extubate by day 3-4 of dexamethasone course

Early systemic steroids (<7 days of age)

Dexamethasone

1. Decreased death/BPD
2. Increased GI bleed and perforation
3. Increased cerebral palsy and death/cerebral palsy

Hydrocortisone

1. Decreased death/BPD
2. Increased GI bleed and perforation
3. Increased cerebral palsy and death/cerebral palsy
4. Not recommended
5. Limited data

Late systemic steroids (≥7 days of age)

Dexamethasone Cochrane systematic review (Doyle)

1. Decreased death/BPD
2. Decreased extubation failure by 28 days
3. Increased transient hyperglycemia and hypertension
4. No increase in cerebral palsy

Start if

1. High BPd risk on NICHD calculator
2. If patient requires mechanical ventilation > 14 days
3. Optimal timing for therapy: 2-6 weeks of age

Ventilation in established BPD

Depends on what type of pathology is there

If there is Marked regional heterogeneity of the lung disease then use

1. Larger tidal volumes (10-12 mL/kg)
2. Longer inspiratory times (≥0.6 s)

If BPD has features of Airways obstruction then use

1. Use Slower rates it allow for better emptying, especially with larger tidal volumes
2. Use higher PEEP for dynamic airway collapse

What do you understand by the term mode of ventilation-?

A mode is a particular pattern of patient ventilator interaction

A patient and a ventilator interact in a particular way, which is referred to as a mode of ventilation. In terms of the flow-time curve, a ventilator cycle consists of a positive flow phase (inflation) and a negative flow phase (expiration).

- What causes the ventilator to provide inflation?
- How is pressure and gas flow controlled during the ventilator cycle,
- How is the inflation stopped?

(pressure-controlled [PC] ventilation) or (volume-controlled [VC] ventilation)

Indications for Mechanical Ventilation

- Absent, weak, or intermittent spontaneous effort
- Frequent (.6 events/hour) or severe apnea requiring PPV
- Marked retractions, severe tachypnea, 90–100/mi
- High oxygen requirement
- Severe respiratory acidosis
- Intestinal obstruction; intestinal perforation; recent gastrointestinal surgery; ileus; CDH
- Postoperative period

CHARACTERISTICS OF IDEAL TRIGGER

• Highly sensitive • Rapid response time • Immune to auto triggering • Proper cycling • Calculation of TV • No added dead space.

Ventilators used in Neonatology – Continuous flow – Time cycled – Pressure limited

Untriggered* CMV (IPPV) and IMV

Triggered*

- A/C (SIPPV, PTV);
- SIMV
- PSV
- PSV+VG

CMV - Untriggered • Ventilatory cycle occurs periodically at fixed intervals

During Continuous Mandatory Ventilation the RR of the ventilator rate is set faster than the spontaneous RR (usually 50-80/min)

IMV –

- Untriggered
- Ventilatory cycle occurs periodically at fixed intervals
- During Intermittent Mandatory Ventilation the RR of the ventilator rate is set lower than the spontaneous RR (usually <30/min)
- In between the 2 control breaths baby can breath spontaneously

SIMV - Ventilator delivers 'mandatory' number of breaths set, Tries to search for inspiratory effort of baby AND match

The RR of the ventilator is fixed to the set rate • Between the ventilator inflations the baby can breath spontaneously on the PEEP level

- The ventilator set RR/min are synchronized with the spontaneous respiration of the baby
- The duration of inspiration (Ti) is fixed and determine by ventilator setting

**ASSIST CONTROL MODE **

Each breath is assisted by the ventilator with a predefined level of pressure

- The duration of Ti is fixed and determined by ventilator setting
- RR can be controlled by patient
- PSV - Patient triggered, pressure limited, flow cycled

What is Non-invasive ventilation?

Delivery of ventilatory support without the use of an invasive artificial airway

What is Noninvasive Ventilation (NIV?)

NIV refers to any method of providing respiratory support, where an endotracheal tube is not used.

MOA of HHHFNC

- Dead space washout
- Reduce inspiratory work of breathing
- Eliminate metabolic work associated with gas conditioning
- Provision of mild distending pressure

Use of HHHFNC

- To prevent extubation failure
- Primary therapy for RDS
- Primary therapy for AOP
- Weaning from cpap
- BPD

HFNC vs CPAP for respiratory support

1. No differences in the rates of death or CLD (4 studies, n= 439)
2. Less nasal trauma/air leak
3. Duration of respiratory support higher in HFNC

HFNC versus NCPAP primary respiratory support;

1. Treatment failure: 25.5% vs 13.3%; $P < 0.001$ (n= 564, GA > 28 w)

Following extubation

- No differences in death, CLD, treatment failure or re-intubation (6 studies, n=934)
- Data is limited for infants born < 26 weeks' GA

When used as a primary mode of respiratory support for RDS, HFNC was found to have higher failure rates compared to Ncpap

In post-extubation settings, HFNC has similar efficacy compared to CPAP,

Bubble CPAP (bCPAP) and ventilator CPAP are the two methods of delivering continuous flow -CPAP

NIPPV

NIPPV is a form of non-invasive ventilation that delivers intermittent positive pressure without using an endotracheal tube.

A Cochrane review from 2017 reported that NIPPV reduces the incidence of extubation failure within 48 hours and up to 7 days after extubation. The number needed to treat with NIPPV to prevent one extubation failure is eight. A new meta-analysis from 2021 showed less risk of developing BPD and a lower extubation failure rate in premature patient's extubated to NIPPV vs CPAP (moderate to low quality evidence

NIPPV INDICATIONS

- Hypoxemic/ hypercarbic respiratory failure
  - Primary mode: Preterms with respiratory distress at delivery
  - Post extubation weaning mode: with shallow respiratory effort
  - Apnoea- self reverting on CPAP
- Cardiac failure

Beneficial physiological effects of NIV in New-borns

Improved respiratory mechanics

- Increased lung volume
- Increased compliance
- Decreased resistance

Improved respiratory timing

- Decreased thoracoabdominal asynchrony
- Decreased obstructive and mixed apnoea

Improved oxygenation

- Decreased pulmonary vascular resistance

•Decreased intrapulmonary shunting

- Increased alveolar volume and less collapse
- Physiologic effects of NIV

EFFECTS OF NIMV/NIV	MECHANISM FOR THESE EFFECTS
Decreased intrapulmonary shunting	Recruits additional alveoli. decreases PVR
Increased compliance, FRC & prevention of atelectasis	Recruits additional alveoli & splints airways
Improved oxygenation	Decreases PVR
• Decreased thoraco-abdominal asynchrony	Splints airways & diaphragm, stabilizes chest wall·
Decreased obstructive & mixed apnea	Regularizes & slows respiratory rate
Conservation of surfactant	• Recruits alveoli, improves pulmonary blood flow & oxygenation
Improved lung growth	Stretches lung tissue

Transition of Support

Stop NIPPV – Rate 15-25 – PIP < 17 – PEEP <6 – FiO2 <35% Transition to CPAP or HHHFNC

- **Intubate** – pH < 7.25 PaCO2 > 60 – Apnea requiring bagging – Frequent As & Bs – Frequent desaturations

What are the causes of increased anion gap acidosis? • Asphyxia • Hypothermia • Severe RDS • Sepsis • Shock • Severe Anemia

Assisted Ventilation

- Defined as movement of gas into and out of the lung by an external source connected directly to the patient
- External Source
  - Resuscitation Bag
  - Continuous Distending Pressure Device
  - Mechanical Ventilator

Indications for MV

1. Respiratory Failure based on ABG
2. Impending Respiratory Failure (Clinical&/ABG)
3. CPAP Failure
4. Prolonged/ Recurrent Apnea

Respiratory Failure Based on ABG

- pH <7.25
- PaO2 < 50mmHg or SpO2<80% with FiO2 of 1.0 (except in neonate with cong cyanotic HD)
- PaCO2 >60mmHg

Impending Respiratory failure

- Clinical Criteria- SAS >7 in PT neonates Downe's >7 in term neonates
- ABG Score of 3 or more

Respiratory Distress Syndrome

- Acute phase • PIP - To achieve TV of 5-6 ml/kg. Usually 15- 20 cm of H2O suffice
- Moderate PEEP – 4-5 cm of H2O • Ti – 0.3-0.4 • Rates- 40-60 /min
- FiO2 – 10% higher than required on hood or CPAP. Adjust according to SpO2
- Target ABG pH:
- 7.25-7.35
- PaO2: 50-70 mm Hg PaCO2: 45-55 mm Hg

X-ray grades of RDS

Grade 1 - fine reticulogranular pattern (Expanded alveoli and terminal airways against a background of atelectasis appear on X-ray as fine reticulogranular pattern), Collapsed alveolar sacs - granular pattern,Air in terminal bronchioles-reticular pattern

Grade 2 - increased air bronchograms (Expanded airways against background of engorged lymphatics, interstitial fluid)

Grade 3 - Complete loss of visualisation of heart borders (Increased opacification as disease progresses as a result of non-expanded alveoli with little or no terminal airway expansion)

Grade 4 - white out lungs S/o severe disease

RDS is seen in Diabetics despite at GA > 34 wks due to

1. Hyperinsulinemia interferes with glucocorticoid induction of surfactant synthesis.
2. Decreased formation of phosphatidylcholine and phosphatidylglycerol
3. Activities of the key enzymes responsible for these phospholipid production is also significantly decreased
4. Inadequate pulmonary glycogen for surfactant synthesis

Ventilator Modes

Set of operating characteristics that control how the ventilator functions" ."The way a ventilator is triggered into inspiration, cycled into exhalation, variables limited during inspiration and whether mandatory or spontaneous or both breaths are allowed.

Harms of asynchrony

- Ineffective ventilation
  - Increased Work of breathing
  - Hypoxia and hypercarbia
- Inadvertent PEEP
  - Air trapping
  - Air leaks (PIE, pneumothorax)
- Interference with CBF
  - IVH

Flow sensors

Measured parametres – flow, pressure and time rest are derived parameters

Flow sensor – Pneumotachometer and Hot-wire anemometers

- Pneumotachometers are between the Y-piece of the ventilator and the endotracheal tube. Has small tubular structure called resistor which measures the pressure difference
- The pressure difference is proportional to flow
- Extremely sensitive even with small flows but may be affected by humidity and secretions

Hot-wire anemometers

- There is a hot wire inside the sensor; any airflow through the sensor will change temperature of hot wire, which affects the electric current through the wire.
- This change in current is detected by microprocessor and it is proportional to the flow.
- Hot-wire anemometers are less sensitive for very small flows and direction of flow.
- Sensors are less prone to gas humidity and condensation in tube

Use of pulmonary graphics

- Helps clinicians to assess a patient's respiratory physiology and Pathophysiology and Helps to adjust the ventilator settings
- Reduce ventilator induced lung injury
- Evaluation of infant's spontaneous effort and Facilitates weaning process
- Therapeutic response to pharmacological agents Detect tube leakage, secretions
- Improve quality of care

Patient triggered ventilation (PTV)

- The patient (neonate) can initiate (trigger) the ventilator breaths
- A sensor detects the inspiratory effort of the neonate and signals the ventilator to initiate the breath

Mean Airway Pressure ($\overline{P}aw$)

$$\overline{P}aw = \frac{(T_I \times PIP) + (T_E \times PEEP)}{Ttot}$$

Types of PTV

1. SIMV (synchronized IMV)
2. A/C – Assist/Control or SIPPV
3. PSV - Pressure support ventilation
4. SIMV + PSV, A/C + PSV

Issues with AC

- Air trapping – compromises expiratory time
- Dangerous hypocarbia – esp. in tachypnoea with normal lungs (shock, CHD, IEM)
- Expiratory asynchrony is still not overcome
- In AC, remember that reducing rates will not help to tackle hypocarbia!

	INSPIRATION ASYNCHRONY	**EXPIRATION ASYNCHRONY**
SIMV	SOME BREATH	ALL BREATH
A/C	NONE	ALL BREATH

PSV

- Flow cycling – baby controls the Ti
- Baby inhales fast, peak flow is reached early, 15% of peak flow reaches early – Ti will be short
- Baby inhales slowly ('sigh' breath), peak flow is reached late, 15% peak flow is late – Ti will be longer

Neonatal HFV:

- Frequencies of 5-15 Hz (1 Hz = 60) = (300-900 breaths per min)
- HFV is use of subnormal TV at supra physiologic rates to provide oxygenation
- Primarily characterized by low TVs < anatomical dead space.

HFOV Mechanisms of Gas Transport

- Direct bulk flow
- Taylor dispersion -The quicker or more energy dense the inspiratory pulse, the sharper the spike & further it extends into airway
- Pendelluft -The back-and-forth currents of gas through lung units with unequal TCs are called Pendelluft. Gas from fast units (short TC) will empty into the slow (long TC) units. Pendelluft: Major mechanism in HFOV
- Movement of gas between adjacent lung units due to differing time constants of alveoli under high frequency & short Ti
- Asymmetric velocity profiles - During inspiration, the high frequency pulse creates a "bullet" shaped profile, with the central molecules moving further down the airway than those molecules found on the periphery of the airway

- Cardiogenic mixing
- Molecular diffusion

Elevating the baseline pressure during HFO, "splints" the airways open while gas is actively withdrawn from alveoli.

During HFOV, inspiration and expiration are both active

The control variables for HFOV are independent adjustment of Paw and pressure amplitude.

Decoupling of oxygenation and ventilation

CO2 ELIMINATION IMPROVES WITH DECREASING VENTILATOR FREQUENCY AS LONG AS I:E IS CONSTANT

Ventilation is proportional to the product of frequency and the square of TV, thus decrease infrequency or increase in TV by means of increase inset amplitude cause increased CO2 REMOVAL.

When the inspiratory-to-expiratory time ratio (I: E) is held constant, a reduction in frequency results in a longer inspiratory time.

Consequently, gas flow occurs over a longer period of time, producing a larger tidal volume at any given pressure amplitude (volume = flow integrated over time)

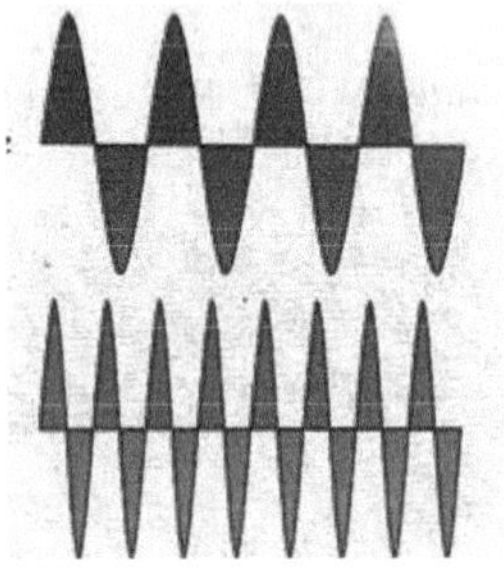

Reasons for HFOV

- To improve gas exchange in severe RF
- To reduce VILI
- Prevention of volutrauma
- Reduced exposure to FiO2
- To decrease pulmonary morbidity
- To allow severe PALs to heal

Using HFV in NICU

- Atelectatic lung disease: RDS
- Restrictive lung disease (Low CL): pneumonia, PIE, CDH, hypoplasia
- Obstructive lung disease: aspiration syndromes
- PALS

Disadvantages of HFOV

- Greater potential for gas trapping & the development of inadvertent PEEP
- Defining optimal mean lung volume is difficult yet crucial
- Lung over-inflation: decreased VR & CO
- Under-inflation: difficult recruitment, lung injury, increased PVR & shunts & hypoxemia

When to initiate?

- Elective vs rescue therapy: although there is marginal improvement in rates of BPD with elective HFOV still it is not recommended as primary mode of support
- Rescue therapy MAP requirement > 12 or OI > 15-20 or Air leaks or Severe MAS or Pneumonia or PPHN or CDH or For delivery of iNO

Major determinants of Lung injury:

1. High TV
2. High End Inspiratory Lung Volume
3. End Expiratory Alveolar Collapse

Basic principles of lung protective ventilation: Optimal lung volume or open lung strategy

- Reducing alveolar over-distension
- Reducing atelectrauma
- Avoiding high oxygen exposure

Lung protective strategies with conventional ventilation:

- Synchronised ventilation
- Volume targeted ventilation
- Open lung ventilation
- Permissive hypercapnia

In conventional ventilation, open lung is achieved by applying optimal PEEP which helps in

- Recruitment of atelectatic units
- Reduces alveolar over-distension
- Minimizes cyclic atelectasis

MECONIUM ASPIRATION SYNDROME

- Respiratory distress and an oxygen requirement in an infant born through MSAF whose symptoms cannot be otherwise explained
- Characteristics of meconium -Sterile, odorless, highly viscous

- Accumulates in the fetal intestine starting around 12 weeks of gestation.
- Formed by a combination of water, lanugo, desquamated cells, vernix, amniotic fluid, pancreatic enzymes, and bile pigment
- Irritant with the potential to cause inflammation and inhibit/displace surfactant.
- Good culture medium, especially for Gram-negative bacilli.
- Meconium has a very high surface tension and is a potent inhibitor of surfactant

PASSAGE OF MECONIUM

- Vagal reflex
- Motilin, produced mainly by the jejunum, stimulates peristalsis, is raised in asphyxiated term babies who pass meconium intrapartum, but is very low in preterm infants and non-asphyxiated term infants
- Post term - rising motilin levels (physiological)
- Preterm and term - vagal response leading to increased peristalsis in fetal gut - usually secondary to head compression or fetal hypoxi

Fresh meconium – green staining of cord

Yellow staining – old meconium

MSAF and outcome:

Fetal hypoxia -> meconium passage [due to increased intestinal peristalsis (motilin receptors), increase vagal tone so relaxation of anal sphincter].

Outcome mainly depends on the timing and quantity of meconium passed.

Timing:

1-early (early light, early heavy) - meconium noted on rupture of membranes before or during active phase of labour. Light or heavy based on the quantity and color.

2- late - after active phase of labour

Interpretation:

1. Early light (constitutes 54% of total MSAF)- no depression in New-born
2. Late - (constitutes 21%)- have APGAR score <7 at 1 & 5 min two to three times more than the control part.
3. Early heavy - (constitutes 25%) - increased likelihood of neonatal depression as well as intrapartum and neonatal death.

MAS severity

- Mild: neonate requires less than 40 % oxygen for less than 48 h
- Moderate: neonate requires more than 40 % oxygen for more than 48 h with no air leak syndromes
- Severe: neonate requires assisted ventilation for more than 48 h. is often associated with PPHN

MECHANISM OF LUNG INJURY in MAS

- Complete or partial obstruction of airways,
- Inflammation, complement activation and cytokine production,
- Inhibition of surfactant synthesis and function,
- Apoptosis of epithelial cells,
- Increased pulmonary vascular resistance

Risk Factors for MSAF

- Advanced gestation
- Small for Gestational Age (SGA)
- Black or South Asian ethnicity
- Vaginal breech delivery
- Intra-uterine infection
- Gestational cholestasis
- Fetal diarrhoea (maternal listeriosis)

X-ray in MAS

- Heterogeneous coarse patchy infiltrates widespread areas of hyper and under-aeration
- Air trapping predominates- hyperinflated chest.
- Pleural effusions
- Increased risk of pneumothorax or pneumomediastinum, (25% of severely affected

Routine endotracheal suction for non-vigorous, meconium-stained babies not suggested

Surfactant in MAS

- Frequently used prior to HFOV and nitric oxide to allow the lung to "open" optimally
- Reduces the duration of mechanical ventilation and duration of hospital stay, need of ECMO
- No reduction in the key outcomes of mortality or air leak

No advantage of routine antibiotic use in the incidence of sepsis or in mortalit

Steroids not recommended.

PPHTN

- Persistence of fetal pulmonary hypertension resulting in severe hypoxia.
- Failure of the normal postnatal fall in pulmonary vascular resistance, which leads to persisting right to left shunts across the fetal channels and resultant hypoxia.
- Crying of infant - opening of lungs - O2 – Fall in pulmonary vascular resistance
- Cutting of the cord – Increase in systemic vascular resistance
- Hypoxemic respiratory failure (HRF) is often associated with PPHN.5
- PPHN and HRF can be primary (no lung disease, also called black-lung PPHN) or secondary to lung disease (such as meconium aspiration syndrome, MAS])
- Cyanosis is secondary to extra-pulmonary right-to-left shunting at the patent foramen ovale (PFO) and patent ductus arteriosus (PDA

SUSPECTING PPHTN

- Hypoxia in neonates disproportionate to chest X-ray
- TR murmur
- ABG suggestive of hypoxemia and normal CO2
- Difference of oxygen saturations between pre and post ductal SaO2 >5%
- Pre and post ductal PaO2 difference >20mmHg
- Cyanosis (differential cyanosis – pink above blue below)
- Single loud S2 (loud with a ringing quality – tambour)
- Systolic murmur at RLSB
- Tricuspid regurgitation
- Prominent precordial impulse
- Labile or fluctuating oxygenation

Cyanotic congenital heart disease is characterized by "fixed" hypoxemia and normal or low PCO2. "Labile" hypoxemia with normal or high PCO2 is seen in PPHN secondary to lung disease

MECHANISM OF PPHTN

Mal-adaptation (Reflex Vasoconstriction)

- Asphyxia, MAS, CDH, Pneumonia, RDS
- Hypoxia, acidosis, hypocalcaemia, Mg
- Hypothermia

(Maldevelopment) Muscularization of Pulmonary Acinar Arteries

- Chronic in-utero hypoxia (IUGR), Post maturity
- Maternal Salicylate or Indomethacin therapy
- Abnormal muscularization of the normally nonmuscular intra-acinar arteries, increases medial thickness of the larger muscular arteries leads to decreased diameter of vascular bed and elevated PVR

Decreased Pulmonary Arterioles (Underdeveloped)

- Hypoplastic lungs, CDH, Alveo-capillary dysplasia

Primary (black lung) PPHN: • Classical definition • Typically presenting soon after birth with hypoxemia • In a baby with clinically and radiologically normal lungs

PATHOPHYSIOLOGY OF PPHTN

- Increased right ventricular afterload initially leads to right ventricular hypertrophy but subsequently causes dilation and poor contractility of the right ventricle (RV).
- Bowing of the interventricular septum and reduced pulmonary venous return lead to reduced left ventricular (LV) preload.
- Diminished systemic perfusion and right-to-left shunts at the patent foramen ovale (PFO) and/or patent ductus arteriosus (PDA) contribute to systemic hypoxemia.
- Systemic hypoxemia and hypoperfusion reduce coronary perfusion pressure and exacerbate myocardial ischemia and ventricular dysfunction

Severe BPD: Incidence of PPHN up-to 50%

Elevated PAP can be the result of three causes

- Elevated Qp: large left-to-right shunt
- Elevated PVR:
- Elevated PCWP

Recent data from lambs with MAS and PPHN suggest that targets in the 93% to 97% range might be associated with lower PVR compared with the 90% to 94% range

Oxygenation Index

Mild <15, Moderate 15 to 25, Severe 25 to 40 and Very Severe > 40

OSI = (FiO2 × Paw / SpO2) × 100

Approximately, OI is 1.8 to 2 times higher than OSI.

ECHO

- Estimation of PAP from tricuspid regurgitation jet

- Transductal shunting
- Morphology of interventricular septum
- TAPSE - TAPSE, 4 mm is associated with increased need for ECMO or death in PPHN.
- Apical view: "eyeballing" reveals Rt vent dilatation with
- Compromised LV, deviation of Interventricular septum to left, TR jet
- Normal TPV/RVET is about 0.2 during early transition and increases to around 0.3 afterward
- Estimating the Effect of Pulmonary Pressure: TPV/RVET
  - Time to peak velocity (TPV) is inversely related to pulmonary pressure
  - TPV is adjusted for the duration of right ventricular ejection time (TPV/RVET)
  - PVR can be estimated by the ratio of pulmonary artery acceleration time (PAAT) to right ventricular ejection time (RVET). The normal value is 0.31 or more, and values under 0.23 are suggestive of elevated PVR

Increased cGMP

- Nitric oxide (arginine, Citrulline)
- PDE 5 inhibitors (Sildenafil)

Increased cAMP

- Prostaglandin (alpostin) and Adenosine
- PDE 3 Inhibitors (Milrinone)

INHALED NITRIC OXIDE

- It reduces the incidence of ECMO/death in PPHN attributed to all etiologies except CDH.
- NO acts by stimulating soluble guanylyl cyclase (sGC) in vascular smooth muscle to produce cyclic guanosine monophosphate (cGMP), which in turn reduces cytosolic concentration of ionic calcium leading to vasodilation.
- The vasodilatory effect of iNO is selective to the pulmonary circulation partly because of its inactivation by combining with hemoglobin to form methemoglobin (MHb) once it diffuses into the circulation. .
- In addition, iNO is microselective to ventilated portions of the alveoli as it only dilated blood vessels adjacent to ventilated alveoli, thereby improving V/Q matching
- initiation of iNO at 20 parts per million (ppm) for HRF with OI of 15 to 20.
- In approximately two thirds of cases, a sustained improvement in oxygenation with an increase in PaO2/FiO2 ratio by 20 mm Hg is seen within 20 minutes or less (the 20-20-20-20 rule.
- Once inspired oxygen is weaned to 60% or less, and PaO2 remains 50 mm Hg or higher or preductal SpO2 consistently is 90% or higher, iNO can be weaned in steps of 5 ppm every 2 to 4 hours (from 20 ppm to 15 ppm, subsequently 10 ppm and 5 ppm)

Indication

- Mechanically ventilated term or near-term infants with HRF with clinical or echocardiographic evidence of PPHN OI >25 (although 15–20 in the presence of echocardiography confirmed PPHN is reasonable and commonly practiced)
- Dose 20 ppm—wean if there is an oxygenation response
- Optimize lung inflation with adequate positive end-expiratory pressure or Paw (high-frequency ventilator) or surfactants in the presence of parenchymal lung disease

Contraindications for iNO

- CDH, left ventricular dysfunction, presence of ductal dependent systemic circulation (e.g., hypoplastic left heart syndrome)

Weaning rate of iNO - 5ppm every 4 hrs till 5ppm - 1ppm every 4hrs

Milrinone

- Treatment of PPHN associated with ventricular dysfunction
- Adjunct to iNO if there is an inadequate oxygenation response to iNO
- Dose IV—50 to 75 mcg/kg load over 1–3 hours
- Carries a risk of systemic hypotension)
- Maintenance—0.33 to 1 mcg/kg/min

Contraindications

- Severe renal dysfunction, shock, or severe hypotension

Sildenafil (IV or Oral) Indication

Treatment of PPHN or BPD associated pulmonary hypertension especially if

- iNO is not available
- Suboptimal response to iNO—especially if associated

with normal blood pressure and good ventricular function

- Difficulties in weaning iNO

Dose IV—0.14 mg/kg/hr for 3 hours followed by 0.07 mg/kg/hr maintenance

Precautions

- Systemic hypotension is common—may need fluid bolus before initiation

Contraindications

- Severe liver dysfunction, Shock or severe hypotension

Prostaglandin E1 Indication

- PPHN with right ventricular failure because of afterload to maintain ductal patency, reduce RV afterload and promote pulmonary vasodilation
- Dose IV—usual dose: 0.01 to 0.05 mcg/kg/min

Definition of PPHTN

Failure of normal postnatal fall in pulmonary vascular resistance, which leads to persisting right to left shunting across the fetal channels resulting in hypoxia.

Suspect PPHTN when following are present

- When hypoxia is disproportionate to the degree of resp distress or radiological sign
- Hypoxemia without hypercapnia
- Labile saturations
- Pre post sats difference of > 5 %
- Pre and post ductal PaO2 difference > 20 mm Hg.

TRIALS

Caffeine Therapy for Apnea of Prematurity Barbara Schmidt N Engl J Med 2006;354:2112-21.

- P- 2006 infants with birth weights of 500 to 1250 g
- I- Received either caffeine or placebo during the first 10 days of life to, until drug therapy for apnea of prematurity was no longer needed.

RESULT

Outcome	Odds ratio (95 % CI)	P value
Death	0.93 (0.63-1.38)	0.73
BPD	0.63 (0.52–0.76)	<0.001
Drug therapy only for closure of patent ductus arteriosus	0.67 (0.55–0.81)	<0.001
Surgical closure of PDA	0.32 (0.22-0.45)	<0.001

- Of 963 infants who were assigned to caffeine 350 (36 percent) received supplemental oxygen, as did 447 of the 954 infants (47 percent) assigned to placebo (adjusted odds ratio, 0.63; 95 percent confidence interval, 0.52 to 0.76; P<0.001)
- Positive airway pressure was discontinued one week earlier in the infants assigned to caffeine (median postmenstrual age, 31.0 weeks; interquartile range, 29.4 to 33.0) than in the infants in the placebo group (median postmenstrual age, 32.0 weeks; interquartile range, 30.3 to 34.0; P<0.001)
- The mean difference in weight gain between the group receiving caffeine and the group receiving placebo was greatest after two weeks (mean difference, –23 g; 95 percent confidence interval, –32 to –13; P<0.001).
- The rates of death, ultrasonographic signs of brain injury, and necrotizing enterocolitis did not differ significantly between the two groups.
- Of the 937 infants assigned to caffeine 377 (40.2%) died or survived with a neurodevelopmental disability, as compared with 431 of the 932 infants (46.2%) assigned to placebo for whom adequate data on the primary outcome were available (odds ratio adjusted for center, 0.77; 95% confidence interval [CI], 0.64 to 0.93; P=0.008). at a corrected age of 18 to 21 months.
- Treatment with caffeine as compared with placebo reduced the incidence of cerebral palsy (4.4% vs. 7.3%; adjusted odds ratio, 0.58; 95% CI, 0.39 to 0.87; P=0.009) and of cognitive delay (33.8% vs. 38.3%; adjusted odds ratio, 0.81; 95% CI, 0.66 to 0.99; P=0.04) at a corrected age of 18 to 21 months.
- The rates of death, deafness, and blindness and the mean percentiles for height, weight, and head circumference at follow-up did not differ significantly between the two groups

Caffeine therapy for apnea of prematurity improves the rate of survival without neurodevelopmental disability at 18 to 21 months in infants with very low birth weight.

Survival without Disability to Age 5 Years after Neonatal Caffeine Therapy for Apnea of Prematurity

- The combined outcome of death or disability was not significantly different for the 833 children assigned to caffeine from that for the 807 children assigned to placebo (21.1% vs 24.8%; odds ratio adjusted for center, 0.82; 95% CI, 0.65-1.03; P=.09).

- The rates of death, motor impairment, behavior problems, poor general health, deafness, and blindness did not differ significantly between the 2 groups.
- The incidence of cognitive impairment was lower at 5 years than at 18 months and similar in the 2 groups (4.9% vs 5.1%; odds ratio adjusted for center, 0.97; 95% CI, 0.61-1.55;P=.89)
- Neonatal caffeine therapy was no longer associated with a significantly improved rate of survival without disability in children with very low birth weights who were assessed at 5 years.

Neurobehavioral Outcomes 11 Years After Neonatal Caffeine Therapy for Apnea of Prematurity

Neurobehavioral outcomes were generally similar for both the caffeine and placebo group. The caffeine group performed better than the placebo group in fine motor coordination (mean difference [MD] = 2.9; 95% confidence interval [CI]: 0.7 to 5.1; P = .01), visuomotor integration (MD = 1.8; 95% CI: 0.0 to 3.7; P < .05), visual perception (MD = 2.0; 95% CI: 0.3 to 3.8; P = .02), and visuospatial organization (MD = 1.2; 95% CI: 0.4 to 2.0; P = .003).

Neonatal caffeine therapy for apnea of prematurity improved visuomotor, visuoperceptual, and visuospatial abilities at age 11 years.

General intelligence, attention, and behavior were not adversely affected by caffeine, which highlights the long-term safety of caffeine therapy for apnea of prematurity in very low birth weight neonates.

Continuous Positive Airway Pressure or Intubation at Birth (COIN) trial

Colin J. Morley NEJM 2008.

P-610 infants who were born at 25-to-28-weeks' gestation

I- CPAP or intubation and ventilation at 5 minutes after birth.

RESULTS

CPAP Group

- Death / BPD- 33.9 % vs 38.9%
- Lower risk of death or need for oxygen therapy- OR- 0.63, 95% CI, 0.46 to 0.88; P = 0.006
- Little difference in overall mortality
- In the CPAP group, 46% of infants were intubated during the first 5 days.
- Surfactant use- half
- Pneumothorax- 9% in the CPAP group, as compared with 3% in the intubation group (P<0.001).
- Fewer days of ventilation.

Conclusion: In infants born at 25-to-28-weeks' gestation, early nasal CPAP did not significantly reduce the rate of death or bronchopulmonary dysplasia, as compared with intubation.

Even though the CPAP group had more incidences of pneumothorax, fewer infants received oxygen at 28 days, and they had fewer days of ventilation.

Early CPAP versus Surfactant in Extremely Preterm Infants SUPPORT

- P- between 24 weeks 0 days and 27 weeks 6 days of gestation.
- I- Infants were randomly assigned to intubation and surfactant treatment (within 1 hour after birth) or to CPAP treatment initiated in the delivery room.
- The primary outcome was death or bronchopulmonary dysplasia as defined by the requirement for supplemental oxygen at 36 weeks

RESULTS

- The rates of the primary outcome did not differ significantly between the CPAP group and the surfactant group (47.8% and 51.0%, respectively; relative risk with CPAP, 0.95; 95% confidence interval [CI], 0.85 to 1.05)
- The results were similar when bronchopulmonary dysplasia was defined according to the need for any supplemental oxygen at 36 weeks (rates of primary outcome, 48.7% and 54.1%, respectively; relative risk with CPAP, 0.91; 95% CI, 0.83 to 1.01).
- Infants who received CPAP treatment, as compared with infants who received surfactant treatment, less frequently required intubation or postnatal corticosteroids for bronchopulmonary dysplasia.

Conclusions: The results of this study support consideration of CPAP as an alternative to intubation and surfactant in preterm infant.

Benefits of Oxygen Saturation Targeting (BOOST) trial

- Oxygen-Saturation Targets and Outcomes in Extremely Preterm Infants Lisa Maree Askie
- P- Double-blind, randomized, controlled trial involving 358 infants born at less than 30 weeks of gestation who remained dependent on supplemental oxygen at 32 weeks of postmenstrual age.
- I- 91 to 94 percent (standard-saturation group) or 95 to 98 percent (high-saturation group); this target was

maintained for the duration of supplemental-oxygen therapy.

- The primary outcomes were growth and neurodevelopmental measures at a corrected age of 12 months.

RESULTS

- There were no significant differences between the groups in weight, length, or head circumference at a corrected age of 12 months.
- The frequency of major developmental abnormalities also did not differ significantly between the standard-saturation group and the high-saturation group (24 percent and 23 percent, respectively, P=0.85)
- The high-saturation group received oxygen for a longer period after randomization (median, 40 days vs. 18 days; P<0.001) and had a significantly higher rate of dependence on supplemental oxygen at 36 weeks of postmenstrual age and a significantly higher frequency of home-based oxygen therapy.

Conclusions: Targeting a higher oxygen-saturation range in extremely preterm infants who were dependent on supplemental oxygen conferred no significant benefit with respect to growth and development and resulted in an increased burden on health services.

Oxygen Saturation and Outcomes in Preterm Infants The BOOST II

- P- infants born before 28 weeks' gestation
- I- effects of targeting an oxygen saturation of 85 to 89%, as compared with a range of 91 to 95%
- O- disability-free survival at 2 years

RESULTS

- 1187 infants whose treatment used the revised oximeter-calibration algorithm, the rate of death was significantly higher in the lower-target group than in the higher-target group (23.1% vs. 15.9%; relative risk in the lower-target group, 1.45; 95% confidence interval [CI], 1.15 to 1.84; P=0.002)
- In all 2448 infants, those in the lower-target group for oxygen saturation had a reduced rate of retinopathy of prematurity (10.6% vs. 13.5%; relative risk, 0.79; 95% CI, 0.63 to 1.00; P=0.045) and an increased rate of necrotizing enterocolitis (10.4% vs. 8.0%; relative risk, 1.31; 95% CI, 1.02 to 1.68; P=0.04)
- Targeting oxygen saturation below 90% with the use of current oximeters in extremely preterm infants was associated with an increased risk of death.

Effects of Targeting Higher vs Lower Arterial Oxygen Saturations on Death or Disability in Extremely Preterm Infants Canadian Oxygen Trial (COT)

- 2 treatment groups with true target saturations of 85% to 89% (n=602) or 91% to 95% (n=599)
- The primary outcome was a composite of death, gross motor disability, cognitive or language delay, severe hearing loss, or bilateral blindness at a corrected age of 18 month

RESULTS

- In lower target range 298 (51.6%) died or survived with disability compared with 283 of the 569 infants (49.7%) assigned to the higher target range (odds ratio adjusted for center, 1.08; 95% CI, 0.85 to 1.37; P=.52).
- The rates of death were 16.6% for those in the 85% to 89% group and 15.3% for those in the 91% to 95% group (adjusted odds ratio, 1.11; 95% CI, 0.80 to 1.54; P=.54).
- Targeting lower saturations reduced the postmenstrual age at last use of oxygen therapy (adjusted mean difference, 0.8 weeks; 95% CI, 1.5 to 0.1; P=.03)

Conclusion: In extremely preterm infants, targeting oxygen saturations of 85% to 89% compared with 91% to 95% had no significant effect on the rate of death or disability at 18 months. These results may help determine the optimal target oxygen saturation.

Association between Oxygen Saturation Targeting and Death or Disability in Extremely Preterm Infants in the Neonatal Oxygenation Prospective Meta-analysis (NeOProM) Collaboration.

- To compare the effects of different target ranges for oxygen saturation as measured by pulse oximetry (SpO2) on death or major morbidity.
- Prospectively planned meta-analysis of individual participant data from 5 randomized clinical trials (conducted from 2005-2014 SUPPORT 1 AND 2, BOOST 1 AND 2, COT) enrolling infants born before 28 weeks' gestation.
- SpO2 target range that was lower (85%-89%) vs higher (91%-95%).
- The primary outcome (death or major morbidity) occurred in 1191 of 2228 infants (53.5%) in the lower SpO2 target group and 1150 of 2229 infants (51.6%) in the higher SpO2 target group (risk difference, 1.7% [95% CI, −1.3% to 4.6%]; relative risk [RR], 1.04 [95% CI, 0.98 to 1.09], P = .21)

- Death occurred in 484 of 2433 infants (19.9%) in the lower SpO2 target group and 418 of 2440 infants (17.1%) in the higher SpO2 target group (risk difference, 2.8% [95% CI, 0.6% to 5.0%]; RR, 1.17 [95% CI, 1.04 to 1.31], P = .01).
- Treatment for retinopathy of prematurity was administered to 220 of 2020 infants (10.9%) in the lower SpO2 target group and 308 of 2065 infants (14.9%) in the higher SpO2 target group (risk difference, "4.0% [95% CI, "6.1% to "2.0%]; RR, 0.74 [95% CI, 0.63 to 0.86], P < .001).
- Severe necrotizing enterocolitis occurred in 227 of 2464 infants (9.2%) in the lower SpO2 target group and 170 of 2465 infants (6.9%) in the higher SpO2 target group (risk difference, 2.3% [95% CI, 0.8% to 3.8%]; RR, 1.33 [95% CI, 1.10 to 1.61], P = .003)

Conclusion: There was no significant difference between a lower SpO2 target range compared with a higher SpO2 target range on the primary composite outcome of death or major disability at a corrected age of 18 to 24 months. The lower SpO2 target range was associated with a higher risk of death and necrotizing enterocolitis, but a lower risk of retinopathy of prematurity treatment.

Randomized Trial Comparing 3 Approaches to the Initial Respiratory Management of Preterm Neonates Vermont Oxford Network DRM Study Group

- To compare 3 approaches to the initial respiratory management of preterm neonates:
  - o prophylactic surfactant followed by a period of mechanical ventilation (prophylactic surfactant [PS])
  - o prophylactic surfactant with rapid extubation to bubble nasal continuous positive airway pressure (intubate-surfactant-extubate [ISX])
  - o Initial management with bubble continuous positive airway pressure and selective surfactant treatment (nCPAP).
- Neonates born at 26 0D 7 to 29 6D 7 weeks' gestation
- Primary outcome was the incidence of death or bronchopulmonary dysplasia (BPD) at 36 weeks' postmenstrual age.
- When compared with the Prophylactic Surfactant group, the relative risk of BPD or death was 0.78 (95% confidence interval: 0.59 –1.03) for the intubate-surfactant-extubate group and 0.83 (95% confidence interval: 0.64 –1.09) for the nCPAP group.
- There were no statistically significant differences in mortality or other complications of prematurity.
- In the nCPAP group, 48% were managed without intubation and ventilation, and 54% without surfactant treatment.
- Preterm neonates were initially managed with either nCPAP or PS with rapid extubation to nCPAP had similar clinical outcomes to those treated with PS followed by a period of mechanical ventilation. An approach that uses early nCPAP leads to a reduction in the number of infants who are intubated and given surfactant.

High-Flow Nasal Cannulae in Very Preterm Infants after Extubation Brett J. Manley, M N Engl J Med 2013; 369: 1425-33.

Infants to receive treatment with either high-flow nasal cannulae (5 to 6 liters per minute) or nasal CPAP (7 cm of water) after extubation.

The primary outcome was treatment failure within 7 days

1. The use of high-flow nasal cannulae was noninferior to the use of nasal CPAP, with treatment failure occurring in 52 of 152 infants (34.2%) in the nasal-cannulae group and in 39 of 151 infants (25.8%) in the CPAP group (risk difference, 8.4 percentage points; 95% confidence interval, –1.9 to 18.7).
2. Almost half the infants in whom treatment with high-flow nasal cannulae failed were successfully treated with CPAP without reintubation.
3. The incidence of nasal trauma was significantly lower in the nasal-cannulae group than in the CPAP group (P=0.01), but there were no significant differences in rates of serious adverse events or other complications

Although the result for the primary outcome was close to the margin of non-inferiority, the efficacy of high-flow nasal cannulae was similar to that of CPAP as respiratory support for very preterm infants after extubation.

Nasal High-Flow Therapy for Primary Respiratory Support in Preterm Infants HIPSTER Trial Investigators

(Gestational age, ≥28 weeks 0 days) with early respiratory distress who had not received surfactant replacement to treatment with either nasal high-flow therapy or nasal CPAP. The primary outcome was treatment failure within 72 hours after randomization

1. Treatment failure occurred in 71 of 278 infants (25.5%) in the high-flow group and in 38 of 286

infants (13.3%) in the CPAP group (risk difference, 12.3 percentage points; 95% confidence interval [CI], 5.8 to 18.7; P<0.001

Conclusion: When used as primary support for preterm infants with respiratory distress, high flow therapy resulted in a significantly higher rate of treatment failure than did CPAP.

Nasal High-Flow Therapy for New-born Infants in Special Care Nurseries e HUNTER Trial Investigators*

(<24 hours of age; gestational age, $\geq$31 weeks) in special care nurseries in Australia. New-born infants with respiratory distress and a birth weight of at least 1200 g were assigned to treatment with either high-flow therapy or CPAP.

The primary outcome was treatment failure within 72 hours after randomization

- Treatment failure occurred in 78 of 381 infants (20.5%) in the high-flow group and in 38 of 373 infants (10.2%) in the CPAP group (risk difference, 10.3 percentage points; 95% confidence interval [CI], 5.2 to 15.4
- Nasal high-flow therapy was not shown to be noninferior to CPAP and resulted in a significantly higher incidence of treatment failure than CPAP when used in nontertiary special care nurseries as early respiratory support for New-born infants with respiratory distress

Early Inhaled Budesonide for the Prevention of Bronchopulmonary Dysplasia e NEUROSIS Trial Group*

(Gestational age, 23 weeks 0 days to 27 weeks 6 days) to early (within 24 hours after birth) inhaled budesonide or placebo until they no longer required oxygen and positive-pressure support or until they reached a postmenstrual age of 32 weeks 0 days.

The primary outcome was death or bronchopulmonary dysplasia, confirmed by means of standardized oxygen-saturation monitoring, at a postmenstrual age of 36 weeks.

- The incidence of bronchopulmonary dysplasia was 27.8% in the budesonide group versus 38.0% in the placebo group (relative risk, stratified according to gestational age, 0.74; 95% CI, 0.60 to 0.91; P=0.004)
- The proportion of infants who required surgical closure of a patent ductus arteriosus was lower in the budesonide group than in the placebo group (relative risk, stratified according to gestational age, 0.55; 95% CI, 0.36 to 0.83; P=0.004)

Conclusion:

Among extremely preterm infants, the incidence of bronchopulmonary dysplasia was lower among those who received early inhaled budesonide than among those who received placebo, but the advantage may have been gained at the expense of increased mortality

Effect of early low-dose hydrocortisone on survival without bronchopulmonary dysplasia in extremely preterm infants (PREMILOC): a double-blind, placebo-controlled, multicentre, randomised trial

Extremely preterm infants inborn (born in a maternity ward at the same site as the NICU) at less than 28 weeks of gestation to receive either intravenous lowdose hydrocortisone or placebo during the first 10 postnatal days.

Infants randomly assigned to the hydrocortisone group received 1 mg/kg of hydrocortisone hemisuccinate per day divided into two doses per day for 7 days, followed by one dose of 0·5 mg/kg per day for 3 day

The primary outcome was survival without bronchopulmonary dysplasia at 36 weeks of postmenstrual age

1. Of the 255 infants assigned to hydrocortisone, 153 (60%) survived without bronchopulmonary dysplasia, compared with 136 (51%) of 266 infants assigned to placebo (odds ratio [OR] adjusted for gestational age group and interim analyses 1·48, 95% CI 1·02–2·16, p=0·04).
2. The number of patients needed to treat to gain one bronchopulmonary dysplasia-free survival was 12 (95% CI 6–200).
3. Sepsis rate was not significantly different in the study population as a whole,
4. But subgroup analyses showed a higher rate only in infants born at 24–25 weeks gestational age who were treated with hydrocortisone (30 [40%] of 83 vs 21 [23%] of 90 infants; sub-hazard ratio 1·87, 95% CI 1·09–3·21, p=0·02).
5. Other potential adverse events, including notably gastrointestinal perforation, did not differ significantly between groups.

Interpretation In extremely preterm infants, the rate of survival without bronchopulmonary dysplasia at 36 weeks of postmenstrual age was significantly increased by prophylactic low-dose hydrocortisone.

Low-dose dexamethasone facilitates extubation among chronically ventilator-dependent infants: a multicenter, international, randomized, controlled trial Doyle 2006

Very preterm (gestational age: <28 weeks) or extremely low birth weight (birth weight: <1000 g)

Ventilator dependent after the first 1 week of life

Dexamethasone (0.89 mg/kg over 10 days) or saline placebo.

Seventy infants were recruited

More infants were extubated successfully by 10 days of treatment in the dexamethasone group (60%, 21 of 35 patients) than in the control group (12%, 4 of 34 patients) (odds ratio [OR]: 11.2; 95% confidence interval [CI]: 3.2-39.0).

Ventilator and oxygen requirements improved substantially, and the duration of intubation was shorter.

- There was little evidence for a reduction in either the mortality rate (dexamethasone group: 11%; control group: 20%; OR: 0.52; 95% CI: 0.14-1.95) or the rate of oxygen dependence at 36 weeks (dexamethasone group: 85%; control group: 91%; OR: 0.58; 95% CI: 0.13-2.66).
- There were no obvious effects of low-dose dexamethasone on blood glucose concentrations, blood pressure, or other complications.
- No infant experienced intestinal perforation.

Conclusions:

Low-dose dexamethasone treatment after the first 1 week of life clearly facilitates extubation and shortens the duration of intubation among ventilator-dependent, very preterm/extremely low birth weight infants, without any obvious short-term complications.

Outcome at 2 Years of Age of Infants From the DART Study: A Multicenter, International, Randomized, Controlled Trial of Low-Dose Dexamethasone Lex W. Doyle, MD

Survivors were assessed at 2 years' corrected age by staff blinded to treatment group allocation to determine neurosensory outcome, growth.

1. There was little evidence for a difference in the major end point, the rate of the combined outcome of death, or major disability at 2 years of age (dexamethasone group: 46%; controls: 43%).
2. Rates of mortality before follow-up (11% vs 20%), major disability (41% vs 31%), cerebral palsy (14% vs 22%), or of the combined outcomes of death or cerebral palsy (23% vs 37%) were not substantially different between the groups.

There were no obvious effects of low-dose dexamethasone on growth or readmissions to hospital after discharge.

Association Between Early Low-Dose Hydrocortisone Therapy in Extremely Preterm Neonates and Neurodevelopmental Outcomes at 2 Years of Age for the PREMILOC Trial Group

After birth, patients were randomly assigned to receive placebo or hydrocortisone (0.5 mg/kg twice per day for 7 days, followed by 0.5 mg/kg per day for 3 days)

The distribution of patients without neurodevelopmental impairment (73% in the hydrocortisone group vs 70% in the placebo group), with mild neurodevelopmental impairment (20% in the hydrocortisone group vs 18% in the placebo group), or with moderate to severe neurodevelopmental impairment (7% in the hydrocortisone group vs 11% in the placebo group) was not statistically significantly different between groups (P = .33).

The mean global developmental quotient score was not statistically significantly different between groups (91.7 in the hydrocortisone group vs 91.4 in the placebo group; between-group difference, 0.3 [95% CI, –2.7 to 3.4]; P = .83).

The incidence of cerebral palsy or other major neurological impairments was not significantly different between groups

Effect of Hydrocortisone Therapy Initiated 7 to 14 Days after Birth on Mortality or Bronchopulmonary Dysplasia Among Very Preterm Infants Receiving Mechanical Ventilation A Randomized Clinical Trial STOP-BPD Study Group

Preterm infants with a gestational age of less than 30 weeks and/or birth weight of less than 1250 g who were ventilator dependent between 7 and 14 days of life

Infants were randomly assigned to receive a 22-day course of systemic hydrocortisone (cumulative dose, 72.5 mg/kg) (n = 182) or placebo (n = 190).

The primary outcome was a composite of death or BPD assessed at 36 weeks' postmenstrual age

- Death or BPD occurred in 128 of 181 infants (70.7%) randomized to hydrocortisone and in 140 of 190 infants (73.7%) randomized to placebo (adjusted risk difference, "3.6% [95% CI, "12.7% to 5.4%]; adjusted odds ratio, 0.87 [95% CI, 0.54-1.38]; P = .54).
- Death at 36 weeks' postmenstrual age (15.5% with hydrocortisone vs 23.7% with placebo; risk difference, "8.2% [95% CI, "16.2% to "0.1%]; odds ratio, 0.59 [95% CI, 0.35-0.995]; P = .048)

Hyperglycaemia requiring insulin therapy was the only adverse effect reported more often in the hydrocortisone group (18.2%) than in the placebo group (7.9%).

CONCLUSIONS AND RELEVANCE

Among mechanically ventilated very preterm infants, administration of hydrocortisone between 7 and 14 days after birth, compared with placebo, did not improve the composite outcome of death or BPD at 36 weeks' postmenstrual age. These findings do not support the use of hydrocortisone for this indication

Effect of Sustained Inflations vs Intermittent Positive Pressure Ventilation on Bronchopulmonary Dysplasia or Death among Extremely Preterm Infants the SAIL Randomized Clinical Trial 2015

Preterm infants 23 to 26 weeks' gestational age requiring resuscitation with inadequate respiratory effort or bradycardia were enrolled.

The experimental intervention was up to 2 sustained inflations at maximal peak pressure of 25 cm H2O for 15 seconds using a T-piece and mask (n = 215); standard resuscitation was intermittent positive pressure ventilation (n = 211)

The primary outcome was the rate of BPD or death at 36 weeks' postmenstrual age

- In the sustained inflation group, 137 infants (63.7%) died or survived with BPD vs 125 infants (59.2%) in the standard resuscitation group (adjusted risk difference [aRD], 4.7% [95% CI, –3.8% to 13.1%]; P = .29).
- Death at less than 48 hours of age occurred in 16 infants (7.4%) in the sustained inflation group vs 3 infants (1.4%) in the standard resuscitation group (aRD, 5.6% [95% CI, 2.1% to 9.1%]; P = .002

CONCLUSIONS

Among extremely preterm infants requiring resuscitation at birth, a ventilation strategy involving 2 sustained inflations, compared with standard intermittent positive pressure ventilation, did not reduce the risk of BPD or death at 36 weeks' postmenstrual age.

These findings do not support the use of ventilation with sustained inflations among extremely preterm infants, although early termination of the trial limits definitive conclusions.

Lung recruitment before surfactant administration in extremely preterm neonates with respiratory distress syndrome (IN-REC-SUR-E Lancet Respir Med 2020)

Preterm infants of 24-27 weeks failing Ncpap during first 24 hrs of life.

Surfactant administered during HFOV with optimal lung volume vs Surfactant administered via INSURE method using conventional ppv

Need for mechanical ventilation

According to the intention-to-treat analysis, the need for mechanical ventilation within the first 72 h of life occurred in 40% in the IN-RECSUR-E group compared to 54% in IN-SUR-E group.

- The absolute risk reduction was 14% (95% CI 1–27) with a number needed to treat of 7·2.

Lower number of infant's req. 2nd dose of surfactant in IN-REC-SUR-E

Lower hospital mortality in IN-REC-SUR-E group (21%) compared to IN-SUR-E (33%) grp, with no significant difference(RR0.64, 95%CI 0.41-1.01;p=0.055)

Early surfactant replacement guided by lung ultrasound in preterm New-borns with RDS: the ULTRASURF randomized controlled trial European journal of paediatrics European journal of paediatrics 2020

Population- Preterm < 32weeks with RDS

Intervention- ultrasound group, administered surfactant based on LUS score and/or FiO2 threshold,

Control- control group, guided by FiO2 only

Outcomes

- Primary- Earlier surfactant therapy (within the first 3hr of life)

Secondary- levels of oxygen exposure in early life, SpO2/FiO2 ratio, need for MV (during the first 3 days of life), duration of invasive and noninvasive mechanical ventilation, ventilator-free days, Length of stay in the NICU and BPD

Surfactant administration occurred earlier in the ultrasound group than in the control group, with statistically significant differences: 1 h of life (IQR 1–2) vs. 6 h (IQR 4– 6.5), with p < 0.001.

Patients in the ultrasound group had better oxygenation after surfactant therapy, with lower FiO2 requirements and a better S/F.

No differences were detected regarding respiratory support (days of non-invasive and invasive mechanical ventilation, ventilator-free days and duration of oxygen therapy) or frequency of BPD.

The frequency of complications after surfactant administration was no different between groups

This study demonstrates that the use of LUS improves the timeliness of surfactant administration without increasing the number of patients requiring surfactant treatment

On an LUS, patients with RDS show an irregular, thickened pleural line, an absence of A lines and coalescent B lines showing white lung.

A Trial Comparing Noninvasive Ventilation Strategies in Preterm Infants NIPPV Study Group* N Engl J Med 2013;369:611-20

Birth weight of less than 1000 g and a gestational age of less than 30 weeks to one of two forms of noninvasive respiratory support — nasal intermittent positive-pressure ventilation (IPPV) or nasal continuous positive airway pressure (CPAP) — at the time of the first use of noninvasive respiratory support during the first 28 days of life.

The primary outcome was death before 36 weeks of postmenstrual age or survival with bronchopulmonary dysplasia

Nasal IPPV, 191 died or survived with bronchopulmonary dysplasia (38.4%), as compared with 180 of 490 infants assigned to nasal CPAP (36.7%) (adjusted odds ratio, 1.09; 95% confidence interval, 0.83 to 1.43; P=0.56).

The frequencies of air leaks and necrotizing enterocolitis, the duration of respiratory support, and the time to full feedings did not differ significantly between treatment groups

CONCLUSIONS

Among extremely-low-birth-weight infants, the rate of survival to 36 weeks of postmenstrual age without bronchopulmonary dysplasia did not differ significantly after noninvasive respiratory support with nasal IPPV as compared with nasal CPAP

Permissive hypercapnia in extremely low birthweight infants (PHELBI) 2015

Between 400 g and 1000 g and gestational age 23–28 weeks plus 6 days,

The high target group aimed at

pCO_2 values of

- 55–65 mm Hg on postnatal days 1–3,
- 60–70 mm Hg on days 4–6,
- 65–75 mm Hg on days 7–14,

Control target at pCO_2

- 40–50 mmHg on days 1–3,
- 45–55 mm Hg on days 4–6,
- 50–60 mm Hg on days 7–14.

The primary outcome was death or moderate to severe bronchopulmonary dysplasia,

The rate of bronchopulmonary dysplasia or death in the high target group (65/179 [36%]) did not differ significantly from the control group (54/180 [30%]; p=0·18).

Mortality was 25 (14%) in the high target group and 19 (11%; p=0·32) in the control group, grade 3–4 intraventricular haemorrhage was 26 (15%) and 21 (12%; p=0·30), and the rate of severe retinopathy recorded was 20 (11%) and 26 (14%; p=0·36)

Interpretation

Targeting a higher pCO_2 did not decrease the rate of bronchopulmonary dysplasia or death in ventilated preterm infants.

The rates of mortality, intraventricular haemorrhage, and retinopathy did not differ between groups.

These results suggest that higher pCO_2 targets than in the slightly hypercapnic control group do not confer increased benefits such as lung protection

NIPPV VS NCPAP for preterm infant after extubation Cochrane review 2017

To compare effects of management with NIPPV versus NCPAP on the need for additional ventilatory support in preterm infants whose endotracheal tube was removed after a period of intermittent positive pressure ventilation?

10 trials enrolling a total of 1431 infants and comparing extubation of infants to NIPPV or NCPAP

Respiratory failure post extubation

Meta analysis showed statistically significant benefit in terms of respiratory failure 48 hours to seven days post extubation for infants extubated to NIPPV: typical risk ratio (RR) 0.70, 95% confidence interval (CI) 0.60 to 0.80; typical risk difference (RD)-0.13, 95% CI 0.17 to -0.08, with eight infants (95% CI 6 to 13) needing to be treated with NIPPV to prevent one extubation failure.

Endotracheal re-intubation

The pooled estimate of rates of endotracheal re-intubation favoured NIPPV (typical RR 0.76, 95% CI 0.65 to 0.88; typical RD -0.10, 95% CI - 0.15 to -0.05; number needed to treat for an additional beneficial outcome (NNTB) 10, 95% CI 7 to 20

No significant reduction in rates of chronic lung disease (typical RR 0.94, 95% CI 0.80 to 1.10; typical RD -0.02, 95% CI -0.08 to 0.03) or death, and no difference in the incidence of necrotizing enterocolitis.

Air leaks were reduced in infants randomised to NIPPV (typical RR 0.48, 95% CI 0.28 to 0.82; typical RD -0.03, 95% CI -0.05 to -0.01; NNTB 33, 95% CI 20 to 100).

Conclusions

- NIPPV reduces the incidence of extubation failure and the need for reintubation within 48 hours to one week more effectively than NCPAP;
- However, it has no effect on chronic lung disease nor on mortality.
- Synchronisation may be important in delivering effective NIPPV.

Effectiveness of Nasal Continuous Positive Airway Pressure vs Nasal Intermittent Positive Pressure Ventilation vs Noninvasive High-Frequency Oscillatory Ventilation as Support After Extubation of Neonates Born Extremely Preterm or With More Severe Respiratory Failure A Secondary Analysis of a Randomized Clinical Trial

OBJECTIVE To clarify whether NHFOV is better than NIPPV and NCPAP in reducing the duration of IMV in extremely preterm neonates or those with severe respiratory failure

1. Born at less than or equal to 28 weeks' (plus 6 days) gestation, (2) invasively ventilated for more than 1 week from birth, and (3) with CO2 greater than 50 mm Hg before or in the 24 hours after extubation
2. The co–primary outcomes were total duration of IMV during the NICU stay, need for reintubation, and ventilator-free days calculated as per the original trial protocol

Both NIPPV and NHFOV were associated with significantly fewer reintubations (risk difference range, –28% [95% CI, –39% to –17%] to –15% [95% CI, –25% to –4%]; number needed to treat, 3-7 infants) and early reintubations (risk difference range, –24% [95% CI, –35% to –14%] to –20% [95% CI, –30% to –10%]) than NCPAP, and these reintubations were less frequently due to refractory hypoxemia

IMV was shorter in the NIPPV and NHFOV groups (mean difference range, –5.0 days ([95% CI, –6.8 to –3.1 days] to –2.3 days [95% CI, –4.1 to –0.4 days]) than in the NCPAP group

Infants in the NHFOV group showed significantly less moderate-to-severe bronchopulmonary dysplasia than infants in the NCPAP group (range, –12% to –10%; number needed to treat, 8-9 infants) and better postextubation gas exchange in all subgroup.

CONCLUSIONS AND RELEVANCE: The subgroup analyses of extremely preterm or more ill infants confirm the results obtained in the whole population: NIPPV and NHFOV appeared equally effective in reducing duration of IMV compared with NCPAP.

Prophylactic surfactant nebulisation for the early aeration of the preterm lung: a randomised clinical trial SUNSET study group 2023 Arch Dis Child Fetal Neonatal Ed

Preterm infants between 26 0/7 and 31 6/7 weeks gestation

Interventions Infants were randomised to receive positive distending pressure alone or positive distending pressure and additional surfactant (200mg/kg; poractant alfa) using a customised vibrating membrane nebuliser.

Surfactant commenced with the first application of a face mask immediately after birth

Primary outcome was the difference in end-expiratory lung impedance from birth to 30 min after birth end-expiratory lung impedance from birth to 30 min correlates well with functional residual capacity

Primary outcome was not different between intervention and control group (median (IQR): 25 (7–62) vs 10 (0–26) AU/kg, p=0.21). End-expiratory lung impedance from birth to 30 min was slightly higher in the intervention group at 6 and 12 hours after birth, particularly in the central areas of the lung. There were no differences in cardiorespiratory and clinical parameter

Conclusions

Prophylactic SN in the DR did not significantly affect end-expiratory lung impedance from birth to 30 min and showed only minimal effects on lung physiology

NASAL HIGH-FLOW THERAPY DURING NEONATAL ENDOTRACHEAL INTUBATION NEJM 2022 SHINE TRIAL

QUESTION: (P) In neonates undergoing endotracheal intubation via the oral route

(I) Does the use of high-flow oxygen

(C) Compared to standard care that is no high flow or supplemental oxygen during the procedure

(O) Increase the number of successful intubation without physiological instability

(T) During the first intubation attempt in the delivery room or on the neonatal intensive care unit?

Intervention:

Neonates in the high-flow group had fitted binasal cannulae

applied on the removal of existing ventilatory support before the application of the laryngoscope.

Oxygen was increased to 100% if saturation dropped to less than 90% during laryngoscopy. High-flow therapy was continued throughout laryngoscopy and discontinued after the completion of intubation.

Primary outcome: Successful first attempt at intubation without physiological instability.

The study defined physiological instability as desaturation or bradycardia during the first intubation attempt.

The authors concluded that the trial showed clinically important improvement in terms of intubation success and the maintenance of physiological stability with high-flow therapy, with greater benefit demonstrated in inexperienced operators who take longer and are more likely to be unsuccessful.

The overall number needed to be treated was 6 for 1 infant to benefit. The intervention was not associated with increased risk.

Detect (ductal echocardiographic targeting and early closure trial)

A randomised placebo-controlled trial of early treatment of the patent ductus arteriosus martin kluckow arch dis child fetal neonatal ed 2014

- Eligible infants born <29 weeks were screened for a large PDA and received indomethacin or placebo before age 12 h

Main outcome death or abnormal cranial ultrasound

- 64 eligible infants were screened before 12 h; of the 92 infants with a large pda, 44 were randomised to indomethacin and 48 to placebo.

There was no difference in the main outcome between groups.

- Infants receiving early indomethacin had significantly less early pulmonary haemorrhage (ph) (2% vs 21%), a trend towards less periventricular/ intraventricular haemorrhage (pivh) (4.5% vs 12.5%) and were less likely to receive later open-label treatment for a pda (20% vs 40%).
- Conclusions early cardiac ultrasound-targeted treatment of a large pda is feasible and safe, resulted in a reduction in early pulmonary haemorrhage and later medical treatment but had no effect on the primary outcome of death or abnormal cranial ultrasound.

PDA TOLERATE trial: an exploratory randomized controlled trial of treatment of moderate-to-large patent ductus arteriosus at 1 week of age ronald i. clyman, j pediatr. 2019

To compare early routine pharmacologic treatment of moderate-to-large patent ductus arteriosus at the end of week 1 with a conservative approach that requires pre specified respiratory and hemodynamic criteria before treatment can be given

- A total of 202 neonates of <28 weeks of gestation age (mean, 25.8 ± 1.1 weeks) with moderate-to-large pda shunts were enrolled between age 6 and 14 days (mean, 8.1 ± 2.2 days) into an exploratory randomized controlled trial

There were no differences between the groups in either our primary outcome of ligation or presence of a pda at discharge (early routine treatment [ert], 32%; conservative treatment [ct], 39%) or

In any of prespecified secondary outcomes of necrotizing enterocolitis (ert, 16%; ct, 19%), bronchopulmonary dysplasia (bpd) (ert, 49%; ct, 53%), bpd/death (ert, 58%; ct, 57%), death (ert,19%; ct, 10%), and weekly need for respiratory support

- Fewer infants in the ERT group met the rescue criteria (ERT, 31%; CT, 62%).
- In secondary exploratory analyses, infants receiving ert had significantly less need for inotropic support (ert, 13%; ct, 25%).
- However, among infants who were ≥26 weeks gestational age, those receiving ert took significantly longer to achieve enteral feeding of 120 ml/kg/day (median: ert, 14 days [range, 4.5-19 days]; ct, 6 days [range, 3-14 days]), and had significantly higher incidences of late-onset non-coagulase-negative staphylococcus bacteremia (ert, 24%; ct,6%) and death (ert, 16%; ct, 2%)

Conclusions—in preterm infants age <28 weeks with moderate-to-large pdas who were receiving respiratory support after the first week, ert did not reduce pda ligations or the presence of a pda at discharge and did not improve any of the prespecified secondary outcomes,

But delayed full feeding and was associated with higher rates of late-onset sepsis and death in infants born at ≥26 weeks of gestation

Early paracetamol (EPAR) trial: a randomized controlled trial of early paracetamol to promote closure

of the ductus arteriosus in preterm infants tim schindler 2021

- Whether early treatment with paracetamol reduces the number of infants requiring intervention for patent ductus arteriosus (pda) and assess the safety profile of paracetamol during the early postnatal period.
- Preterm infants born at 0.9 mm at 6 h of life were randomized to either (1) intravenous paracetamol (15 mg/kg initially and then 7.5 mg/kg every 6 h) or (2) intravenous dextrose for 5 days. the primary outcome was the need for any intervention for pda
- Secondary outcomes included ductal closure at 5 days, ductal size at 48 h, ductal reopening, mortality, and significant morbidities
- Less infants in the intervention group required intervention for pda up to 5 days (6 [21%] vs. 17 [59%] infants [p = 0.003]; relative risk reduction 0.35 [95% ci 0.16–0.77; nnt 2.6]).
- The intervention group had a higher rate of ductal closure (20 [69%] vs. 8 [28%] infants [p = 0.002]) and smaller ductal size (1.0 mm [±0.8] vs. 1.4 mm [±0.9]; p = 0.04)

Conclusion: early paracetamol treatment reduced the number of infants requiring intervention for pda

Comparative study of the efficacy and safety of paracetamol, ibuprofen, and indomethacin in closure of patent ductus arteriosus in preterm neonate's abd el-rahman el-mashad

- Three hundred preterm neonates with hemodynamically significant pda (hs-pda) admitted at our neonatal intensive care unit were enrolled in the study.
- They were randomized into three groups. group i (paracetamol group) received 15 mg/kg/6 h iv paracetamol infusion for 3 days. group ii (ibuprofen group) received 10 mg/kg iv ibuprofen infusion followed by 5 mg/kg/day for 2 days. group iii (indomethacin group) received 0.2 mg/kg/12 h indomethacin iv infusion for three dose
- There was no significant difference between all groups regarding efficacy of pda closure (p = 0.868).
- There was a significant increase in serum creatinine levels and serum blood urea nitrogen (bun) in the ibuprofen and indomethacin groups (p < 0.001).
- There was a significant reduction in platelet count and urine output (uop) in both ibuprofen and indomethacin groups (p < 0.001).
- There was a significant increase in bilirubin levels in only the ibuprofen group (p = 0.003).
- No significant difference of hemoglobin (hb) level or liver enzymes in all groups (p > 0.05). ventilatory settings improved significantly in patients with successful closure of pda than those with failed pda closure (p < 0.001)
- The rate of closure after the first treatment course was 80% in paracetamol therapy, 77% in the ibuprofen group, and 81% in the indomethacin group.
- The cumulative closure rate was increased after the second treatment course to be 88% in paracetamol group, 83% in ibuprofen group, and 87% in indomethacin group with no statistically significant difference between the three groups.
- Number of neonates who underwent ductal ligation was nearly the same in the three group

Expectant management or early ibuprofen for patent ductus arteriosus beneductus trial investigators. expectant management or early ibuprofen for patent ductus arteriosus. NEJM 2022

Inclusion criteria:

- GA < 28 weeks
- PDA confirmed by echocardiogram with a diameter of > 1.5 mm and transductal left-to-right shunt between 24- and 72-hours postnatal age

Intervention:

- Ibuprofen administrated intravenously: 10mg/kg/dose for the first dose followed by 5 mg/kg/dose for the subsequent two doses 24 and 48 hours after first dose. a second dose of ibuprofen could be given if closure has not been achieved (defined as ductus that could not be visualized or had a diameter <0.5 mm).

Outcomes:

Primary outcome: composite of necrotizing enterocolitis, moderate-to-severe bronchopulmonary dysplasia, or death at 36 weeks postmenstrual age.

- The composite primary outcome occurred in 63 of 136 infants (46.3%) in the expectant-management group and 87 of 137 infants (63.5%) in the early-ibuprofen group, with an absolute risk difference of -17.2 percentage p<0.001)
- No differences in necrotizing enterocolitis and death were observed regarding the secondary outcomes. Moderate-to-severe bronchopulmonary dysplasia was

diagnosed in 29 of 117 infants (33.3%) in the expectant-management group and 57 of 112 infants (50.9%) in the early-ibuprofen group.

CONCLUSION - expectant management of pda in preterm infants was non-inferior to early-ibuprofen treatment for a combined primary outcome of: necrotizing enterocolitis (stage bell 2a or higher), moderate to severe broncho-pulmonary dysplasia, or death at 36 weeks pma.

Randomized Trial of Liberal Versus Restrictive Guidelines for Red Blood Cell Transfusion in Preterm Infants Bell et al, Pediatrics 2005 IOWA trial

Study Population (P)

•100 hospitalized preterm infants with birth weights of 500 to 1300 g

Result:

- Infants in the liberal-transfusion group received more RBC transfusions
- Infants in the restrictive transfusion group were more likely to have intraparenchymal brain hemorrhage or periventricular leukomalacia, and they had more frequent episodes of apnea, including both mild and severe episodes

The premature infants in need of transfusion (pint) study: a randomized, controlled trial of a restrictive (low) versus liberal (high) transfusion threshold for extremely low birthweight infants Haresh Kirpalani, 2006

Population

•Infants weighing <1000 g birth weight

•assigned within 48 hours of birth

Intervention

- To a transfusion algorithm of either low or high hemoglobin transfusion thresholds

Outcome

- Composite primary outcome was death before home discharge or survival with any of severe retinopathy, bronchopulmonary dysplasia, or brain injury on cranial ultrasound

Results

- Rates of the primary outcome death before home discharge or survival with any of either severe retinopathy, bronchopulmonary dysplasia, or brain injury on cranial ultrasound were 74.0% in the low threshold group and 69.7% in the high (P = .25; risk difference, 2.7%; 95% CI –3.7% to 9.2%)
- In extremely low birth weight infants, maintaining a higher haemoglobin level results in more infants receiving transfusions but confers little evidence of benefit.

Effects of Liberal vs Restrictive Transfusion Thresholds on Survival and Neurocognitive Outcomes in Extremely Low-Birth-Weight Infants The ETTNO Randomized Clinical Trial Axel R. Franz, M 2020

To compare the effect of liberal vs restrictive red blood cell transfusion strategies on death or disability

- The primary outcome, measured at 24 months of corrected age,
- Was death or disability, defined as any of cognitive deficit, cerebral palsy, or severe visual or hearing impairment
- Secondary outcome measures included individual components of the primary outcome, complications of prematurity, and growth

Results -Among infants in the liberal vs restrictive transfusion thresholds groups, respectively, incidence of any transfusion was 400/492 (81.3%) vs 315/521 (60.5%);

- Median volume transfused was 40 mL (IQR, 16-73 mL) vs 19 mL (IQR, 0-46 mL);
- And weekly mean hematocrit was 3 percentage points higher with liberal thresholds.
- The primary outcome was not significantly different between groups, nor was the secondary outcomes of death, cognitive deficit, or cerebral palsy.
- In the liberal vs restrictive thresholds groups, respectively
- Necrotizing enterocolitis requiring surgical intervention occurred in 20/492 (4.1%) vs 28/518 (5.4%);
- Bronchopulmonary dysplasia occurred in 130/458 (28.4%) vs 126/485 (26.0%);
- Treatment for retinopathy of prematurity was required in 41/472 (8.7%) vs 38/492 (7.7%)

Conclusions and relevance among infants with birth weights of less than 1000 g, a strategy of liberal blood transfusions compared with restrictive transfusions did not reduce the likelihood of death or disability at 24 months of corrected age.

Randomized Trial of Platelet-Transfusion Thresholds in Neonates for the PlaNeT2 MATISSE Collaborators

Population

- Infants born at less than 34 weeks of gestation
- In whom severe thrombocytopenia developed to receive a platelet transfusion

Intervention

- At platelet-count thresholds of 50,000 per cubic millimeter (high-threshold group) or 25,000 per cubic millimeter (low-threshold group)

Outcome and results

- The primary outcome was death or new major bleeding within 28 days after randomization
- A new major bleeding episode or death occurred in 26% of the infants (85 of 324) in the high-threshold group and in 19% (61 of 329) in the low-threshold group (odds ratio, 1.57; 95% confidence interval [CI], 1.06 to 2.32; P=0.02).
- There was no significant difference between the groups with respect to rates of serious adverse events (25% in the high threshold group and 22% in the low-threshold group; odds ratio, 1.14; 95% CI, 0.78 to 1.67

CONCLUSIONS

Among preterm infants with severe thrombocytopenia, those randomly assigned to receive platelet transfusions at a platelet-count threshold of less than 50,000 per cubic millimeter had a significantly higher rate of death or major bleeding within 28 days after randomization than those in the group that received less than 25,000 per cubic millimetre

TOP trial Transfusion Of Prematures tri N Engl J Med 2020;383:2639-51

Population

- Infants with a birth weight of 1000 g or less,
- A gestational age between 22 weeks 0 days and 28 weeks 6 days,
- And a postnatal age of 48 hours or less.

Outcome and results

- The primary outcome was composite of death or severe neuro developmental impairment at 22 to 26 months of postmenstrual age
- Among extremely-low- birth-weight infants, the risk of death or neuro-developmental impairment at 22 to 26 months of age, corrected for prematurity, was not significantly lower with a higher hemoglobin transfusion threshold level than with a lower hemoglobin transfusion threshold level
- No other effects of transfusions on beneficial or adverse outcomes, including stage 2 or 3 necrotizing enterocolitis, BPD ROP or severe IVH

Early EPO in preterm and LBW infants Cochrane Ohlsson and aher

- Early EPO significantly reduced the proportion of infants who received one or more RBC transfusions (typical risk ratio (RR) 0.79 umber needed to treat for an additional beneficial outcome (NNTB) 7
- A high dose of EPO given with a high dose of iron significantly reduced the proportion of infants who received one or more RBC transfusions (typical RR 0.84, 95% CI 0.77 to 0.92; typical RD -0.11, 95% CI -0.16 to -0.05; NNTB 9, 95% CI 6 to 20).
- A high dose of EPO and a low dose of iron significantly reduced the proportion of infants who received one or more RBC transfusions (typical RR 0.71, 95% CI 0.62 to 0.82; typical RD -0.21, 95% CI -0.29 to -0.14; NNTB 5, 95% CI 3 to 7).
- A low dose of EPO combined with a low dose of iron did not significantly reduce the proportion of infants who received one or more RBC transfusions (typical RR 0.80, 95% CI 0.60 to 1.07; typical RD 0.12, 95% CI -0.26 to 0.03)
- The significant weighted mean difference (WMD) was a reduction of 6.8 mL/kg of blood transfused per infant
- Data show no significant difference in the incidence of ROP (all stages or stage not stated by trial authors)
- A total of eight studies enrolling 1283 infants reported on severe ROP (stage 3). Data show no significant differences in ROP (stage 3) between groups
- Analysis of 15 studies reporting on 2639 infants any outcome stated as NEC. EPO significantly reduced the rate of NEC (typical RR 0.69, 95% CI 0.52 to 0.91; typical RD -0.03, 95% CI -0.05 to 0.01)
- EPO did not significantly change the rate of IVH (all grades)

39 Developmental Case

Name, Age (post-natal, corrected age, DOB), Sex,

Residing at

Primary caretaker / Informant: Relationship, History Reliability

Any family history of seizure, developmental delay or MR.

Chief complaints (Presenting complaints):

Examples:

1. Delayed milestones since birth
2. Abnormal tightening of limbs since
3. Paucity or preferential movement of any side
4. Hearing /vision complaints /abnormal deviation of eyes noted
5. Seizures since 6 month of age
6. Feeding difficulty
7. floppiness)
8. Contracture

History of present illness:

Delayed millstones

Developmental age should be mentioned in each domain (gross motor, fine motor, social adaptive, and language)

Best attained milestones in each domain

According to history developmental age of the child corresponds to:

There is no history of regression of attained milestones

2-Seizures since birth:

When was the first seizure noted (NICU or after discharge)

Frequency, what medications were given, controlled or not. Any change in pattern or frequency of seizure noted. Any precipitating factor. Any specific type of seizure noted.

Progression, frequency, associated events (loss of consciousness, bowel and bladder incontinence, Postictal drowsiness Residual weakness, tongue bite, injuries),

Severity (hospitalization, status epilepticus, medication needed for control),

3-Abnormal movements:

If present onset, type (twisting suggestive of dystonia, or tremors) frequency and medication.

Type, onset, duration, progression, aggravating factors (sound, touch), relieving factors (spontaneously, drugs) Relation to sleep

Gross motor	Fine motor	Language	Personal social
Head holding (5)	Opening of fist (3)	Vocalisation (2)	Social smile (2)
Roll over (P-S 6, S-P 7)	Hand regard (3)	Laughs aloud (4)	Recognizing mother (3)
Sitting with support (7)	Midline play (4)	Razzing, Ah-goo (5)	Mirror play (5)
Sitting without sup (9)	Reaching for objects (5)	Monosyllable(7)	Responds to name (7)
Standing with sup (10)	Bidextrous approach (5)	Bisyllable (8)	Reacts to 'No' (8)
Standing without sup (11)	Transfer of objects (6)	One meaningful word (12)	Stranger anxiety (7)
Cruising (11-12)	Unidextrous approach (7)	4-6 meaningful words (15)	Waves bye-bye (10)
Walking (13)	Palmar grasp (6)		Mimicry (15)
	Index finger approach (10)		Indicates wet pants (15)
	Pincer grasp (9)		Names one body (15)
	Scribbling (15)		Dry by day (15)
	Feeds self with spoon(18)		Dry by night (50% 2 yrs, 75% 3 yrs, 90% 5 yrs)

Involuntary movements- If present onset, type (twisting suggestive of dystonia, or tremors) frequency and medication

4-Feeding difficulty:

Noted since when.

What was the feeding pattern of baby at the time of discharge from NICU. What's the current feeding pattern, difficulty more for Solid/ liquid. Is there any abnormal Tongue of jaw movement. Any H/O spitting, Regurgitation, aspiration, poor weight gain.

5-Tone abnormality (stiffness / floppiness): time on notice

Stiffness (tightness, scissoring, difficult to put on clothes/ diaper), more in UL or LL. Any difference on both sides in stiffness.

Floppiness (head lag, slipping from the hand), floppiness of any specific limb.

Upper/ lower limb, Right / left, Proximal / distal

Antenatal History:

Born to gravida 3 mother at 29 weeks of gestation with birthweight of 998 gms.

Booked, Mother age, age at marriage, consanguinity, birth order,

Previous pregnancy details (including abortion, still birth, congenital anomaly, ND),

Chronic illness details (Hypertension, diabetes, thyroid, epilepsy, SLE etc.),

Nutrition disorders (anaemia, malnutrition, etc.), preconception folic acid,

Nature of conception (Natural or ART), MBG, number of antenatal visit

1st Trimester:

LMP, When confirmed, how confirmed (UPT/ Ultrasound scan),

Product of conception (Single/ multiple),

Iron and folic acid, weight gain,

Bleeding per vagina, fever with rash, drug intake or radiation (better to avoid), smoking, and alcohol

2nd Trimester:

Quickening, Iron and calcium taken, Inj TT,

Anomaly scan,

Gestational hypertension (when diagnosed, severity, medication, scan anomaly)

Gestational diabetes (when diagnosed, severity, medication, scan anomaly),

If twins (Chorionicity, discordance, co-twin death, TTTS), weight gain

3rd Trimester:

Liquor (Increased/ decreased),

Foetal moments (increased/ decreased),

Growth (over/ restricted),

Doppler anomaly,

Placental anomaly (placenta previa),

Bleeding or leaking per vagina, preterm labour, PPROM, chorioamnionitis

Perinatal infection including UTI

Natal History:

Labour details: Duration of leaking, duration of stage I& II, Spontaneous/ Induced

Intrapartum monitoring details, Place of delivery, Meconium stained liquor

Mode of delivery (Vaginally, instrumentation, LSCS ±elective/emergency)

Sentinel events (Foetal distress, cord prolapse or rupture, abruptio placenta),

Maturity (Term/preterm),

Duration of leaking PV, Lie of the fetus,

Resuscitation details: APGAR, first cry, intubation, chest compression, epinephrine, delayed cord clamping, cord gas, placenta.

Transfer to NICU details: inborn/outborn, shifted to NICU immediately after birth of after few days. Mode of transport, Reason of NICU admission (prematurity, poor activity, breathing difficulty, cyanosis, feeding difficulty, reduced urine output, jaundice, Hypoglycaemia, seizure)

Postnatal history (NICU Couse):

When did the mother first see the baby? How many days baby was admitted in NICU.

When given to mother whether she noticed any paucity of movements, tone abnormality.

What was the Sensorium, tone, any seizures?

Treatment details - drugs, therapeutic hypothermia, IVH, shunt) any LP done. Any low blood sugar value or bilirubin level which mother remember.

Associated problems which impact neurodevelopment (Duration of ventilation/ Pneumothorax Hypotension Meningitis Jaundice, phototherapy Hypoglycemia, Traumatic delivery / bleeding Dysmorphism / anomalies/ neurometabolic tests), timing of initiation of oral feeding and breast feeding.

Discharge details- what was the sensorium, sleep, and cry, activity at the time of discharge.

Seizures at the time of discharge controlled/ Drugs/ Any investigation- MRI, EEG

Feeding at discharge - mode of feeding, problems during feeding, Weight at discharge

Timing of initiation of oral feeding and breast-feeding

History continued:

HMF:- **H/O cortical function:**

Interacts with mother/ surroundings, Quality of sleep, cry, consolability.

H/O cranial nerve involvement

CN 2- eye to eye contact, hand regard, fixation and tracking

CN 3, 4, 6- any abnormal deviation of eyes

CN 5- difficulty in sucking/ chewing food

CN 7- any deviation of angle of mouth, wide palpebral fissure, absence of nasolabial fold

CN 8- Response to sound; and startle

CN 9, 10- pooling of saliva, choking, regurgitation, drooling of saliva

CN 12- Any abnormal movements of tongue

H/O sensory dysfunction

Responds to pain

H/O bowel and bladder involvement

H/O Complications

Mental retardation; Features of autism (eye contact, stereotypy)

Visual impairment (strabismus, nystagmus, optic atrophy, refractive error)-

Hearing problems

Speech (articulation disorders)

Poor weight gain, head size,

Contractures, scoliosis, hip subluxation, equinus deformity

Treatment history:

Drugs, physiotherapy, occupational therapy, speech therapy-when started and any improvement noted.

Investigation: MRI, EEG, BERA, VEP etc.

Feeding/ nutrition history:

Calculate calorie and protein intake based on recall feeding history of last 1 day, when child was not sick. Calculate actual need and deficit as per his age.

Type of feed, mode of feed- since birth

Problems faced during feed -long time for feeding, regurgitation, constipation, spitting.

What age weaning was started

Weight gain or recent weight loss.

Immunization History:

Immunized up to the age, when was the first and last shot was taken, no adverse events or complication during immunization

Birth (BCG, OPV-0, Hep B), 6 weeks (Pentavalent-1, OPV-1, fIPV-1, Rota VV-1, PCV-1*), 10 weeks (Pentavalent-2, OPV-2, Rota VV-2), 14 weeks (Pentavalent-3, OPV-3, fIPV-2, Rota vac-3, PCV-2*), 9-12 month (Measles or MR-1, PCV booster, JE-1**), 16-24 month (MR-2, JE-2**, DPT booster, OPV-booster)

Family History:

Consanguineous/ Non-consanguineous marriage

H/O developmental delay in other family members

Age and health details of parents, siblings, other family members;

history of previous abortion, still birth, death due to unknown course; inherited disease in the family, long standing illness in parents; history of developmental delay in family

Socio economic status & environmental history:

Mention socioeconomic status based on Kuppuswamy classification.

Total members, house, are they getting enough social support. Are they getting enough social support? Kuppuswamy classification

Occupation of the head of the family (A):

Legislators, Senior Officials & Managers (10),
Professionals (9),
Technicians and Associate Professionals (8),
Clerks (7),
Skilled Workers and Shop & Market Sales Workers (6),
Skilled Agricultural & Fishery Workers (5),

Craft & Related Trade Workers (4),
Plant & Machine Operators and Assemblers (3),
Elementary Occupation (2),
Unemployed (1)

Education of the head of the family (B):

Profession or Honours (7),
Graduate (6),
Intermediate or diploma (5),
High school certificate (4),
Middle school certificate (3),
Primary school certificate (2),
Illiterate (1)

Total monthly income of the family (c):

≥199,862 (12),
99,931–199,861 (10),
74,755 –99,930 (6),
49,962–74,755 4),
29,973– 49,961 (3),
10,002–29,972 (2),
≤ 10,001 (1)

Total score (A+B+C):

26–29 (Upper	I),
16–25 (Upper middle	II),
11–15 (Lower Middle	III),
5–10 (Upper lower	IV),
<5 (Lower	V)

Summary:

Baby XYZ, corrected age, sex, born to cons/ non-cons with significant antenatal history in the form of ....

With delayed milestones (predominantly or global), with developmental age of ...,

With static or progressive encephalopathy,

With spasticity involving (UL or LL or both),

With cranial nerve (Involvement),

With seizure disorder ± controlled with or without drugs,

Comorbidities of feeding difficulty/ sleep disturbance/ emotional disturbance / constipation / bony abnormalities / microcephaly /FTT /contracture/

On treatment (drugs, physiotherapy, speech therapy)

Anatomical-(cortical, White matter, basal ganglia, thalamus, brainstem)

Pathological-(Hypoxic-ischemia, vascular, haemorrhagic, structural)

Etiology- (Perinatal asphyxia, IU infection, IEM, Chromosomal abnormality, Kernicterus, Meningitis, Hypoglycemia, IVH)

EXAMINATION

GENERAL EXAMINATION:

Opening statement (General comment):

The child is sitting/lying -Awake or sleeper, Alertness, Orientation (Interaction with mother), Ill looking, emaciated, Wasting, any specific Posture or gait if you can see him walking.

Vitals:

Temperature: at axilla

Pulse: rate, rhythm, volume, character, radio femoral delay, all peripheral pulse.

Respiration: rate, rhythm

Blood pressure:

SpO2:

Pallor, icterus, cyanosis, clubbing, oedema, lymphadenopathy

Head to foot examination:

Head: Size and shape, AF size, Sutural separation/overriding, receding forehead, Low hairline

Face: Dysmorphic faces, eye, nose, ear, signs of vitamin A and B deficiency

Oral cavity: Drooling of saliva, Oral hygiene, Dental caries, dentition (delayed or appropriate), signs of vitamin B and C deficiency.

Neck: Short, webbing

Chest: Pectus carinatum or excavatum, Harrison grove, rachitic rosary

Abdomen: size, shape, Umbilical hernia

Limbs: Deformity, contracture

Skin: Neurocutaneous markers, signs of vitamin deficiency, ulcer, pigmentation, bed sore

Genitalia & Perineum: Ambiguity, hygiene, inguinal area;

Anthropometry:

Weight: Kg, Length: in cm, Head circumference (OFC): in cm, Chest circumference: in cm, Mid arm circumference: in cm

Expected/ current/ growth chart - classify what stage of malnutrition

WHO classification:

Weight for height: Wasting (b/w -2 to -3), Severe wasting (> -3)

Height for age: Stunting (b/w -2 to -3), Severe stunting (> -3)

Developmental Assessment:

Formal assessment only needed

SYSTEMIC EXAMAINATION:

Nervous System Examination:

Higher mental functions:

Interacting with mother, surroundings and examiner, Indicates basic needs

Alertness level: Normal, stupors, coma (appearance, arousal response, quantity, quality),

Behavioural state: (Deep sleep, Light sleep, drowsy, light awake, active awake, and cry)

Cry: Quality, Character

Consolable: (1. spontaneously, 2. by talking, 3. Putting a hand on abdomen, 4. by being picked up & held, 5. May not get consoled)

Habituation: Normal or abnormal

Cranial nerve examination:

1st (olfactory): Difficult to test

Difficult to test, so could not do it. Bring some items (coffee, asafoetida ....) with you, if you get an older child

2nd (optic): Pupillary response direct and consensual both; visual fixation and tracking; blink, dazzle and menace reflex; fundus examination.

Appearance and reaction: tell about the size of the pupil and reaction to light

Normal size of pupil is 3-4 mm and normal reaction to light

For tracking response use fluffy ball of red yarn

By 34 weeks nearly 90% of infants will track.

By term visual fixation and tracking are well developed.

Keep the red wool at 25cm from the eye

Blink comes at 26 weeks: consistently blinks to light

Dazzle (of pieper) comes at 32 weeks: keeps eyes closed as long as light is present

Menace comes at 2-3 months Color vision by 2 months; Binocular vision by 3 months

3rd, 4th, 6th (Oculomotor, trochlear, abducent): position, extra ocular movement, abnormal movements.

Assess the squint:

Paralytic and non-paralytic squint

Paralytic squint: complain of diplopia if bigger child, always manifest, no movement in dolls eye

Non paralytic squint: due to abnormal or little innervations of muscles

May be manifest or latent

Do cover uncover test

5th (Trigeminal): Sensory (Rooting, sucking), motor (Jaw jerk)

Check the sucking of the neonate; Jaw jerk, tightening of masseter muscle

7th *(facial):* Nasolabial fold, palpebral fissure, angle of mouth, glabellar tap

8th (Auditory): Response to sound (1 month-startle, 2 month-cease of activity, 3 month- head turn) , ring bell test

Startle response: Loud noise

Ring a bell at a distance of 45 cm (18 inches) and not in sight of the baby

9th, 10th: Swallowing, gag reflex, pooing of secretion

Gag reflex and movement of the palate, pooling of the secretions

Pseudobulbar palsy: (it a supranuclear type of lesion)

Gag reflex will be present but pooling of secretions will also be present

11th: Hanging of the head of baby by bringing in sitting position

12th: Symmetry of tongue, fasciculation

Mention the size of the tongue and fasciculation if any.

Good sucking response: intact 5th, 7th and 12th nerve is required.

Motor system:

Describe the posture of the upper limbs and lower limbs

Bulk: palpate and inspect

Tone: Make sure the head of the infant is held in midline before assessing tone or eliciting any reflex.

Posture, flappability, passive tones (Amiel Tison angle-Scarf sign, adductor angle, popliteal angle, dorsiflexion angle), active tone (Flip 180)-assess neck flexor and extensors, ventral suspension, *righting,*

1. Posture
2. Flappability- increased or decreased
3. **Passive tone** (Passive tone is extensibility of muscles when the child is not moving and at rest)

(See Table Below)

Active tone (Active tone refers to active movements of the infant in reaction to certain situations imposed by the examiner)

Neck flexors and extensors

Ventral suspension

Righting

Tone assessment in older children

Examine the axial tone by pull to sit maneuver for neck flexors and extensors, dorsal or ventral incurvation.

Appendicular tone in flexor and extensor group of muscles in UL and LL

At the end of the tone assessment, mention whether spasticity or rigidity is predominant.

Spasticity is more in UL or LL or asymmetric

Power: Testing individual actions at various joints (Shoulder, elbow, wrist, hip, knee and ankle)

Mobility: Movements Paucity of movements, Cramped synchronized movements- all muscle groups come into play instead of specific muscles, or Poor repertoire of movements

Involuntary movements:

Reflex: Biceps, triceps, supinator, knee jerk, ankle reflex

Deep tendon reflexes

Biceps reflex (C5, C6)

Supinator reflex (C6, C7)

Triceps reflex (C7, C8)

Knee reflex (L2, 3, 4)

Ankle reflex (S1, S2)

Look for clonus in a child with spasticity. Sustained clonus is abnormal (When the clonus persists until the withdrawal of manoeuvre) .

Primitive reflex: Rooting, sucking, Moro reflex, ATNR, Palmar grasp, crossed extension, Galant reflex

Postural reflex: Parachute, righting

Cerebellum, meninges, Skull and spine:

Coordination

Other System:

Respiratory System: RR, AEBE, No added sounds

CVS: PR, BP, S1 and S2 normal, No murmur

GIT: Soft, bowel sound heard normal

Diagnosis:

1 year old male child with global developmental delay with asymmetric spastic quadriparesis or diplegic cerebral palsy

Probably due to bilateral cortical and deep nuclear involvement due to perinatal asphyxia with seizures (type……)

With vision and hearing impairment and microcephaly, behavioral problems with feeding difficulties and contractures.

AXIAL tone		**APPENDICULAR tone**	
ACTIVE	**PASSIVE**	**ACTIVE**	**PASSIVE**
Neck flexors	Lateral rotation of head	Palmar grasp	Scarf sign
Neck extensors	Ventral suspension	Pull to sit	Arm recoil
	Perez reflex	Axillary suspension	Square window
	Volmer's reflex	Plantar grasp	Adductor angle
	Gallant's reflex	Magnet reflex	Popliteal angle
		Crossed extensor reflex	Heel to ear
			Dorsiflexion of foot

Bladder and bowel incontinence and

Currently on drugs for seizures and contractures

With PEM grade 2/anemia/ Vitamin D deficiency

Relevant theory for a developmental case

Myelination progresses from:

1. Central to peripheral
2. caudal to rostral
3. dorsal to ventral
4. Sensory then motor

Myelinated area at term birth: brainstem, cerebellum, posterior limb of the internal capsule, optic tract, perirolandic region

Wernicke's aphasia – fluent aphasia with impaired comprehension and repetition

Broca's aphasia – non fluent aphasia with impaired repetition and intact comprehension

Toilet training – dry by day in 18 months

Dry by night 50 % by 2 yrs of age /75 % by 3 yrs / 90 % by 5 yrs

Developmental quotient = developmental age/chronological age × 100

DQ	Interpretation
>=85	Normal
71-84	Mild to moderate delay
<=70	Severe delay

Developmental dissociation –refers to discrepancy between the developmental rates of two streams of development with one stream significantly more developed

Developmental deviance –refers to nonsequential unevenness in the achievement of milestones within one or more streams of development

Global developmental delay – significant delay in 2 or more developmental domains.

Significant delay – 2 SD more than mean age appropriate

Age in years	Calorie requirement	Protein requirement
1	1000	10-13 gm
2	1100	18 gm
3	1200	20 gm
4	1300	20 gm
5	1400	25 gm

Protein 0-6 month 2-2.5 gm/kg/day

6-12 month -1.5 gm/kg/day

Other method - Upto 10 kg -100 cal/kg - 10-20 kg – 50 cal/kg

Nutritive value of common food items

Food item	Quantity	Calorie	Protein
Poori	1	65	1
Chapatti	1	70	2
Bread	1 slice	70	1
Biscuit	1	20	0.5
Milk	100 ml	60	3
Sugar	1 teaspoon	20	
Banana	1	80	1
Boiled egg	1	80	6
Cooked rice	1 cup	175	4
Daal	1 cup	30	1.5

Calculation of weight

3 month to 1 year –(age in months + 9) / 2

1 – 6 year - age in years × 2 + 8

Birth Weight double by 5 month/ triple by 12 month/ quadruple by – 30 month/ 5 times by 3 year/ 6 times by 5 years

IAP classification based on W/A

W/A	Grade
>80 %	Normal
71-80 %	Grade 1 malnutrition
61-70 %	Grade 2 malnutrition
51-60 %	Grade 3 malnutrition
<50 %	Grade 4 malnutrition

Height for age classification by waterlow

H/A	Grade
>95 %	Normal
90-95 %	1st degree stunting
85-89 %	2nd degree stunting
<85 %	3rd degree stunting

Water low classification of weight for height

W/H	Interpretation
>90 %	Normal
80-90 %	Grade 1 wasting
70-80 %	Grade 2 wasting
<70 %	Grade 3 wasting

Stunting – H/A 2 SD below the mean

Wasting – W/H 2 SD below the mean .

W/A ;80 % of standard correspond to < 3 rd centile and <-2 SD

W/H : 80 % of standard corresponds to < 3 rd centile and <-2 SD

H/A : 90 % of standard corresponds to < 3 rd centile and <-2 SD

MUAC (between 1- 5 yrs)

15- 17 cm	Normal
<12.5 cm	Severe malnutrition
12.5 – 13.5 cm	Moderate malnutrition

Shakir tape

- Green 13.5 – 16 cm
- Yellow 12.5 – 13.5 cm
- Red < 12.5 cm

Rate of increase of head circumference – microcephaly -> 3 SD below mean

0-3 month	2 cm/month
3-6 month	1 cm/month
6-12 month	0.5 cm/month

Dentition (primary teeth rule – rule of four and lower before upper)

Secondary dentition – rule of three and lower before upper

Central incisors – 7 month

Lateral incisor – 11 month

First molar – 15 month

Canine – 19 month

Second molar – 23 month.

Acute brief total asphyxia damages

- Brainstem
- Thalamus
- Basal ganglia
- Spares cortex

Areas involved in Kernicterus	**Areas involved in HIE**
Globus Pallidus	Cerebral Cortex and PVWM
Sector CA 2, 3 of Hippocampus	Caudate and Putamen
Subthalamic Nuclei	Sector CA 1 of Hippocampus
Reticulata Layer of Substantia Nigra	Anterior an Dlaternal Nuclei of Thalamus
Cochlear and Dentate Nuclei	Compacta Layer of Substantia Nigra

Spasticity	**Rigidity**
Velocity dependent	Not velocity dependent
Tone in antigravity muscle is more	Equally affected
Clasp knife phenomenon	Cogwheel/lead pipe
Pyramidal disease	Extra pyramidal disease
Exaggerated reflexes	Normal reflexes

DTR grading

0. Absent
1. Diminished
2. Normal
3. Exaggerated
4. Clonus

Root values

- Biceps –C5 C6
- Triceps C7 C8
- Supinator –C5 C6
- Knee –L234
- Ankle S1 2
- Anal S 4 5

Extensor plantar response

- Dorsiflexion of great toe
- Fanning out and extension of great toe
- Dorsiflexion of ankle
- Flexion of hip and knee

Other methods of eliciting plantar response

- Gordon – squeeze the calf muscle
- Oppenheim – firm stroke on either side of anterior end of tibia
- Chaddock –light stroke below the lateral malleolus on the outer side of foot.

UMN VS LMN LESIONS

Intellect	Deficit may be found if cortical involvement present	Normal
Cranial nerve	Abnormalities usually involve brainstem dysfunction	May be involved, but may indicate a neuropathy
Power	Slightly decreased but most severely affected because of impaired tone	Markedly reduced
Tone	Spasticity in pyramidal lesions/rigidity in extrapyramidal lesions	Reduced/floppy
Coordination	Impaired when cerebellum is involved	May be hindered by weakness
Reflexes	Exaggerated	Difficult to elicit
Sensation	Usually intact	Impaired with lesions that affect the nerve
Fasciculations	None	Present with ant horn cell disease

Neurological examination In young infant- 360 degree assessment

•Ventral suspension – look for head position compared to spine

•Axillary suspension – look for scissoring

•Pull to sit

•Held in sitting position

•Held in standing position

Features	**Bulbar palsy**	**Pseudobulbar palsy**
Site	LMN of CN 9, 10 and 12 nerve or nuclei involved	Corticobulbar fibres – UMN lesions of 9, 10 and 12.
Causes	GBS, polio, tumors	Cerebral palsy
Gag reflex	Absent	Exaggerated
Jaw jerk	absent	Exaggerated
Speech	Hypernasal	Monotonous, slurred, high pitched
Tongue	Fasciculations	Spastic

Non paralytic squint	**Paralytic squint**
Concomitant squint	Incomitant squint
Eye movement are full and equal in both eyes, but only one eye is directed towards the object being viewed	Affected eye has restricted/limited range of movement due to underaction of one or more extra ocular muscle
Angle of deviation between the two eyes is constant regardless of the direction of gaze.	Dependent of direction of gaze and increase in the direction of action of affected muscle
Cerebral palsy is etiology	Cranial N palsy

Waveforms of BERA remembered as pneumonic: "ECOLI" MA

1. Wave I: Eighth nerve
2. Wave II: Cochlear nucleus
3. Wave III : Superior Olivary nucleus
4. Wave IV: Lateral lemniscus
5. Wave V Inferior colliculus
6. Wave VI: Medial Geniculate Body
7. Wave VII: Auditory cortex

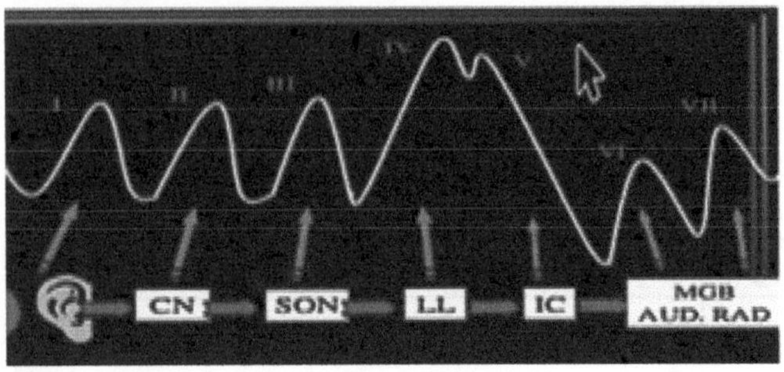

BERA

Small amplitude, delayed or absent:

- Wave I: cochlear lesion
- Wave V: upper brain stem lesion

Prolongation of interpeak latencies:

- I-III Lower brainstem lesion
- III-V Upper brainstem lesion
- I-V Whole brainstem lesion

Role of MRI in HIE

Conventional MRI - Detects changes in 3-4 days

• DWI in 24-48 hours

MAJOR ASPECTS OF MRI IN DIAGNOSIS OF HIE

1. Cerebral cortical gray-white differentiation lost (T1W or TW2)
2. Cerebral cortical high signal in parasagittal Perirolandic cortex (T1W and FLAIR)
3. Basal ganglia/thalamus high signal (TIW and FLAIR)
4. Parasagittal cerebral cortex, subcortical white matter, high signal (TIW and FLAIR)
5. Posterior limb of internal capsule decreased signal (TIW) or increased signal (T2W)
6. DWI- Increased signal

Definitions of perinatal asphyxia

World Health Organization - Failure to initiate and sustain breathing

NNPD Network-

- Moderate PA: Slow/gasping breathing or an Apgar score of 4 to 6 at 1 minute
- Severe PA: No breathing or an Apgar score of 0-3 at1 minute of age

American Academy of Pediatrics and American College of Obstetrics and Gynecology"

Presence of all of following criteria:

- Profound metabolic or mixed academia (pH< 7.0) in umbilical cord blood
- Persistence of low Apgar scores less than 3 for more than 5 minutes
- Signs of neonatal neurologic dysfunction (e.g., seizures, encephalopathy, tone abnormalities)
- Evidence of multiple organ involvement (such as that of kidneys, lungs, liver, heart and intestine).

Cerebral palsy

First described in 1862 by William John Little an orthopedic surgeon • Cerebral Palsy was known as Little's Disease for decades

Cerebral palsy (CP) is a group of permanent disorders of movement and posture causing activity limitation that are attributed to nonprogressive disturbances in the developing fetal or infant brain. • The motor disorders are often accompanied by disturbances of sensation, perception, cognition, communication, and behavior as well as by epilepsy and secondary musculoskeletal problems.

Persistent but not necessarily unchanging disorder disorder of movement and posture due to non progressive disorder of immature brain.

It is caused by a non progressive damage to the brain before during or shortly after birth

Developmental, genetic, metabolic, ischemic, infectious, and other acquired etiologies

Only 10 % CP cases can be attributed to neonatal asphyxia.

80% of cases, antenatal factors could be identified and < 10% had evidence of intrapartum asphyxia.

Intrauterine exposure to maternal infection lead to a significant increase in the risk of CP.

Soft Sign of CP in Neonates

1. Abnormal behaviour- Excessive cry, poor sleep, excessive irritability, feeding problems, poor sucking, poor swallowing
2. Difficulty in handling- Difficulty in handling (excessive stiffness), difficult to wear diapers difficult to dress or undress;
3. Abnormal stiffness or abnormal twisting of limbs & trunk
4. Tone changes -Hypotonia; Spasticity; Dystonia;
5. Unusual fidgety movements; Jerky or abrupt or slow twisting
6. Asymmetry of movements OR Paucity of movements;

Clinical classification based upon on tone

- Spastic – cortex
- Dyskinetic – basal ganglia (extrapyramidal system)
- Hypotonic/ataxic – cerebellum
- Mixed – diffuse

Anatomical classification

- Hemiplegia – upper and lower extremity on one side of body
- Diplegia – four extremities, legs more affected than the arms
- Quadriplegia – four extremities plus the trunk, neck and bulbar muscle involvement
- Double hemiplegia – four extremities, arms more affected than the legs
- Triplegia – both lower extremity and one lower extremity

Spastic diplegia

- Bilateral spasticity of the legs > arms.
- Damage to the immature white matter immature oligodendroglia between 20-34 wk of gestation
- (commando crawl)
- Excessive adduction of the hips. Scissoring posture on suspension by shoulders.
- Paraspinal muscle involvement, the child may be unable to sit.
- Walking is significantly delayed, child walks on tiptoe.
- Disuse atrophy and impaired growth of the lower extremities.
- Prognosis for normal intellectual development is good
- Likelihood of seizures is minimal.
- Often have learning disabilities & vision problems.

Spastic quadriplegia

- Severest, marked motor impairment of all extremities
- Intellectual disability and seizures.
- Swallowing difficulties due to supranuclear bulbar palsies.
- Increased tone and spasticity in all extremities decreased spontaneous movements, brisk reflexes, and plantar extensor responses.
- Flexion contractures of the knees and elbows by late childhood.
- Speech and visual abnormalities

Spastic hemiplegia

- Decreased spontaneous movements on the affected side
- Hand preference at a very early age.
- The arm is often more involved than the leg.
- Walking delayed until 18-24 months,
- Seizure disorder (1/3rd).
- Cognitive abnormalities including mental retardation (25%)

Athetoid CP

- Choreoathetoid, extrapyramidal, or dyskinetic CP
- Characteristically hypotonic with poor head control and marked head lag.
- Increased tone with rigidity and dystonia over several years.
- The upper extremities are generally more affected.
- Feeding difficulties prominent.
- Speech is delayed because the oropharyngeal muscles are involved.
- Intellect is preserved

Problems Associated with CP

Problem Frequency (%) Remarks

1. Mental retardation 50-75 - Most often in spastic quadriplegia and ataxic CP
2. Seizure 25-33 - Most often in spastic hemiplegia and spastic quadriplegia; least in dyskinetic CP

3. Hearing and speech problems 15-20 - Most common in dyskinetic CP and spastic quadriplegia
4. Ocular 50-70 - Refractory errors, strabismus
5. Behaviour problems 30-50 - Stubbornness, aggressiveness, lack of attention and hyper kinetic behaviour

Risk Factors for hearing loss in NICU graduates

- Family H/O of hearing loss
- Admission in NICU-5days with ventilation
- Jaundice requiring - ET
- Meningitis
- Use of Aminoglycoside-5days
- IU infection

Clusters of Sings Useful for Early Identification of CP

Warning signs

- Lack of alertness
- Decreased spontaneous motility
- Stereotyped abnormal movements

Abnormal sign

- Reduced head circumference/fall off in growth
- Constant fisting with adduction of thumb beyond 2 months
- Delayed social smile
- Primitive reflexes persisting beyond 6 months
- Obligatory ATNR
- Delayed appearance of postural reflexes and developmental milestones
- Persistent tone abnormalities
- Persistent asymmetry in posture, movement and reflexes

Developmental screening Tools of Indian Origin

a. Trivandrum developmental screening chart (TDSC)
b. Baroda developmental screening test (BDST)
c. Developmental observation cards up to one year
d. Developmental observation cards 3-6years by MoHFW
e. ICMR psychosocial developmental screening test

HAMMERSMITH INFANT NEUROLOGICAL EXAMINATION

3 months HINE score

- <57 is 96% predictive of cerebral palsy
- <40 never occurs in children with normal outcomes1^
- 50-73 indicates likely unilateral cerebral palsy
- <50 indicates likely bilateral cerebral palsy

HINE scores at 3-6 months:

- 40-60 indicates likely GMFCS I-II
- <40 indicates likely GMFCS III-V

HINE scores at (6, 9, 12 months):

- 90% predictive of cerebral palsy
- <73 predictive of cerebral palsy
- <40 almost always indicates cerebral palsy

Abnormal GM's

- Poor-Repertoire GM's
- Cramped-Synchronized GM's
- Chaotic GM's
- Abnormal Fidgety Movements
- Absence of Fidgety Movements

Follow up schedule of NICU Graduates

- Growth and development- 6, 10, 14 weeks, 3,6, 9 months, yearly till 5 years
- Neuromotor assessment -3, 6, 9 months, 1, 2 year
- Hearing 1-3-6 rule must before 6 months
- Speech and language Assessment before 2 years
- Ophthalmic assessment Intense follow up till 6 months, 2, 3 years
- Assessment of feeding, immunisation, ongoing morbidities - All visits

HAMMERSMITH NEONATAL NEURO EXAMINATION

It has 34 items

- Posture
- Tone patterns
- Reflexes
- Movements
- Abnormal signs
- Orientation and behaviour

Optimum score for term is >30.5 and for preterm at term equivalent age >26

HAMMERSMITH INFANT NEURO EXAMINATION

Age group 3 to 24 months

- Assessment of cranial nerve function
- Posture
- Movements
- Tone
- Reflexes and reactions
- Motor
- Behaviour

AMIEL TISON SCALE includes

- Neuromotor – axial and appendicular tone
- Neurosensory - Hearing and vision
- Neuro behavioural - Arousal pattern, quality of cry, suckling, swallowing
- Head growth - Head circumference and also skull for sutures, size of anterior fontanel

DIFFERENCES BETWEEN PRETERMS AT TERM AND FULL TERM

PRETERM AT CGA TERM EQUIVALENT	TERM
Less flexor tone in limbs	Normal tone as per GA
Lower median scores for both flexor and extensor neck tone	Normal Neck muscle tone as per GA
Preterms were more hyperexci -table- Brisk reflexes, startles & tremors, strong palmar grasp.	Normal excitability
When held in walking position, tends to walk on toes	Walk on whole foot
Good quantity but poor quality of spontaneous movement	Good quality of movements
More visual tracking than term	

VISUAL DEVELOPMENT

- At birth follow a moving target
- 3-4 weeks fixates, watch mother intensely
- 4 weeks can follow bright object in a range of 90 degrees
- 4-6 weeks begins to smile at mother's face
- 3 months follow a target in range of 180 degrees.
- 4 months binocular vision begins at 6 weeks and is well established by 4 months
- 12-20 weeks - hand regard
- 6 months - adjusts his position to see objects

NIDCAP First NIDCAP-Boston in 1982

1. New-born Individualized care and assessment program
2. Implemented right from birth
3. Assessment of need of infant and family is based on regular naturalistic behavioural observations before (baseline), during and after caregiving procedure.
4. Decisions are taken based on maturational stage, current medical condition, psychosocial situation of family.
5. Findings are discussed with parents and staff before recommendations are taken

Definition of Early intervention

Early intervention is defined as "multidisciplinary services provided to children from birth to 5 years to promote child health and wellbeing, enhance emerging competencies, minimize developmental delays, remediating existing/ emerging disabilities, prevent functional functional deterioration and promote adaptive parenting and family function.

It Harness the neuroplasticity in developing brain.

Screening NSG

All infants < 32 weeks or, 1.5kg

- 32-34 weeks or 1.5kg to < 1.8kg –
  1. need for extensive resuscitation,
  2. ventilation or exchange transfusion or
  3. had illness
  4. such as sepsis, NEC.

Routine screening of well preterm babies for intraventricular haemorrhage

1. 1st scan - 48 to 72 hours
2. 2nd scan - 1 to 2 weeks
3. 3rd scan- 3 to 4 weeks
4. 4th scan at term equivalent age depending on clinical condition
5. sick symptomatic / preterm neonates Immediately after birth

IVH as per percentage occurrence on each postnatal day

1. Post natal day 1 =50%

2. Post natal day 2 =25%
3. Post natal day 3 =15%
4. Post natal day 4 =10%

Parameters to be monitored in NSG

1. Ventricular index (levene index)
2. Thalamo occipital distance
3. Anterior Horn width
4. Ventricular height
5. Resistive index

Ventricular index: the distance between the flax and the lateral wall of the anterior horn in the coronal plane at the level of 3rd ventricle.

AHW: The diagonal width of the anterior horn measured at its widest point in the coronal plane.

TOD: distance between the outermost point of the thalamus at its junction with the choroid plexus and the outermost part of the occipital horn in the parasagittal plane normal value 7mm-24mm.

The AHW and TOD measures can indicate the "ballooning" shape of the lateral ventricles

IVH causes brain injury due to following effects

1. Disruption of the ventricular zone with reactive astrogliosis in areas of ependymal loss;
2. Impairment of proliferation of oligodendroglial precursor cells and neuronal precursor cells in the sub-ventricular zone of the ganglionic eminence, and in the cerebral white matter;
3. Impairment of pre-OL maturation;
4. Axonal injury;
5. Microglial activation.

ELVIS trial (Early versus Late Ventricular Intervention Study)

126 infants born preterm at ≤34 weeks of gestation with progressive PHVD following severe IVH.

Low threshold (LT) (VI >97th percentile and AHW >6 mm and/or TOD >25 mm),

High threshold [HT]) (VI >97th percentile +4 mm and AHW >10 mm).

There was no significant difference between the 2 groups for the primary outcome of death and or VP-shunt placement (30% infants in the LT group and 37% for infants in the HT group).

A VP shunt was inserted in 12 of 64 (19%) infants in the LT and in 14 of 62 (23%) infants in the HT group, the lowest rates reported thus far in the literature.

Follow up study of ELVIS trial in which brain injury was assessed by the Kidokoro score on MRI performed at term-equivalent age.

The total Kidokoro score was lower in the infants in the LT group (n = 44) than in the HT group (P < .001).

Ventricular volumes were smaller in the LT group (P = .03).

At 2 years of age, the risk of developmental impairment was low among both study groups, with 75% of all infants tested achieving a cognitive composite score of 85.

There was no significant difference for adverse outcome (composite outcome: death/cerebral palsy/developmental test score <70) between the 2 groups.

In the post-hoc multivariable analysis, children in the LT group had a decreased risk of composite adverse outcome, after correcting for gestational age and hemorrhage severity (P = .03).

These findings support the conclusion that timely intervention with reduction of the extent of ventricular dilatation may mitigate brain injury associated with ventricular dilation

Intervention in PVHD

Ventricular size with the following VI >97 percentile & AHW >6 mm &/or TOD >25 mm

And

Absence of the following clinical criteria:

- HC growth >2cm per week • Separated sutures .Bulging fontanelles

Management:

- Consider LP 2-3 times
- CUS 2-3 × a week until stable for 2 weeks then every 1-2 weeks till 34 weeks PMA
- Neurosurgical intervention when no stabilization occurs MRI at Term Equivalent

How does Therapeutic hypothermia works

- Decrease energy consumption
- Decrease accumulation of extracellular glutamate
- Decrease generation of reactive oxygen & nitrogen
- Inhibits inflammation
- Inhibition of platelet-activating factor and inflammatory cascade

- Suppression of free radical activity
- Attenuation of secondary energy failure
- Inhibition of apoptosis (cell death)

Therapy for cerebral palsy

Neurodevelopmental treatment (NDT Bobath neurodevelopmental therapy –

This was developed by Karl and Berta Bobath hence called Bobath principles.

- It is most popularly practised principles for CP in the world
  - Aims to normalize muscle tone, inhibit primitive reflexes and promote postural responses
  - Primitive reflexes – extinction by repeated stimulation Range of motion exercises, encouraging normal motor patterns
  - The aim of NDT is to facilitate normal motor development and prevent the development of secondary impairments due to contractures and deformities.
  - Bobath used various techniques to inhibit abnormal tone and reflexes- this helped to facilitate normal righting reflexes and movement patterns

Rood sensory motor treatment approach

Vojta method

Peto conductive education technique

Therapeutic Modalities Used to Reduce Spasticity

Non-pharmacologic Modalities

- Physiotherapy
- Occupational therapy
- Use of adaptive equipment
- Use of orthoses
- Various orthopedic surgical procedures
- Selective dorsal rhizotomy

Physiotherapy

- Goals Activity Motor Enrichment (GAME) is a specific early intervention program that involves goal-directed activities and parental coaching and has been shown in a randomized trial to improve motor and cognitive skills of children with CP at 1 year of age compared with usual care
- Infants with hemiplegic cerebral palsy who receive early constraint induced movement therapy (CIMT) have better hand function than controls in the short term and long term.

Ankle-foot orthoses are most commonly prescribed to assist the child with positioning of the ankle and foot during gait

Gait trainer

Pharmacologic Modalities

- Oral drugs
  - Baclofen
  - Benzodiazepines: valium, clonazepam
  - Dantrolene
  - Alpha2-adrenergic agonists: tizanidine, clonidine
- Local injections
  - Phenol injections
  - Botulinum toxin injections
- Intrathecal baclofen

Baclofen

- Baclofen acts at the level of the neurones in the spinal cord, enhancing gamma aminobutyric acid (GABA) activity as a GABA agonist.
- It inhibits some of the excess excitatory activity responsible for spastic tone.
- Its effect will be global, rather than targeted, which may produce undesirable hypotonia of truncal muscles

Botulinum toxin A (BTA

- Is a paralyzing agent derived from Clostridium botulinum. It causes muscle relaxation by chemically blocking acetylcholine release.
- Its effect reverses over 3–6 months as affected nerve roots sprout forming new junctions.
- Multiple site injections, selected after clinical and video assessment by a multidisciplinary team, are most effective

Three groups of patients may benefit:

- Ambulant children with a dynamic equinus throughout the gait cycle with knee flexion > 20 degrees or scissoring;
- Children who are losing ability to get to standing or maintain standing;
- Children of any functional category who are in pain or discomfort around the hip, or where adductor spasm Seriously hampers care and hygiene

Hearing assessment

9 M to 2 ½ years	OAE/ABR/visual reinforcement audiometry
2- 5 yrs	Conditioned play audiometry
5 yrs	Pure tone audiometry

TRIALS OF THERAPEUTIC HYPOTHERMIA

Whole-Body Hypothermia for Neonates with Hypoxic–Ischemic Encephalopathy Seetha Shankaran (NIHCD trial) N Engl J Med 2005; 353:1574-84

This was the first trial for therapeutic hypothermia for HIE.

Inclusion criteria:

- Those babies who are > 36 weeks GA with moderate to severe encephalopathy if full filling the prescribed criteria were given TH.
- PH of 7.0 or less or BE -16 mmol/l in cord gas or within 1 hr after birth.
- OR PH 7.01 - 7.15 OR base deficit -10 to 15.9 mmol/L then needed additional criteria such as acute perinatal event (e.g., late or variable decelerations, cord prolapse, cord rupture, uterine rupture, maternal trauma, hemorrhage, or cardiorespiratory arrest)
- And either a 10-minute Apgar score of 5 or less or assisted ventilation initiated at birth and continued for at least 10 minutes.
- Encephalopathy was defined as the presence of one or more signs in at least three of the following six categories:
- Level of consciousness, spontaneous activity, posture, tone, primitive reflexes (suck or Moro), and autonomic nervous system (pupils, heart rate, or respiration).
- The number of moderate or severe signs determined the extent of encephalopathy; if signs were equally distributed, the designation was based on the level of consciousness.

Intervention

- Usual care (control group) or whole-body cooling
- Oesophageal temperature of 33.5°C for 72 hours

Outcome studied

- Primary outcome was a composite outcome of death or moderate or severe disability
- Neurodevelopmental outcome at 18 to 22 months of age.

Participants - 239 eligible infants, 102 - hypothermia group, control group -106

Results

- Death or moderate or severe disability 45/102 infants (44 percent) in the hypothermia group and 64/103 infants (62 percent) in the control group (risk ratio, 0.72; 95 percent confidence interval, 0.54 to 0.95; P=0.01).
- 24 % died in the hypothermia group and 37 percent died in the control group- not statistically significant P=0.08.
- Cerebral palsy 19 % hypothermia group VS 30 % control group (risk ratio, 0.68; 95 percent confidence interval, 0.38 to 1.22; P=0.20).
- Neuromotor disability assessment based on cerebral palsy, and functional disability was graded according to the Gross Motor Function Classification System (GMFCS)
- Cognitive outcome was assessed with the use of the BSID II.

Conclusion - Whole-body hypothermia reduces the risk of death or disability in infants with moderate or severe hypoxic–ischemic encephalopathy

Selective head cooling with mild systemic hypothermia after neonatal encephalopathy Cool cap trial Peter D Gluckman Lancet 2005; 365: 663–70

Population

- Included 234 term infants
- With moderate to severe neonatal encephalopathy and abnormal amplitude integrated electroencephalography (aEEG)

Intervention

- Selective head cooling for 72 h, within 6 h after birth, with rectal temperature maintained at 34–35°C (n=116)
- Conventional care (n=118)

Outcome

- Primary outcome was death or severe disability at 18 months.
- 73/110 (66%) allocated conventional care and 59/108 (55%) assigned head cooling died or had severe disability at 18 months (odds ratio 0·61; 95% CI 0·34–1·09, p=0·1).
- Head cooling had no effect in infants with the most severe aEEG changes (n=46, 1·8; 0·49–6·4, p=0·51),

but was beneficial in infants with less severe aEEG changes (n= 172, 0·42; 0·22–0·80, p=0·009).

Conclusion - Improve survival without severe neuro-developmental disability in infants with less severe aEEG changes.

Effects of Hypothermia for Perinatal Asphyxia on Childhood Outcomes Denis Azzopardi TOBY Study Group* Total Body Hypothermia for Neonatal Encephalopathy Trial (TOBY) 2008 BMC paediatrics.

Population

- 325 New-borns with asphyxial encephalopathy
- Gestational age of 36 weeks or more

Intervention

- Standard care alone (control) or standard care with hypothermia to a rectal temperature of 33 to 34°C for 72 hours within 6 hours after birth

Outcome

- The primary outcome survival with an IQ scores of 85 or higher.
- A total of 75 of 145 children (52%) in the hypothermia group versus 52 of 132 (39%) in the control group survived with an IQ score of 85 or more (relative risk, 1.31; P=0.04).
- The proportions of children who died were similar in the hypothermia group and the control group (29% and 30%, respectively).
- More children in the hypothermia group survived without neurologic abnormalities (65 of 145 [45%] vs. than in the control group 37 of 132 [28%]; relative risk, 1.60; 95% confidence interval, 1.15 to 2.22).
- Among survivors, children in the hypothermia group, had significant reductions in the risk of cerebral palsy (21% vs. 36%, P=0.03)
- Children in hypothermia group had lower risk of moderate or severe disability (22% vs. 37%, P=0.03);
- They also had significantly better motor-function scores
- Moderate hypothermia after perinatal asphyxia resulted in improved neurocognitive outcomes in middle children

Moderate hypothermia within 6 h of birth plus inhaled xenon versus moderate hypothermia alone after birth asphyxia (TOBY-Xe): a proof-of-concept, open-label, randomised controlled trial Denis Azzopardi

- Administration of xenon within the delayed timeframe used in this trial is feasible and apparently safe, but is unlikely to enhance the neuroprotective effect of cooling after birth asphyxia.

Whole-Body Hypothermia for Term and Near-Term New-borns with Hypoxic-Ischemic Encephalopathy A Randomized Controlled Trial Infant Cooling Evaluation Collaboration

Participants:

- New-borns of 35 weeks' gestation
- Indicators of peripartum hypoxia-ischemia and moderate to severe clinical encephalopathy, randomly allocated to hypothermia (n=110) or standard care (n=111)

Intervention:

- Whole-body hypothermia to 33.5°C for 72 hours or standard care (37°C)

Main Outcome Measures:

- Death or major sensorineural disability at 2 years of age

Results:

- Therapeutic hypothermia reduced the risk of death or major sensorineural disability at 2 years of age: 55 of 107 infants (51.4%) in the hypothermia group and 67 of 101 infants (66.3%) in the control group died or had a major sensorineural disability at 2 years (risk ratio, 0.77 [95% confidence interval, 0.62-0.98]; P=.03).
- The mortality rate decreased, and the survival rate free of any sensorineural disability increased.
- Adverse effects of hypothermia were minimal

Therapeutic hypothermia for neonatal hypoxic ischaemic encephalopathy in India (THIN study): a randomised controlled trial Karoline Aker

Objective to evaluate the neuroprotective effect of therapeutic hypothermia (TH) induced by phase changing material (PCM) on MRI biomarkers in infants with hypoxic-ischaemic encephalopathy (HIE) in a lower source setting

Patients

- 50 term/near-term infants
- Admitted within 5 hours after birth with
- Predefined physiological criteria and signs of moderate/severe HIE.

Interventions

- Standard care (n=25) or standard care plus 72 hours of hypothermia (33.5°C±0.5°C, n=25) induced by PCM

Main outcome measures

- Primary outcome was fractional anisotropy (FA) in the posterior limb of the internal capsule (PLIC) on neonatal diffusion tensor imaging

Results

- Diffusion tensor imaging showed significantly higher Fractional Anisotropy in the cooled than the non-cooled infants in left Post Limb of Internal Capsule and several white matter tracts.
- Conventional MRI was available for 46 infants and demonstrated significantly less moderate/severe abnormalities in the cooled (n=2, 9%) than in the noncooled (n=10, 43%) infants.
- There was no difference in adverse events between groups.

Conclusions

- This study confirmed that TH induced by PCM reduced brain injury detected on MRI in infants with moderate HIE in a neonatal intensive care unit in India

A Randomized Trial of Erythropoietin for Neuroprotection in Preterm Infants S.E. Juul PENUT Trial Consortium*

Population

- 24 weeks 0 days to 27 weeks 6 days of gestation

Intervention

- High-dose erythropoietin within 24 hours after birth

Outcome

- The primary outcome was death or severe neuro-developmental impairment at 22 to 26 months of postmenstrual age

Results

- There was no significant difference between the erythropoietin group and the placebo group in the incidence of death or severe neurodevelopmental impairment at 2 years of age.
- There were no significant differences between the groups in the rates of retinopathy of prematurity, intracranial hemorrhage, sepsis, necrotizing enterocolitis, bronchopulmonary dysplasia, or death or in the frequency of serious adverse events

CONCLUSIONS

- High-dose erythropoietin treatment administered to extremely preterm infants from 24 hours after birth through 32 weeks of postmenstrual age did not result in a lower risk of severe neurodevelopmental impairment or death at 2 years of age

Feeding during neonatal therapeutic hypothermia, assessed using routinely collected National Neonatal Research Database data: a retrospective, UK population-based cohort study

- Necrotising enterocolitis is rare in babies receiving therapeutic hypothermia.
- Enteral feeding during hypothermia is safe and associated with beneficial outcomes compared with not feeding, although residual confounding could not be completely ruled out.
- Our findings support starting milk feeds during therapeutic hypothermia

Effect of Therapeutic Hypothermia Initiated after 6 Hours of Age on Death or Disability among New-borns with Hypoxic-Ischemic Encephalopathy A Randomized Clinical Trial Abbot R. Laptook 2017

- The composite of death or disability (moderate or severe) at 18 to 22 months adjusted for level of encephalopathy and age at randomization occurred in 19 of 78 hypothermic infants (24.4%) and 22 of 79 noncooled infants (27.9%)
- Hypothermia initiated at 6 to 24 hours after birth may have benefit but there is uncertainty in its effectiveness

Effect of Depth and Duration of Cooling on Death or Disability at Age 18 Months among Neonates with Hypoxic-Ischemic Encephalopathy A Randomized Clinical Trial

- A total of 364 neonates were randomly assigned to
- 4 hypothermia groups: 33.5°C for 72 hours (n = 95),
- 32.0°C for 72 hours (n = 90),
- 33.5°C for 120 hours (n = 96), or
- 32.0°C for 120 hours (n = 83)

Main outcomes and measures

- The primary outcome was death or moderate or severe disability at 18 to 22 months of age adjusted for center and level of encephalopathy
- Death or disability occurred in 56 of 176 (31.8%) cooled for 72 hours and 54 of 171 (31.6%) cooled for 120 hours

- And in 59 of 185 (31.9%) cooled to 33.5°C and 51 of 162 (31.5%) cooled to 32.0°C

Conclusions and relevance

- Among term neonates with moderate or severe hypoxic-ischemic encephalopathy, cooling for longer than 72 hours, cooling to lower than 33.5°C, or both did not reduce death or moderate or severe disability at 18 months of age

Prediction of outcome from MRI and general movement's assessment after hypoxic-ischaemic encephalopathy in low-income and middle-income countries: data from a randomised controlled trial Karoline Aker

Population

Fifty infants with HIE

- Therapeutic hypothermia (25 cooled and 25 noncooled).

Outcome

- All infants underwent brain MRI at day 5, GMA at 10–15 weeks
- Outcome assessments including Bayley Scales of Infant and Toddler Development, third edition, at 18 month

Conclusion(s)

- Neonatal MRI and GMA predicted outcomes with high accuracy in infants with HIE.
- The GMA is a feasible low-cost method which can be used alone or complementary to MRI in low-resource settings to prognosticate and direct follow-up

STUDY	DEATH/DIABILITY AT 18 MONTH (OR)
COOL CAP	0.61
NICHD	0.72
TOBY	0.86
ICE	0.77

STUDY	CP AT 18 MONTH (OR)
COOL CAP	0.75
NICHD	0.68
TOBY	0.67
ICE	0.92

Cooling for New-borns with hypoxic ischaemic encephalopathy Jacobs 2013 cochrane

To determine the effect of therapeutic hypothermia in encephalopathy asphyxiated New-born infants on mortality, long term neurodevelopmental disability and clinically important side effects

11 randomised controlled trials

Comprising 1505 term and late preterm infants with moderate/severe encephalopathy and evidence of intrapartum asphyxia.

Therapeutic hypothermia resulted in a statistically significant and clinically important reduction

- In the combined outcome of mortality or major neurodevelopmental disability to 18 months of age (typical RR 0.75 (NNTB) 7.
- Reductions in mortality (typical RR 0.75 NNTB 11)
- Reduction in neurodevelopmental disability in survivors (typical RR 0.77) NNTB 8
- Some adverse effects of hypothermia included an increase sinus bradycardia and a significant increase in thrombocytopenia.

Effect of Therapeutic Hypothermia on the Outcome in Term Neonates with Hypoxic Ischemic Encephalopathy- A Randomized Controlled Trial R Christina Catherine Jipmer study

- Term infants with moderate to severe HIE
- Normothermia or hypothermia.
- Mortality, neurological abnormality or normal outcome was recorded at hospital discharge or 28 days of age, whichever was earlier, and at 18 months of age.
- The 78 infants in the hypothermia group had more normal survivors at discharge (38%) than the 84 infants in the normothermia group (30%), ratio 1.29 (95% confidence interval 0.84-1.99), and at 18 months of age (65% vs. 42%), ratio 1.54 (1.13-2.10).
- When these results were combined with those of a previous randomized trial in the same neonatal unit, there were significantly more normal survivors with hypothermia compared to normothermia at discharge, ratio 1.49 (1.18-1.88) and at 6-18 months of age, ratio 1.37 (1.17-1.60).
- **Conclusion:** In term infants with HIE, therapeutic hypothermia reduced mortality and neurological abnormalities, and resulted in more normal survivors.

Therapeutic hypothermia in neonates with Hypoxic Ischemic Encephalopathy in low-middle-income countries (HELIX trial)

To determine whether therapeutic hypothermia that is initiated within 6 h of birth and continued for 72 h reduces death or disability at 18–22 months when compared with usual care, in full-term babies with moderate or severe neonatal encephalopathy who have been admitted to tertiary neonatal units in LMIC.

- Cerebral MRI done at 1–2 weeks after birth (3 Tesla scanners)
- A neurodevelopmental paediatrician masked to the allocation, assessed each infant at 18–22 months using the BSID III and did a detailed neurological examination.

	Hypothermia	Control	P value
Death or mod severe disability	50 %	47 %	0.55
Death upto 18 month	42 %	31 %	0.022
Gastric bleeding	31 %	17 %	0.0007
Persistent hypotension	22%	12 %	0.006
Pulmonary HGH	21 %	14 %	0.054
Prolonged blood coagulation	39 %	25 %	0.0027
Severe thrombocytopenia, persistent metabolic acidosis, cardiac arrhythmia.			

- TH with optimal neonatal intensive care couldn't reduce the composite outcome of death/moderate or severe disability, but resulted in increased mortality irrespective of the place of delivery, perinatal sentinel events, growth restriction, or coexistent sepsis
- Secondary outcomes were worse in the cooled infants like persistent hypotension, metabolic acidosis, thrombocytopenia, prolonged blood coagulation and gastric bleeding.

Increased incidence of death in this group might be related to the hypothermia induced suppression of hepatic metabolism in an already compromised liver, leading to persistent metabolic acidosis and myocardial depression

The MRI biomarker data do not suggest any beneficial effect of hypothermia on brain injury

80% infants in HELIX trial had a white matter injury, suggesting a subacute or partial prolonged hypoxia, which might explain the absence of hypothermic neuroprotection

- Done in only Government tertiary care hospitals
- Enrolled neonates in hypothermia group were more sick and required more inotropes, more sedation and were more acidotic and hyperglycaemic and this indicates the important role of supportive care in such patients
- High proportion of out born patients that emphasises the role of optimising post-resuscitation care and transport facilities in such patients

Levetiracetam versus Phenobarbital for Neonatal Seizures: A Randomized Controlled Trial

Population

- Term infants **between 36 and 44 Weeks**
- Suspicion of clinical seizures, HIE and at-risk neonates

Intervention

- Levetiracetam group C- Phenobarbitone group

Outcome

- Complete seizure freedom for 24 hours, Seizure control at 24 & 48 hrs

Results

- Greater efficacy of 20 to 40 mg/kg of phenobarbital than 40 to 60 mg/kg of levetiracetam.
- Eighty percent of patients (24 of 30) randomly assigned to phenobarbital remained seizure free for 24 hours, compared with 28% of patients (15 of 53) randomly assigned to levetiracetam (P, .001; relative risk 0.35 [95% confidence interval: 0.22–0.56]; modified intention-to-treat population)
- More adverse events occurred with phenobarbital

Effect of treatment of clinical seizures vs electrographic seizures in full-term and near-term neonates: a randomized clinical trial

- In a group of neonates with acute symptomatic seizures,
- Treatment of electrographic and clinical seizures with currently used anticonvulsants did not significantly reduce the risk of death or disability at 2 years compared to treatment of only clinical seizures.

Interventions to Reduce Severe Brain Injury Risk in Preterm Neonates A Systematic Review and Meta-analysis JAMA Netw Open. 2023 Apr; 6(4): e237473.

Perinatal interventions in the development of severe intraventricular hemorrhage and cystic periventricular leukomalacia in neonates born before 37 weeks' gestation.

Which perinatal interventions associated with reducing the risk of severe intraventricular hemorrhage (sIVH) in neonates born at less than 37 weeks' gestation.

- Showed with moderate certainty that antenatal corticosteroids were associated with small reduction in sIVH risk (risk ratio [RR], 0.54 [95% CI, 0.35-0.82] number needed to treat [NNT], 80
- Indomethacin prophylaxis was associated with moderate reduction in sIVH risk (RR, 0.64 NNT, 20
- Volume-targeted ventilation was associated with large reduction in risk of sIVH (RR, 0.51 NNT, 11
- Early erythropoiesis-stimulating agents (RR, 0.68 NNT, 34
- Prophylactic ethamsylate (RR, 0.68 were associated with moderate reduction in sIVH risk (low certainty).
- The meta-analysis also showed with low certainty that compared with delayed cord clamping, Umbilical cord milking was associated with a moderate increase in sIVH risk (RR, 1.82 NNT, –30)

NEONATAL REFLEXES STATION

The primitive reflexes (or primary reflexes) are stereotypic motor responses to various stimuli that develop before birth and disappear during early infancy in a predictable pattern.

Classification of reflexes

- Automatic
- Spinal cord
- Brain stem
- Midbrain
- Cortex

Automatic reflexes – Moros/gallant/landau/parachute.

Reflexes	Appears	Disappears
Moros	28 weeks	3-6 M
Gallant	32 weeks	2 m
Landau	3-4 M	12-18 M
Parachute	6-8 M	Lifetime

Automatic Reflexes

1. MORO A -28wks DA- 3-6 mo/ Incomplete Moro before 36 weeks
2. GALLANT A-32 weeks DA - 2 mo / Persists / Exaggerated Athetoid CP
3. LANDAU A -3-4 mo DA 12-18 mo
4. PARACHUTE A 6-8 mo DA – Never

Spinal Reflexes / Primitive Reflexes

1. Palmar grasp A- 10 weeks GA DA - 4-6 mo
2. Plantar reflex A-18 weeks GA DA -6mo
3. Rooting A -28 weeks DA-3 mo
4. Sucking A -28 weeks DA 3 mo
5. Flexor withdrawal A-Birth DA -2 mo
6. Stepping Reflex A -37 weeks DA 2 mo

Spinal reflex /primitive reflexes

Reflexes	Appears	Disappears
Palmar	10 weeks GA	4-6 M
Plantar	18 weeks GA	6 M
Rooting	28 weeks	3 M
Sucking	28 weeks	3 M
Flexor withdrawal	Birth	2 M
Extensor thrust	Birth	4 M
Stepping reflex	37 weeks	2 M

BRAIN STEM REFLEXES

Brainstem level reflexes

1. Symmetric Tonic Neck Reflexes A- 0-4 mo DA 8-12 mo/ helps in Quadrupled Crawling
2. Asymmetric Tonic Neck A -0-2 DA 4-6 mo/Prevents body from Rolling side ways
3. Tonic labyrinthine A –Birth DA 4 mo

STNR	0-4 M	8-12 M
ATNR	0-2 M	4-6 M
Tonic labyrinthine	Birth	4 M

Mid brain reflex

Optical righting 1- 2 yrs – persist

4 permanent reflexes

- Parachute
- Optical righting
- Pupillary
- Corneal /blink reflex

Moro's reflex

Can be elicited in 3 ways

1. Holding the infant in a way so that the trunk of the infant is supported in the forearm and the head in the palm of the examiner's hand. Drop the head by 45° and look for the response. Normal response consists

of abduction of the shoulders, extension at the elbow, opening of the hands and audible cry.

2. Lifting the head of the child from the cot up to 45° and dropping suddenly.
3. Lifting the baby by holding at the wrist for 45° and dropping.

Normal response is Moro reflex

Hand opening- 28 weeks

Abduction& audible cry- 32 weeks

Anterior flexion /Adduction-37 weeks

Habituation

- Term- habituates after 3 attempts
- Preterms- habituates after 10 attempts

Normally disappears by 3 months. It is considered to be abnormal if persists beyond 6 months

Abnormal moro's reflex

- Exaggerated: CNS infection, Tetanus.
- Decreased: Hypotonic baby, HIE.
- Asymmetrical: Erb's Palsy, # clavicle, #humerus, Hemiplegia, splinting.
- Persistence: Cerebral Palsy

Palmar grasp

Head should be in midline

If not, more easily elicited in the direction to which occiput is directed.

The dorsum of hand should not be touching the bed or any other surface

Asymmetrical palmar grasp: Klumpke's palsy Hemiplegia HIE.

Startle Reflex

Startle responses – Elicited either by noise or movement or spontaneously. With a sudden, loud noise or by tapping on the sternum.

Difference from the Moro reflex is that this reaction involves flexion of the elbows with hands remain closed (in moros there is extension of elbow and opening of hand), but there should be a total body reaction.

Habituation after repeated stimulus and last showing anger with crying

Asymmetrical Tonic Neck Reflex

Baby should be in Light sleep or awake but not crying, lying supine, head mid-line, and shoulders horizontal.

The head is gently turned to one side until the jaw is over the same shoulder,

Keep in that position for 15 seconds, and then release.

Note the position of the extremities.

A normal response is chin extension and occipital flexion.

The arm and leg on the side toward which the face is turned will be extended.

The extremities on the side opposite the face will be flexed.

The response may be stronger in the lower extremities, especially in premature infants.

Repeat by turning the head to the other side

Elicited response is a passive reflex;

Active reflex occurs spontaneously as the infant turns his or her own head.

Complete ATNR seen in 50 %

Leg ATNR seen in 25 %

Arm ATNR seen in 4 %

One sided ATNR seen in 15 % of cases

Perez Reflex

Apply pressure upward over the spine from the sacrum towards the head while the baby is suspended ventrally. This will cause the arms and legs to flex and the neck to extend.

Perez reflex stimulates more response from the upper extremities with its upward stroke.

Vollmer Reflex

Stroke the infant's spine down after firmly holding it in ventral suspension. This reaction tends to cause increased activity in the lower trunk with flexion of the leg and extension of lower back.

Galant's Response (Incurvation of the Trunk)

With the infant in the prone position either lying on the mattress or in suspension, rub lightly along either side of the spinal column from the shoulder toward the buttocks, first On one side and then the other.

A normal response is strong incurvation of the whole vertebral column with concavity on the stimulated side. Running the stimulation from the shoulders to the buttocks stimulates all the skin segments on the trunk.

Modified Sarnat Neurological Examination

Six categories to determine three levels of encephalopathy.

1. Level of consciousness

2. Spontaneous activity
3. Posture
4. Tone
5. Primitive reflexes
6. Autonomic nervous system: pupils, heart rate, respiration

Start with observation first like posture, spontaneous movement/activity, limb position then things, which require minimal handling such as, examine for heart rate and respiration.

For Spontaneous Activity: Observe for at least one minute and don't disturb the baby

Normal – good amount of limb movements with good variability, movements are asynchronous

Mild - decreased activity movements have Poor variability

Moderate – baby may appear sleepy

Severe – no activity noted

Posture

Supine position and the head in the midline

No – flexed at knees, hips and elbows.

Mild – abducted hips/ mildly flexed knees and elbows / adducted, flexed and opposed thumb.

Moderate – Complete extension of legs and arms Strong flexion of distal joints. -thumb in fist

Severe – decerebrate and decorticate posture

Level of consciousness

Give light tactile stimuli to trunk and check for response

Mild – Hyper-alert: Exaggerated response to stimuli. Eyes wide open with Jitteriness.

Moderate – Lethargic: sleepy delayed response to stimuli

Severe – Stupor / Coma

Tone

Traction is the most sensitive measure of tone

Head lag, ventral suspension, arm recoil, arm traction, leg recoil, leg traction

In ventilated infants, only arm and leg traction and recoil can be performed

Mild Normal resistance but slightly increased peripheral tone

Moderate Hypotonia (focal or general) or hypertonia

Severe – Flaccid (like a rag doll) or Rigid (stiffness or inflexibility

Primitive reflexes (suck and Moro)

Suck – look for strength and quality of suck and note the feeling os striping of the baby's tongue on your fingers

Mild – weak suck

Moderate – bite

Severe – no suck

Moros

Mild – low threshold for moros (hyperactive moros)

Mod – incomplete moros

Severe – absent moros

Pupils – average pupil size of a New-born in darkness is roughly 3.5 mm.

Mild – dilated pupil

Mod – miosis

Severe – no reactive

If the severity is equally distributed, use the level of consciousness to determine the outcome

40 Growing Preterm Case

- **Case allotted**
- **Relevant Examination done**
- **Relevant history to be asked in presence of examiner**
- **Examination finding presentation**
- **Discussion on case**

Case details given as Fch Neha currently 42 days of life born at 28 weeks of gestation with a birth weight of 1026 gms current weight 1346 gms admitted in transitional care unit.

In a DM exam at my centre the usual process is that you will be given a one line history of the baby. You are supposed to do a detailed examination of the baby in the allotted time.

After finishing your examination, the examiners will come and will ask you to ask relevant history about the case from the doctor managing the baby.

You have to ask specific and relevant questions based on your examination of the baby.

If you ask questions, which are not relevant, at this point you will be questioned for the purpose of that question.

When you are done with the relevant questions examiner with ask you to tell the examination findings .Usual pattern is the examiner asks what relevant history would you like to ask retrospectively.

Relevant questions to be asked which can vary case by case

1. Most important question is to find out why this baby is still admitted in NICU.
2. Maternal age/Primi/multi para / registered or unregistered pregnancy/ regular follow up /twin, singleton. Product of spontaneous conception/assisted/ IVF.
3. Any known significant medical history in mother / periconceptional medication if any. Any h/o renal, endocrine, cardiac disease.
4. Any complications in first trimester- there is no history of any, fever, rash or Bleeding PV
5. Second trimester - calcium and iron supplementation and had 2 doses of tetanus toxoid. Any abnormal scan
6. Cause for prematurity PIH, GDM, APH, placenta previa/pprom/spontaneous preterm labour. Any h/o aph, pih, dm, leaking pv, any signs of chorioamnionitis /bleeding pv/ precipitous labor/spont onset of labor/ Doppler changes leading to preterm delivery . no h/o of gestational hypertension/ gestational diabetes, BPV/ LPV or h/o of decreased fetal movements, excess or decreased amniotic fluid
7. Mother blood group/father blood group - HIV ELISA, Hep B, VDRL. TORCH profile
8. Antenatal steroid – Magnesium sulphate for neuro protection Iv antibiotics – if any
9. Mode of delivery Resuscitation details, Delivery room CPAP/ Surfactant, Place of delivery

In NICU

1. Duration of ventilation, type of ventilation, highest pressure required/medication required surfactant/ INO/ sildenafil. Post natal steroid , diuretics , nebs
2. Complication of ventilation like Pneumothorax, VAP, BPD
3. CVS – hypotension & Inotropes, PDA, blood transfusion
4. CNS- IVH, hydrocephalus, seizures, medication
5. Jaundice – PT DVET,IVIG
6. Nutrition – TPN, when was feed started, when baby reached full feeds, type of milk, fortification , regain birth weight, current weight, rate of growth Current status – volume, mode of feeding, calories, protein. Calculate calories and protein appropriate or not.

   Day of reaching birth weight

   - Episodes of feed intolerance/ nil per oral
   - Feeding transition – tube/paladai/direct feeding
   - Weight gain in the past 3 days/1 week

7. Sepsis – any history of infection, meningitis, duration of antibiotics, ventriculitis.
8. Screening – ROP, AOP, OOP, USG cranium, Thyroid profile, BERA, CAH, metabolic Immunization if done
9. Developmental supportive care/OMS/NNS/KMC/Hind milk feeding/involvement of OT.
10. Details about other twin

By the end of this history, you should be able to tell the reason for baby still admitted in NICU. Most probable causes are

1. BPD
2. On-going sepsis/infection /fungal
3. Not on full oral feeding
4. Not gaining weight
5. Heart diseases
6. Still on caffeine
7. Direct hyperbilirubinemia
8. Treatment of congenital infection
9. Post haemorrhagic hydrocephalus with shunt or in monitoring
10. Social issues

Vitals – same as venti case but less detailed

Anthropometry – weight /weight gain last 3 days/ length gain/head gain / plot him on fenton chart (most important). Label EUGR if fitting in criteria.

General examination – detailed head to toe examination with special emphasis on OOP/AOP/ any abnormal facies, over all activity. Accessories attached to the baby.

Systemic examination – not in detail but examine all systems. Especially basic tone examination.

Summary

Diagnosis

Target Growth Parameters For Preterm Babies

- >1500 grams: weight gain of 10-20g/kg/day
- <1500 grams: weight gain of 15-20 g/kg/day
- 1 cm/week of length
- 0.8-1 cm/week of head circumference

Strategies Aimed At Prevention of EUGR

1. Prevention of IUGR and preterm delivery – good antenatal care
2. Early initiation of TPN in VLBW neonates to prevent energy and protein deficiency
3. Early trophic feeding (MEN) in VLBW neonates
4. Early target to achieve full feeds with adequate fortification of preterm milk
5. Regular monitoring of length, weight and HC
6. NICU environment to support premature infant growth and development
7. Lung protective ventilation strategies to prevent CLD
8. Avoid postnatal systemic steroids and diuretics
9. Prevention and early treatment of neonatal morbidities like IVH, NEC
10. Appropriate post-discharge nutrition and monitoring

Multi-nutrient fortification of human milk (cochrane)

1. ↑ in-hospital rate of weight gain (MD 1.76 g/kg/d)
2. ↑ in-hospital rate of body length (MD 0.11 cm/week)
3. ↑ in-hospital rate of head circumference (MD 0.06 cm/week)
4. No increase in NEC
5. Inadequate evidence on long term growth or NDO

Neolact MMF

- Per 100 ml-
- energy 14 kcals,
- fats-0.08g,
- proteins 0.48 g,
- Ca 10 mg, Mg 2.36 mg, P 6.8mg

KMC COCHRANE 2016 Conde-Agudelo A, Díaz-Rossello JL. Kangaroo mother care to reduce morbidity and mortality in low birthweight infants. Cochrane Database of Systematic Reviews 2016

1. ↑ weight gain (MD 4.1 g/d; 11 trials, 1198 infants)
2. ↑ length gain (MD 0.21 cm/week; 3 trials, 377 infants)
3. ↑ HC gain (MD 0.14 cm/week; 4 trials, 495 infants)

Nutrition in established BPD

1. Fluid restriction <150 ml/kg/d. ideally upto 135ml/kg/day
2. Optimise enteral energy intake 120-150kcal/kg/day
3. Optimise enteral protein intake <1kg: 4-4.5g/kg/d / >1-1.8kg: 3.5-4g/kg/d
4. Optimise enteral lipid intake

5. Optimise Calcium, Phosphorus intake Ca 130-140 mg/kg/day ; P 60-90 mg/kg/day
6. Optimise sodium intake if diuretics are used
7. Provide Na supplementation to keep Na >135 meq/L
8. Optimise Vit A intake 1330-3300IU/kg/d
9. Optimise Vit E intake 2.2-11 mg/kg/d
10. Supplemental Iron 4 mg/kg/d,

Supportive strategies for encouraging BF

1. Early initiation, stimulation within 24 hours of delivery
2. Frequent expression from day 1, esp at night
3. KMC
4. Family centred NICU care
5. Family support
6. Adequate nutrition and rest for mother
7. Good lactation support right from antenatal period
8. Availability of Donor human milk

Grading Severity of GMH/IVH

Papile (CT BASED)

- I -Isolated GMH (no IVH)
- II- IVH without ventricular dilatation
- III-IVH with ventricular dilatation
- IV -IVH with parenchymal haemorrhage

Volpe

- I-GMH with no or minimal IVH (<10% ventricular volume)
- II-IVH occupying 10%-50% of ventricular area on parasagittal view
- III-IVH occupying >50% of ventricular area on parasagittal view, usually distends lateral ventricle (at time of IVH diagnosis)
- Separate notation Periventricular echodensity (location and extent)

De Vries Classification of PVL

Grade 1: Transient periventricular echogenicity persisting for > 7 days

Grade 2: Transient periventricular echogenicity evolving into small, localized frontoparietal cysts

Grade 3: periventricular echogenicity evolving into extensive periventricular cystic lesions

Grade 4: Extensive leukomalacia involving deep cortical white matter

PRESENTATION OF IVH

- Hypotension
- Metabolic acidosis
- Bradycardia
- Bulging anterior fontanelle
- Falling haematocrit
- Sudden onset pallor
- Temperature derangements
- Abnormal glucose homeostasis
- Abnormal water homeostasis

IVH and definite neurological sequel

Grade I 15 %

Grade II 25%

Grade III 50 %

Grade III and apparent periventricular haemorrhagic infarction 75%

Indication of intervention in PVHD

(If $\geq$ 2 features are noted- perform a therapeutic lumbar puncture)

1. Head circumference - >14 mm/ week or > 2mm/day for 2 weeks
2. Ventriculomegaly: Levene index greater than action line (>97% centile +4mm)
3. Features of raised intracranial pressure like bulging fontanelle, splayed sutures or neurological signs (lethargy, poor feeding, tone abnormalities or seizures)
4. Resistive index > 0.85 on Doppler of intracranial vessels

Following neonates should be screened for Retinopathy of Prematurity (ROP): NNF

- Born at less than 34 weeks of gestation, OR
- If gestation at birth is not known conclusively, birth weight below 2000 g, OR
- Born at 34-36 weeks of gestation, AND

Having ANY of the following risk factors:

- need of respiratory support,
- oxygen therapy for more than 6 h,
- sepsis,
- episodes of apnea and need of blood transfusion,
- exchange transfusion or

- Unstable clinical course as determined by paediatrician.
- In absence of reliable records, admission in neonatal intensive care unit (NICU) or Special Care New-born Unit (SCNU) can be taken as a surrogate risk factor.

KOOs Radiological classification of osteopenia of prematurity (OOP).

- Grade 0- The normal density of the bone cortex along the shaft with a normal dense white line at metaphysis and normal band of lucency, and thinning of the cortex
- Grade 1- Loss of dense white line at the metaphysis increased submetaphyseal lucency and thinning of the cortex
- Grade 2- Changes in grade 1 plus irregularity and fraying of the metaphysis, with splaying and cupping that is indicative of rickets
- Grade 3 associated with the presence of spontaneous fractures

Daily accretion rate per kg body weight is 120 mg of calcium and 70 mg of phosphorous during the last trimester of pregnancy. (80% of total transfer)

AT RISK INFANT for OOP

1. Born at <27 weeks' gestation
2. Birth weight <1000 g
3. Unsupplemented human milk.
4. Excessive fluid restriction
5. Long-term parenteral nutrition.
6. Usage of formulas not designed for preterm infants.
7. Furosemide therapy (BPD)
8. Long-term steroid use.

Clinical signs of OOP

- Respiratory insufficiency or failure to wean off from ventilator.
- Hypotonia
- Pain on handling (pathological fracture)
- Decreased linear growth with sustained head growth
- Frontal bossing
- Enlarged anterior fontanel
- Widened cranial sutures
- Craniotabes
- Rachitic rosary (swelling of costochondral junction)
- Harrison grooves (indentation of ribs at the diaphragmatic insertions)
- Enlargement of wrist, knees and ankle
- Enamel hypoplasia.

DEXA is currently the most widely used modality to assess BMD. It correlates well with fracture risk and, in both term and preterm Infants,- but not feasible to do easily

ALP >900 IU/l with serum phosphorus levels <5.6 mg/dl (<1.8 mmol/l) yields 100% sensitivity with 70% specificity for diagnosis of rickets.

Serum calcium is not a useful screening test as infants can maintain a normal calcium level at the expense of a loss of bone calcium.

Brain imaging abnormalities and neurological outcomes in severe Neonatal Hypoglycaemia

Major imaging findings-

- Occipital with or without parietal lesions (75%)
- Corticospinal tract involvement (15%)
- Watershed pattern (10%)

Neurological sequelae-

- Developmental delay/ mental retardation 84%
- Seizures 66%
- Visual impairment 37%
- Microcephaly 32%

Primary TSH based screening

I. More sensitive and specific for the diagnosis of CH
II. May miss central hypothyroidism or delayed rise of TSH

Primary T4 based screening

I. Can identify both primary and central hypothyroidism
II. Will miss compensated (subclinical) hypothyroidism
III. Higher false positive results

Primary TSH based screening adopted by most centres worldwide and is recommended for India

Supplemental Therapeutic Oxygen for Pre threshold Retinopathy of Prematurity (STOP-ROP), A Randomized, Controlled Trial. I: Primary Outcomes JAMA 2000

To determine the efficacy and safety of supplemental therapeutic oxygen for infants with pre threshold retinopathy of prematurity (ROP) to reduce the probability of progression to threshold ROP and the need for peripheral retinal ablation

Use of supplemental oxygen at pulse oximetry saturations of 96% to 99% did not cause additional progression of pre threshold ROP but also did not significantly reduce the number of infants requiring peripheral ablative surgery.

FINAL RESULTS OF THE EARLY TREATMENT FOR RETINOPATHY OF PREMATURITY (ETROP) RANDOMIZED TRIAL BY William V. Good MD,* on behalf of the Early Treatment for Retinopathy of Prematurity Cooperative Group 2006

Methods: Infants with bilateral high-risk pre threshold retinopathy of prematurity (ROP) (n = 317) had one eye randomized to early retinal ablative treatment and the fellow eye managed conventionally (control eye).

In asymmetric cases (n = 84), the eye with high-risk pre threshold ROP was randomized to early or to conventional management.

The primary outcome was visual acuity assessed by masked testers using the Teller acuity card procedure. Structural examinations were performed at 6 and 9 months

Grating acuity results showed a reduction in unfavorable visual acuity outcomes with earlier treatment, from 19.8% to 14.3% ($P < .005$).

Unfavorable structural outcomes were reduced from 15.6% to 9.0% ($P < .001$) at 9 months. Further analysis supported retinal ablative therapy for eyes with type I ROP, defined as zone I, any stage ROP with plus disease; zone I, stage 3 ROP without plus disease; or zone II, stage 2 or 3 with plus disease.

The analysis supported a "wait and watch" approach to type II ROP, defined as zone I, stage 1 and 2 without plus disease, or zone II, stage 3 without plus disease. These eyes should be considered for treatment only if they progress to type I ROP or threshold.

Conclusion: Early treatment of high-risk pre threshold ROP significantly reduced unfavorable outcomes in both primary and secondary (structural) measures

Efficacy of Intravitreal Bevacizumab for Stage 3+ Retinopathy of Prematurity BEAT-ROP Cooperative Group NEJM 2011

Assess intravitreal bevacizumab monotherapy for zone I or zone II posterior stage 3+ (i.e., stage 3 with plus disease) retinopathy of prematurity.

Infants were randomly assigned to receive intravitreal bevacizumab (0.625 mg in 0.025 ml of solution) or conventional laser therapy, bilaterally.

- The primary ocular outcome was recurrence of retinopathy of prematurity in one or both eyes requiring retreatment before 54 weeks' postmenstrual age.
- Retinopathy of prematurity recurred in 4 infants in the bevacizumab group (6 of 140 eyes [4%]) and 19 infants in the laser-therapy group (32 of 146 eyes [22%], P=0.002).
- A significant treatment effect was found for zone I retinopathy of prematurity (P=0.003) but not for zone II disease (P=0
- Intravitreal bevacizumab monotherapy, as compared with conventional laser therapy, in infants with stage 3+ retinopathy of prematurity showed a significant benefit for zone I but not zone II disease.

Development of peripheral retinal vessels continued after treatment with intravitreal bevacizumab, but conventional laser therapy led to permanent destruction of the peripheral retina

Ranibizumab versus laser therapy for the treatment of very low birthweight infants with retinopathy of prematurity (RAINBOW): an open-label randomised controlled trial LANCET 2019

We evaluated the efficacy and safety of intravitreal ranibizumab compared with laser therapy in treatment of ROP.

Randomised patients equally (1:1:1) to receive a single bilateral intravitreal dose of ranibizumab 0·2 mg or ranibizumab 0·1 mg, or laser therapy.

The primary outcome was survival with no active retinopathy, no unfavourable structural outcomes, or need for a different treatment modality at or before 24 week.

Treatment success occurred in 56 (80%) of 70 infants receiving ranibizumab 0·2 mg compared with 57 (75%) of 76 infants receiving ranibizumab 0·1 mg and 45 (66%) of 68 infants after laser therapy.

Using a hierarchical testing strategy, compared with laser therapy the odds ratio (OR) of treatment success following ranibizumab 0·2 mg was 2·19 (95% Cl 0·99–4·82, p=0·051), and following ranibizumab 0·1 mg was 1·57 (95% Cl 0·76–3·26); for ranibizumab 0·2 mg compared with 0·1 mg the OR was 1·35 (95% Cl 0·61–2·98)

Findings.

In the treatment of ROP, ranibizumab 0·2 mg might be superior to laser therapy, with fewer unfavourable ocular outcomes than laser therapy and with an acceptable 24-week safety profile

41 Neonatal Jaundice

Questions are based to find answers of below mentioned questions in a NNH case

- Etiology of jaundice
- Extent of jaundice
- Complication of jaundice
- Treatment received

Sample case

Fch Neha currently 4 days of life with GA 38 weeks with Birth weight of 2.9 kg currently under intensive phototherapy.

Questions to elicit the etiology of NNH

1. When was the jaundice noticed
2. How fast was the progression of jaundice
3. MBG/FBG/BBG/DCT
4. If rh negative – then what ICT, anti D status, previous baby jaundiced .MCA PSV value in MOM. Any intrauterine Blood transfusion
5. Any scan suggestive of hydrops in baby
6. Cord bilirubin, corb CBC.
7. G6pd status/ consanguinity/any h/o splenectomy in family
8. H/O Rh ABO and minor blood group incompatibility), erythrocyte biochemical abnormalities such as glucose-6-phosphate dehydrogenase (G6PD) or pyruvate kinase deficiencies, or abnormal erythrocyte morphology such as hereditary spherocytosis (HS
9. Poor feeding
10. infants of diabetic mothers and with congenital hypothyroidism, galactosemia, and other inherited metabolic dis
11. impaired intestinal motility due to intestinal atresia's, meconium ileus, or Hirschsprung's disease
12. Family history
13. A family history of jaundice, anemia, splenectomy, or early gallbladder disease suggests hereditary haemolytic anemia (e.g., spherocytosis, G6PD deficiency).
14. A family history of liver disease may suggest galactosemia, α1-antitrypsin deficiency, tyrosinosis, hypermethioninemia, Gilbert's disease, Crigler–Najjar syndrome types I and II, or cystic fibrosis.
15. c. Ethnic or geographic origin associated with hyperbilirubinemia (East Asian, Greek, and American Indian
16. A sibling with jaundice or anemia may suggest blood group incompatibility or breast milk jaundice.
17. Vacuum extraction (cephalohematoma).
18. Birth trauma may be associated with extravascular bleeding and hemolysis.
19. Oxytocin use may be associated with neonatal hyperbilirubinemia, although this is controversy

Extent of jaundice

1. Progresssion in how many hrs/days
2. Involvement of conjunctiva sclera
3. Palm and sole involvement
4. Rate of rise per hr or per day

Complications of NNH

1. History suggestive of encephalopathy—poor feeding, excessive sleepiness, and temperature instability increase the risk of bilirubin-induced neurologic injury and may be early signs of kernicterus. In either case, urgent ET may be critical.
2. Abnormal movement, eye deviation, retro Collis. Alternate period of hypo or hypertonia
3. Fever or hypothermia

Treatment received

1. When was the phototherapy started
2. Any dose of IVIG given
3. DVET
4. Feeding

After this history you should be able to tell the possible aetiology and BIND status of the baby

Examination

Weight/GA/DOL/head circumference

Describe the environment around the baby

Baby is nursed under radiant warmer with intensive phototherapy with interventions done for increasing the effectives of phototherapy. Skin patch applied, eyes and genitalia covered

Head to toe examination

Purpose if to look for findings relevant to a case of NNH

1. Lower gestational age/ Small for gestational age (SGA
2. Microcephaly may be associated with congenital infections.
3. Extravascular blood—bruising, cephalohematoma, or other enclosed haemorrhage
4. Pallor associated with haemolytic anemia or extravascular blood loss
5. Petechiae may suggest congenital infection, sepsis, or erythroblastosis.
6. Polycythaemia, icterus, purpura, sclerema.
7. Omphalitis or other sign of infection
8. Chorioretinitis associated with congenital infection
9. Evidence of hypothyroidism- protrude tongue, umbilical hernia

Systemic examination

Abdominal system – hepatomegaly, splenomegaly

CNS – sensorium, tone, posture, eye movement

Resp and cvs – basic examination

Jaundice in first <24 hours

I. Look for hemolysis Rh incompatibility, ABO incompatibility,
II. Criggler Najjar- severe form

2nd day- 3rd week

- Physiological jaundice
- Haemolytic jaundice
- Breast milk jaundice
- Polycythaemia
- Cephalohematoma
- Sepsis, DIC
- Genetic

Persistent jaundice

- Cholestasis jaundice
- Hypothyroidism
- Galactosemia
- Pyloric stenosis
- Sepsis
- Breast milk jaundice

Life of RBC as per age

Adult -110-120

Term New-born -60-90

Preterm New-born 35-50*

42 FAQs

When should a Radiant warmer used in manual mode?

- Initial preparation of bed for the baby
- Rapid rewarming of severely hypothermic infant
- Prior to resuscitation in delivery room before the birth of the baby.
- Only to be used in the continuous presence of nurse who is monitoring the skin temperature of the baby

How Disinfection of radiant warmer is done?

- Once everyday/after discharge/shifting of baby
- First clean thoroughly using sterile cloth soaked in soap water-then dry with sterile cloth.
- Disinfect with 1% virkon solution or 0.5% bacillocid solution may be used.
- All approachable internal and external surfaces should be cleaned including corners, side-panels and mattress.
- Spirit should not be used to clean the glass panels as the transparency will be affected.
- Adhesive materials like micropore or dynaplast should not be stuck on the glass panels the surface becomes rough which encourages dirt and microorganisms to adhere to it

PULSE OXIMETER

- If equipment is visibly dirty, clean with sterile cloth moistened with soap water and remove visible contamination. Then wipe with sterile moist cloth using 0.5% bacillocid or use bacillol spray.
- Do not use virkon/hypochlorite solution

Phototherapy machine

- Jean Ward in 1956, with one of the first infants given phototherapy at Rochford General Hospital
- Should be cleaned once daily.
- If equipment is visibly dirty, clean with sterile cloth moistened with soap water and remove visible contamination.
- Then wipe with sterile moist cloth using 0.5% bacillocid or use bacillol spray.
- Do not use virkon/hypochlorite solution
- No use of spirit or organic solvents as they reduce the transparency of the glass used

Steps in purchasing equipment for NICU

- Background search
- General specification
- Technical specification
- Details of minimum 3 companies providing the equipment
- Multiple response letter
- Justification letter
- AMC AND CMC
- Biomedical engineer committee

What are the General specifications of a NICU EQUIPMENT?

- A total of 3 years comprehensive warranty to be followed by 5 years AMC.
- Technical support, required spares and consumables should be assured for two years after initial 3 + 5 years period is over.
- It should be CE Certified by European notified body along with declaration of conformity and US FDA approved.
- Demonstration of quoted model is compulsory.
- Power supply : 230 V + 15%, 50 Hz + 3%.
- Service Training to MEC Engg. & Operational training to user department.
- Operating and detail service manual should be provided.
- Tropicalization : Operating Temperature : 40 O C
- Storage Temperature: 60 O C

Cost for Annual maintenance contract (AMC)

- Cost of the Annual Maintenance Contract (AMC) for each year is fixed to 3% of the ordered value of the equipment
- AMC for at least 5 years after the completion of guarantee period of 36 months.
- Rate is fixed for 5 years
- Includes repair and maintenance of equipment & all accessories supplied by the tenderer as a part of tender

Cost For comprehensive maintenance contract

- Cost of the Comprehensive Maintenance Contract (CMC) for each year is fixed to 8% of the ordered value of the equipment
- Includes the equipment & all accessories supplied by the tenderer as a part of tender.
- Assures an "up-time" guarantee of at least 96% (calculated on the basis of 24 hours a day and seven days a week).
- If this is not done, a penalty @ 1% per day of contract cost of equipment is imposed on the tenderer & same is recovered from contract deposit or payment due if any.
- Rate quoted for spares are freezed for 8 years
- Rate quoted for consumables are also freezed for 8 years

Fluconazole

Fluconazole is a highly selective inhibitor of fungal cytochrome P-450 sterol C-14 α-demethylation, thus inhibiting ergosterol synthesis. Ergosterol is an essential component of the fungal cell membrane, and instability of the cell membrane results in cell death.

Fluconazole prophylaxis can be considered when baseline incidence of invasive fungal disease is > 10 %

Prophylaxis

- Decreases invasive fungal infections
- No differences in mortality
- No impact on neurodevelopment at 18-22 months

Aminoven

- Contain fewer amounts of conditionally essential amino acids tyrosine, glutamine, and cysteine.
- pH: 5.5 – 6.0 , Osmolality: 885 mosm/L
- What should be the Calorie: Protein ratio in TPN for VLBW infants 20 NP calories/kg: 1 gm protein/kg

SMOF lipid contains a mixture of 4 different lipid sources

- Soybean oil, which provides essential fatty acids (30%)
- Olive oil which is high in monounsaturated fatty acids (that are less susceptible to lipid peroxidation) (30%)
- Medium-chain triglycerides, which show a faster metabolic clearance than long-chain triglycerides (25%)
- Fish oil, which provides the supply of omega-3 fatty acids. (15%)
- Less Hepatic Inflammation (Cholestasis), provides DHA & EPA (fish oil)
- 2kcal/ml
- Heparin at 0.5 IU/ml to TPN infused through a neonatal long line reduces the incidence of culture-positive sepsis- CLABSI (HILLTOP).

Sildenafil

- Selective phosphodiesterase type 5 (PDE5) inhibitor. PDE5 is found in the smooth muscle of the pulmonary vasculature. Sildenafil increases cGMP within pulmonary vascular smooth muscle cells resulting in smooth muscle relaxation.
- Used in Persistent Pulmonary Hypertension of the Neonate (PPHN) which are
  - o Refractory to inhaled nitric oxide (iNO) and other conventional therapies
  - o Neonate persistently unable to be weaned off inhaled nitric oxide
  - o Where inhaled nitric oxide not available
  - o Severe Ebstein's Anomaly
- Loading dose: 0.4 mg/kg IV over 3 hours, maintenance 1.6mg/kg/day.
- Hypotension, Retinopathy, Pulmonary Hemorrhage.

Inhaled nitric oxide

- Started at an OI of 20 at a dose of 20 ppm and will show a response of PaO2:FiO2 > 20.
- After 6 hours of stability, inspired oxygen concentration is first weaned below 60%, and then iNO is weaned only if Pao_2 can be maintained at 60 mm Hg or higher (or preductal oxygen saturation as measured by pulse oximetry ≥90%) for 60 minutes (60-60-60 rule of weaning iNO).

- Optimize lung recruitment, rule out CHD, correct LV dysfunction, shock, baseline Methemoglobin before starting inhaled nitric oxide

Magnesium Sulphate for neuroprotection

- Indication -Women with imminent preterm birth between 24 and 32 weeks of gestation. Antenatal magnesium sulfate is to be administered as a 4-g IV loading dose, over 30 minutes, followed by a 1 g/ hour maintenance infusion until birth (for a maximum of 24 hours).
- Mechanism of action – anti-excitatory amino acid [impairs release, blocks the N -methyl- d -aspartate (NMDA) receptor], antioxidant [essential for glutathione biosynthesis], anti-cytokine [decreases levels of inflammatory cytokines], and antiplatelet [decreases platelet aggregation] effects)
- Result - When given with neuroprotective intent decreased CP (relative risk [RR], 0.71; 95% confidence interval [CI], 0.55–0.91) and reduced the total occurrences of death and cerebral palsy (summary RR, 0.85; 95% CI, 0.74–0.98).

SURFACTANT

- **Curosurf Vial –**
  - Porcine minced lung
  - 120mg/1.5 ml 80 mg/ml
- **Neosurf -**
  - BLES – Bovine Lipid extract – Lung lavage
  - 137/ 5 ml- 27 mg/ml
- Survanta –
  - Bovine Minced Lung
  - 25 mg/ml

100 ml of 0.9 % Normal saline =15.4 mEq of Sodium

100 ml of 3 % Normal saline =51.3 mEq of Sodium

100 ml Isolyte P =2.5 mEq Na, 2 mEq K

1 ml KCL (15 %) =3.8 mEq Potassium

1 ml conc. Ringer's lactate = 3 mEq of Sodium

$PAO_2 = 7X\ FiO2 - PaCO2$

Alveolar(A)-arterial(a)oxygen gradient: ($AaDO_2$)

$AaDO_2 = PAO_2 - PaO_2$ ($PAO_2 = 7 \times FiO_2 - PaCO_2$)

New-borns on room air $AaDO_2$ of 10-25 mmHg is normal

Normally it ranges between 5-15, if breathing room air. A-aDO2 is considered to be abnormal if more than 40

> 250 - Need for assisted ventilation

>400 - Shunt situation/PPHN

>600 - Need for ECMO

Oxygenation index: (OI)

OI = Mean airway pressure (MAP) × FiO_2 × 100 / Post ductal PaO_2

Pressure cost of achieving certain level of oxygenation

>15 – Severe respiratory compromise

30-35 – Failure of existing mode of ventilation

>40 – 80% risk of mortality- ECMO indication

a /A ratio: Ratio of PaO2 to PAO2

. It is considered to be a better indicator of gas exchange as the ratio is usually not affected by changes in FiO2

Interpretation:

a) Greater than 0.8: Normal

b) Less than 0.6: indicates need for O2 therapy

c) Less than 0.15: severe hypoxemia

O2 HOOD

While using oxygen hood, change in the flow rate will not alter the FiO2 much. If one wants to decrease the FiO2, more mixing with air has to be allowed through portholes. Occlusion of these holes increases the O2 concentration by preventing air entrainment.

Approximate FiO2 delivered with a flow rate of 5-8 Lpm:

- With all portholes closed: 60-70%
- With one port hole opened – 40-50%
- With both the portholes opened – 30-40%

Hypocarbia of less than 30 mmHg has been shown to be associated with periventricular leukomalacia (PVL) and a poor long-term neurodevelopmental outcome

Prerequisites for weaning from acute ventilation (up to 7 days of ventilation) include

a) Clinically & hemodynamically stable

b) Effective respiratory efforts

c) Basic lung pathology / disease improving

d) No significant co-morbidity

e) Optimum blood gases

Prerequisites for weaning from chronic ventilation (> 7 days of ventilation):

a) All the above features for acute ventilation

b) Adequate and consistent weight gain (over the last 5-7 days)

c) Normal serum electrolytes (especially potassium)

d) Acceptable hematocrit

General principles of weaning:

a) Decrease the most potentially harmful parameters first (PIP & FiO2).

b) Limit changes to one parameter at a time.

c) Avoid changes of a large magnitude.

d) Document the infant's response to each change in the ventilation parameter.

Nasal cannula

- Depth of insertion -Nares to the inner margin of the eyebrow
- Flow rate - 1-2
- FiO2 delivered - 25-45

Nasal prongs

- 0.5-1 cm
- Flow rate - 1-2
- FiO2 delivered - 25-45

What is the target population for cranial USG?

- Preterm for e/o GMH-IVH & follow up
- HIE
- Neonatal seizures
- Unexplained CCF (r/o vascular abn)
- Evaluation of congenital anomaly
- Suspected subgaleal hematoma

What is Thompson' scoring of PNA?

- Total 9 signs: LOC, Posture, Tone, Seizures, Moro, Grasp, Suck, Respiration, & Fontanel.
- Each scored from 0-3
- Maximum score: 22 Mild: < 10 Moderate: 11-14 Severe: > 14
- Score 3 is attributed to only 4 signs: LOC: comatose Tone: flaccid Posture: decerebrate Respiration: IPPV (apneic) That's how the maximum score is 22.

What is hyperoxia test?

- Predictable PaO2 on room air & > 10 mins of 100% O2 administration via a hood or ET tube. > 300: normal
- < 100: cardiac conditions Parallel circulation
- > 100 & < 150: PPHN, TAPVC
- 150 & < 300: pulmonary lesions CNS disorders

What is the mechanism of action of ANS?

- Animal studies: ANS bind specific receptors on fetal lung cells & leads to FPF (Fibroblast Pneumocyte Factor) production by lung fibroblasts.
- FPF acts on type II pneumatocysts & increase production of surfactant & associated proteins
- ANS also accelerates morphological maturation of fetal lung by increasing surface area for gas exchange, maturing alveolar lining cells, decreasing capillary leak, accelerated synthesis of lung collagen.

What is blueberry muffin baby? Which diseases may cause blueberry muffin?

- Skin resembles blueberry muffin - diffuse, dark to violaceous purpuric macules & papules. Represent dermal hematopoiesis & sign of serious systemic disease.
- Most common congenital rubella. • Congenital infections: rubella, CMV, toxoplasmosis, herpes, coxsackie B2, parvovirus B19 • HDN •. Neoplasms: Leukaemia Neuroblastoma Congenital Rhabdo-myosarcoma with cutaneous metastasis • Langerhans histiocytosis

What is FGR & SGA?

- FGR is a deviation in the rate of growth of a fetus that is < its genetically predetermined growth potential.
- SGA refers to an infant whose birth weight is < 10th centile for that GA.
- IUGR & FGR is same.
- Because of nature of the term retardation, it is replaced by restriction.
- FGR is pathological etiology

What are the humidity values for infants nursed in incubators?

- For GA < 28 weeks
- Commence with humidity of 80%
- Maintain humidification at 70-80% for first 7 days.
- Wean by 5% daily from day 8 if temperature & fluid balance stable.
- Discontinue when 40% is achieved or at 21 days whichever is reached first.

Dr. Rangasamy Ramanathan, neonatologist, Los Angeles CA.... Inventor of RAM cannula.

Which twin is the better candidate for foeticide in TTTS?

Recipient twin due to

- Ease of cord visualisation & access
- Less risk - intraop uterine wall injury
- Increased risk of developing cardiac dysfunction & hydrops.

Donor twin is selected if

- Presence of severe cardiac anomaly or brain injury.
- Increased thickness of the recipient's cord.

What are the major causes of heart failure in a fetus?

- Severe anemia
- Arrhythmia
- Infection
- Large systemic AV fistula (vein of Galen AV malformation)
- Severe AV valve insufficiency

When do the 5 senses develop in the fetus?

1. Touch: 8-15 weeks GA 32 weeks: consistently responds to temperature, pressure & pain
2. Taste: 13 weeks GA 24 weeks: gustatory response +
3. Hearing: 20 weeks GA (cochlea fun +) 25 weeks: response to VA stim +
4. Vision: 29 weeks GA (pupillary resp + 32 weeks: consistent response
5. Smell: 28-32 weeks GA

In response to hypoxia, how do the components of BPS get affected?

- Components disappear in the inverse of their appearance
- FHR activity: 1st sign of fetal compromise
- Followed by FBM, GBM, & lastly tone.
- Oligohydramnios is a feature of chronic fetal hypoxia.

What is furcate insertion of cord?

Topographic site of insertion is central but umbilical vessels lose their protective Wharton's jelly shortly before they insert. Covered only by an amnion sheath. Prone for compression, twisting & thrombosis.

Which areas of the brain are stained by bilirubin during ABE?

- Basal ganglia: GP & subthalamic nuclei
- Hippocampus: sectors H2-3
- S. Nigra
- CN nuclei: 3, 7, 8
- Reticular formation of pons
- Inferior Olivary nuclei
- Cerebellar nuclei: dentate
- AH cells of spinal cord

What fetal findings are a/w good postnatal renal functions?

- Normal level of AF
- Normal renal parenchymal echogenicity by fetal USG.
- Fetal urine values: Na: < 100 mEq/ L Cl: < 90 mEq/ L Osmolarity: < 210 mOsm
- UO: > 2 mL/hr

What is Fetomaternal hemorraghe ?

- FM hge is caused by a disruption of the normal barrier at placental-decidual interface.
- It may occur with
- Abruptio placentas
- Abruption with maternal trauma
- Maternal trauma without abruption
- Spontaneously without apparent cause

What are the heart lesions that can present with heart failure in the first week of life?

- Duct dependent lesions • HLHS with large PDA • TA • COA with VSD • Critical AS • IAA type B
- Non duct dependent • TAPVR • ECD • Cardiomyopathy • SVT

What is ankyloglossia?

- A congenital midline anomaly in which the bottom of the tongue is attached to the floor of the mouth by a membrane (lingual frenulum)
- 2-5% of infants
- Typically heart shaped appearance of the tongue tip.
- Isolated/ familial/ syndromic
- May impair breastfeeding in some.
- Frenotomy: office procedure
- Frenulectomy & frenuloplasy: for significant ankyloglossia.

What is red reflex?

- Quick screening tool during eye examination in Newborns.
- Elicited by using an ophthalmoscope using its wide beam.
- The light should be shown on both eyes from a distance of 45-50 cms.
- Adjust the focus to bring the glow at the level of pupils.
- Normal eye: presence of a red choroidal reflex in both eyes.
- Absent: cataract, corneal clouding, vitreous hemorrhage, or retinal detachment.

Why photo protection is necessary during TPN?

- To prevent or reduce peroxide formation.
- Peroxide interferes with lipid metabolism causing hypertriglyceridemia & impair glucose uptake in muscle & fat: hyperglycaemia.
- Peroxides disrupt cell membrane integrity, mediate tissue injury, and change quality of PN.

Photo protection

- Reduces peroxide load.
- Incidence of BPD
- Done by wrapping infusion lines with aluminium foil or by using special infusion sets.

Sources of peroxide in PN

- Amino acids: tryptophan, tyrosine, methionine, cysteine & phenylalanine •
- MV: riboflavin
- Trace elements
- Lipid emulsion: PUFA
- Additives used for stabilisation

What is Ventricular Index of Levene?

- Flax to lateral wall of ventricles in mm.
- (Horizontal expansion) 4 mm aver the 97th centile for VI is considered as action line for PHVD.

Endotracheal suction

1. Two appropriately skilled staff to perform the procedure. 2. Hand hygiene. 3. Wear personal protective equipment. 4. Assemble suction equipment, suction catheter size (2× endotracheal tube (ETT) internal diameter size). 5. Disconnect patient from the ventilator. 6. Use clean hand/dirty hand technique, perform suction using dedicated clean hand. 7. Insert suction catheter only to a depth of 0.5 cm past the end of the ETT (length is determined using centimetre markings on the ETT).

Total suction procedure should be less than 15 s. 9. Suction is only applied (70mm Hg) during catheter withdrawal and for no longer than 5 s

Prevention strategies for CLABSI in the NICU

- Education, training, and staffing
- To prevent CLABSI, an intervention bundle is recommended for insertion and maintenance of CVC
- When using an intervention bundle, it is better to use a checklist to encourage compliance with medical staff training and recommendations.
- In a United States study, the incidence of CLABSI was reduced by about 40% after the administration of a bundle compared to before
- Before inserting a peripheral venous catheter, it is recommended to disinfect the skin using 70% alcohol, tincture of iodine or alcoholic chlorhexidine gluconate (CHG) solution
- It is recommended that transparent dressing used on short-term CVC sites be changed every 7 days, except when infants are more likely to lose their catheter while replacing dressings
- It is recommended that low-doses of heparin (0.25–1.0 U/mL) be added to the fluid injected into the UA catheter to maintain its patency.
- If UA and UV catheters are no longer needed, they should be removed as soon as possible.
- An umbilical catheter can be replaced if it malfunctions and there is no other indication for removal.
- The total period of catheter use should not exceed 5 days for UA catheter, or 14 days for UV catheter.
- When CRBSIs occur or signs of vascular insufficiency or thrombosis are seen, UA or UV catheters should be removed and never be replaced
- The tubing set used to administer blood, blood products, or IVFEs should be replaced within 24 hours of initiating the infusion

Hand hygiene is the most effective method of decreasing health care–related infections

Before entering the NICU, a 3- to 5-minute scrub (surgical, washing up to the elbows) or rub is typically necessary.

A 30-second hand wash or shorter alcohol-based hand rub is indicated before and after each patient contact

Recommended maximum duration of use:

UAC < 5 days

UVC < 7 day

Umbilical Artery Catheterization

Indications

- Frequent measurements of arterial blood gases.
- Continuous arterial blood pressure monitoring.
- Access for exchange transfusion (to withdraw blood).

UAC recommendation. 3.5 F if 1.2 or 1.5 kg

- UAC with a single lumen is advised.
- Catheters with multiple lumens are only advised for use with UVCs.
- When compared to side-hole catheters, end-hole catheters had a lower risk of aortic thrombosis.
- Cochrane review notes that there is no benefit of using a heparin bonded polyurethane catheter versus the standard polyvinyl chloride (PVC) catheter.
- Heparin (as little as 0.25 U/mL) should be used, according to Cochrane studies, to reduce the likelihood of catheter blockage and extend the life of the catheter.
- Intermittent heparin flushes not recommended
- AAP recommends the umbilical artery catheter should be used to administer low dosages of heparin (0.25–1.0 U/L).
- Low UAC catheters are associated with an increased risk of vasospasms. Cochrane review now recommends high catheters exclusively.
- High catheter/line.
- UAC tip lies above the diaphragm at the level of T6–T9.
- This position is above the celiac artery (T12), the renal arteries (L1), and the superior mesenteric artery (T12–L1)
- When using a catheter for a longer period of time, high positioning is linked to fewer vascular complications, a lower incidence of blanching and cyanosis of the extremities, and no statistically significant increase in hypertension, intraventricular haemorrhage, necrotizing enterocolitis (NEC), or hematuria.

Low UAC catheter/line.

UAC tip lies between the level of L3 and L4 (above the L4–L5 aortic bifurcation) and is associated with more episodes of lower extremity vasospasm.

Methods to estimate UAC length for insertion

Dunn method.

- Uses the shoulder-to-umbilicus length (SUL) and a nomogram to determine the insertion length.

Shukla and Ferrara method.

- Uses the birthweight (BW) UAC length (cm) = (birthweight in kg × 3) + 9 cm

Wright formula

- For LBW UAC length (cm) = (birthweight in kg × 4) + 7 cm

The most common cause of failure to catheterize an umbilical artery is inadequate dilation of the artery.

Pull the catheter slowly for last 5 cm of UAC while removing (1 cm/min).

Complications of UAC

1. Infection (septic emboli, cellulitis, omphalitis, sepsis)
2. Vasospasm, thrombosis, embolism, and infarction can occur Air embolism
3. Arterial vasospasm. If the leg blanches, warm the other leg (reflex vasodilatation).
4. Femoral artery thrombosis.
5. Renal artery thrombosis.
6. Mesenteric artery thrombosis.
7. Aortic thrombosis
8. Vessel perforation.
9. Intestinal necrosis (embolization to the gut), or localized perforation
10. Hypertension secondary to renal artery embolus

Emergency needle aspiration (tension pneumothorax).

Needle aspiration is done at the second intercostal space at the midclavicular line on the suspected side of the pneumothorax. The needle is inserted above the third rib.

For pneumothorax

- The chest tube should be at the fourth or fifth intercostal space between the anterior axillary line and midaxillary line (modified Buelau position)
- The chest tube should be inserted 2–3 cm for a small, preterm infant and 3–4 cm for a term infant

- The fifth or sixth rib is where the skin is cut.
- The pleura is punctured above the fifth rib in the fourth intercostal space if the skin incision is at the fifth rib.
- The pleura is punctured above the sixth rib in the fifth intercostal space if the skin incision is at the sixth rib.
- The tube should be inserted anteriorly, towards the apex.

Nasal endotracheal intubation.

More commonly performed in elective settings or if surgery rules out the oral route. An endotracheal tube can be used through the nose in excessive activity in New-borns or in New-borns with excessive secretions. it provides tube stability but can be bonded associated with an increase in postextubation atelectasis and a risk of nasal damage.

MEDICATIONS FOR PREMEDICATION FOR NONEMERGENCY INTUBATION

1. Administer oxygen.
2. Vagolytic agent to prevent bradycardia. Atropine preferred.
3. Analgesic (fentanyl preferred) and/or sedative/ hypnotic. None preferred.
4. Muscle relaxant. Vecuronium or rocuronium preferred

Analgesic Fentanyl

Hypnotic/sedative Midazolam

Muscle relaxant Pancuronium Vecuronium

To limit hypoxia, limit each intubation attempt to < 20 sec

Length of ET for insertion

- 7-8-9 rule (Tochen rule).
- Nasal tragus length (NTL) and sternal length (STL

Orotracheal route. NTL or STL plus 1.

Nasotracheal route. NTL or STL plus 2

Caution is necessary as breath sounds heard over the anterior part of the chest can come from the stomach or oesophagus

Lidocaine, atropine, naloxone, and epinephrine can be given through the ETT

Exchange Transfusion

Double-volume exchange blood transfusion. Refers to 2 times the estimated blood volume at ~85% of infant's blood volume

Infants with Rh incompatibility. The blood must be type O, Rh-negative, low titer anti-A, anti-B blood. It must be cross-matched with the mother's plasma and RBCs. 2.

Infants with ABO incompatibility. The blood must be type O, Rh-compatible (with the mother and the infant) or Rh-negative, low-titer anti-A, anti-B blood. It must be cross-matched with both the infant's and mother's blood

Normal Neonatal Chest X-ray

- Vascular markings
- Well seen central 2/3rd
- Not visualised in the peripheral 1/3rd Air bronchogram" appearance
- In left lower lobe behind the cardiac silhouette – normal
- Thoracic vertebrae are clearly visualised
- Normal for vertebral bodies to have a central defect

Correct exposure on AP view

- Examine vertebral column behind the heart
- You can see the detailed spine and pedicle through heart
- You can see the pulmonary vessels in peripheral lung

Evidence-Based Consensus Recommendations for Skin Care in Healthy, Full-Term Neonates in India

Neonatal skin care at birth

- Clean gloves need to be worn to handle the New-born
- Remove blood, meconium, or amniotic fluid from the baby's skin.
- Leave the vernix intact. Do not scrub it off as it protects the skin and favors appropriate colonization.
- Use cotton swabs soaked in water boiled and cooled to an appropriate temperature to gently clean the skin and then gently dry the skin.
- Establish skin-to-skin contact during the first hour after birth as it supports timely breastfeeding, thermoregulation, survival, establishment of a healthy skin microbiome, and mother-baby bonding

Bathing the New-born

- The first bath should be given once the New-born has achieved cardiorespiratory and thermal stability; the ideal time-period may range between 6 and 24 hours after birth.
- For neonates born to an HIV-positive mother, the first bath should occur at the earliest.
- Keeps the bath time short, lasting not more than 5–10 minutes.
- The frequency of bathing should not exceed twice or thrice a week.

- Bathing should not occur immediately after feeding.
- Bathing should preferably be carried out 45 minutes to 1 hour following the last feed.
- The tub swaddle bath is considered the ideal modality of bathing. However, the traditional method of placing the neonate between the knees is required to be explored, and may be recommended as an alternative.
- Use lukewarm water (at around 38°C) and maintain room temperature (between 26°C-28°C). Also, a mild gentle cleanser which has been demonstrated appropriate for New-borns could be used.29,30 The cleanser should be formulated to be pH neutral to mildly acidic and to not disturb the normal pH of the baby skin.1

Skin care practices within the hospital

- Neonatal skin assessment should be a part of routine New-born care. The skin should be assessed at the earliest following birth, on a continuous basis, or, at least once daily using valid and reliable tools; increase frequency, if needed.
- Umbilical cord care: Follow dry cord care. If cord gets soiled with urine or feces, it may be cleaned with water, or a mild cleanser.
- Diaper area cleansing and care: Use a soft cloth, water, and a mild cleanser or disposable diaper wipes to gently clean the perianal area and buttocks after each diaper change.
- Appropriately, formulated emollients for baby skin are recommended at the first signs of dryness, fissures or cracking of the skin and can be employed to maintain or enhance the skin barrier function.
- It may also be considered in high-risk infants to prevent occurrence of Atopic Dermatitis. Additionally, emollients may be applied on the scalp in New-borns with cradle cap.
- Appropriately formulated baby oils can be lightly applied to the neonate skin before bath for transitory dryness only. Oils meant for cooking or sourced from the kitchen should not be used on the baby's skin.

Critical congenital heart disease screening

CCHDs are congenital heart defects requiring surgery or catheter intervention within the first year

Pulse oximetry screening likely to help diagnose the following seven CCHDs:

a. Hypoplastic left heart syndrome
b. Pulmonary atresia
c. Tetralogy of Fallot
d. Total anomalous pulmonary venous return
e. d-Transposition of the great arteries
f. Tricuspid atresia
g. Truncus arteriosus

Diseases not detected by CCHD screening are coarctation of the aorta, double-outlet right ventricle, Ebstein anomaly, interrupted aortic arch, single ventricle, and l-transposition of the great arteries

Impact of pulse oximetry screening on the detection of duct dependent CHD : a Swedish prospective screening study in 39821 New-borns BMJ 2008;337: 3037

Results:

- **29 babies in well baby nurseries had duct dependent circulation undetected before neonatal discharge examination.**
- In 13 cases, oxygen saturations $\leq$ 90%. Of the remaining 16 cases, physical examination alone detected 10 (63%).
- **Combining physical examination with pulse oximetry screening had a sensitivity of 24/29 (82.8% (95% CI 64.2% to 95.2%)) and detected 100% of the babies with duct dependent lung circulation.**
- Five cases were missed (all with aortic arch obstruction).
- False positive rate with pulse oximetry was substantially lower than that with physical examination alone (69/39 821 (0.17%) *v* 729/38 413 (1.90%), P<0.0001), and 31/69 of the "false positive" cases with pulse oximetry had other pathology.

Thus, referral of all cases with positive oximetry results for echocardiography resulted in only 2.3 echocardiograms with normal cardiac findings for every true positive case of duct dependent circulation

- **Introducing pulse oximetry screening before discharge improved total detection rate of duct dependent circulation to 92%.**

Adverse effects of prostaglandin E1 infusion in neonates

Common Adverse Effects

- Apnea (usually occurs within 1st hour and with increasing dosing)

- Hypotension (due to vasodilatation consider fluid bolus)
- Fever
- Tachycardia
- Flushing

Less Common and Rare Adverse Effects

- Hypothermia
- Bradycardia
- Convulsions
- Diarrhoea
- Cardiac arrest

Adverse Effects due to Prolonged Use

- Gastric outlet obstruction syndrome
- Cortical hyperostosis

Causes of deterioration after administration of PGE1

I. TAPVC with obstruction of common pulmonary vein
II. TGA with intact VSD and a restrictive foramen oval.
III. HLHS with restrictive foramen oval and IAS
IV. MA with a restrictive foramen oval

Limitations of Pulse Oximetry

1. Hypovolemic states or low perfusion states.
2. Dyshemoglobinemias-COHb, Meth Hb.
3. Dyes and pigments including nail polish, henna
4. Optical interference from external light sources (phototherapy)
5. Excess movement artifacts.
6. As software varies between manufactures, inter-use of sensors by different manufacturers gives false results

Limitations of pulse oximetry

- Shape of oxygen dissociation curve
- Dyshemoglobins
- - Carboxyhemoglobin
- - Methemoglobin
- Dyes
- Low perfusion state
- Skin pigmentation
- Anemia
- Nail polish
- Motion artifact
- Limited knowledge of the technique

Pitfalls and Precautions in pulse oximetry

1. The accuracy of pulse oximetry is about +4 to 5% at or above 80% saturation. Accuracy declines below 80%.
2. Less accurate in severe anemia
3. Unable to distinguish different types of hemoglobins.
4. No value in estimation of adequacy of ventilation
5. Lag monitor phenomenon often a fall in partial pressure of oxygen precedes the fall in oxygen saturations
6. If probe does not fit properly, the light can be shunted from the LEDs directly to photodetector affecting the accuracy of the measurement

Definition /Normal value and some percentage of common and uncommon things

Normal values

– S calcium- 9-11 mg/dl
– S phosphorus- 4.3 to 7.1 mg/dl

Serum magnesium – 1.9 ±0.3 mg/dl

UA PI –

– 2nd TM- 2-1.5
– 3 rd TM – 1.5 -1

DIVING REFLEX /diving seal reflex

- Named based on the Reflex activated in animals like seals/penguins when they dive into cold water.
- Initiated on contact of face with the cold water-bradycardia, peripheral vasoconstriction preferentially preserves circulation to brain, heart and adrenals at cost of gut, liver, kidneys, skin, and muscle.
- Similar reflex happens in perinatal asphyxia
- Brain heart and adrenals blood supply is preserved at the cost of other organs - Explains situations with multiorgan dysfunction with relative sparing of brain.
- May fail in situations of acute total asphyxia- because no time for diving reflex to activate .

What are sentinel events?

- Prolapsed umbilical cord ›
- Uterine rupture
- › Abruptio placentae
- › Acute blood loss from cord

- › Any condition causing an abrupt decrease in maternal cardiac output and/or blood flow to the fetus

Patho Physiology of Brain Damage In Perinatal Asphyxia

Primary Energy Failure: minutes

- Acute stage of HI insult affecting ATP dependent Na-K pump, intracellular entry of Na, and Cl, H2O cell swelling & death – Necrosis

Secondary Energy Failure: 6-72 hrs after insult

- During the reperfusion phase -
- Glutamate induced NMDA, AMPA receptor over activation
- Opening of voltage dependent Ca2+ channels
- Influx of Ca2+ and generation of ROS & NOS death by Apoptosis
- Latent Phase in first six hours post birth- Utilize therapeutic 'window of opportunity

High Tech Cooling Systems Available

1. Cooling blankets: Blanketrol III, Criticool
2. Tecotherm: TS Med 200 N:,Tecotherm servo, tecotherm Neo

Low Cost Options

- PCM – MIRA CRADLE - Passive cooling or heating substances made of salt hydride, fatty acid, and esters of paraffin, PCM melting point 32°C
- In contact with a warm object, absorbs heat and slowly melts, thus reducing the temperature of the object.
- Completely passive, but behaves like a servo-automated cooling device.

DWI in HIE

Early – restricted diffusion

7-10 days – pseudonormalization of diffusion

>7-10 days – increased diffusion

Trimester cut off for TSH

- 1 tm – 0.1 to 2.5
- 2 tm 0.2 to 3.0
- 3 rd tm 0.3- 3.0

Risk of congenital malformation in

- Pregestational Type 1 Diabetes is roughly 3% to 7.5%
- In pregestational type 2 diabetes risk is 2% - 12%

Incidence of large for gestational age babies in diabetes is 35 to 45%

Features of NICU design

- 120 square feet per bed space
- 165 square feet per single patient room
- Feet distance between two bed
- Light between 10 to 600 lux
- Procedure light 2000 lux
- Noise level 45 decimal
- Temperature 22 to 26 degree
- Humidity 30- 60%
- Minimum 6 year exchange per hour which includes two changes from outside air

Status marmoratus

- Patchy marble like appearance of basal ganglia and thalamus develops after 6 months of HIE due to abnormal myelination of glial bundle

Definition of live Birth

- Complete expulsion or extraction of a product of human conception irrespective of duration of pregnancy, which show breathing, or any other sign of life after birth.

Nucleated RBCs

- Upper limit 3000/ul at birth
- Should be < 500/ul after 3-4 days
- Usually higher in preterms

Doppler indices

S/D ratio –

- < 4 before 30 weeks
- < 3 after 30 weeks

RI –

- <0.8 in umbilical artery
- >0.8 in MCA

PI- 1 to 1.5

PSV –

- mean of 23.3 at 18 weeks
- 64.4 at 40 weeks

GOLDEN HOUR IN NEONATOLOGY

The first 60 minutes of postnatal life are referred to as the

"Golden Hour" in neonatology. It has been demonstrated that applying standardised protocols and evidence-based therapies within the first hour of life can enhance long-term outcomes for preterm infants.

Golden hour in term babies three main goals by the World Health Organization direct, immediate skin-to-skin contact between the mother and New-born, delayed cord clamping, and early initiation of breastfeeding

Intervention	Time
Birth	0
Resuscitation	10
Transport to nicu	5 (15)
UAC/UVC/PICC	40 (55)
TPN/fluids	5 (60)

The Golden Hour practises for clinical management of premature infants includes

- prompt and appropriate resuscitation,
- temperature control, minimising transcutaneous fluid losses,
- timely administration of surfactant if indicated,
- early initiation of intravenous fluids containing dextrose and amino acids, and
- administration of oxygen only when or as needed

"Critical sample" during a hypoglycemic episode

1. Insulin
2. Free fatty acids
3. Growth hormone
4. Lactate/pyruvate
5. Bicarbonate
6. Ammonia
7. Ketones
8. Cortisol

AWaRe classifies antibiotics into three stewardship groups: **Access, Watch and Reserve**, to emphasize the importance of their optimal uses and potential for antimicrobial resistance. (WHO 2019)

TRANSPORT PEUMONICS

STABLE

1. Sugar
2. Temperature
3. Airway
4. Blood pressure
5. Lab investigations
6. Emotional support

SAFER

1. Sugar
2. Airway
3. Fluids
4. Emotional support
5. Reports

TOPS

1. Temperature
2. Oxygenation
3. Pulse
4. Sugar

NSCS neonatal skin condition score

Criteria Dryness:

1 = Normal, no signs of dry skin

2 = Dry skin with visible scaling

3 = Very dry skin with cracking and/or fissures present

Erythema:

1 = No evidence of erythema

2 = Visible erythema (<50% body surface)

3 = Visible erythema (>50% body surface)*

Breakdown:

1 None evident

2 Small and/or localized areas

3 Extensive

Interpretation of the results

The relevant medical team must be notified if a neonate scores a single score of 3 in one area or a combined score of 6 and above. A dermatology referral may also be appropriate.

NRP Key Behavioral Skills

1. Know your environment.
2. Use available information.
3. Anticipate and plan.
4. Clearly identify a team leader.
5. Communicate effectively.

6. Delegate workload optimally.
7. Allocate attention wisely.
8. Use available resources.
9. Call for additional help when needed.
10. Maintain professional behavior.

MODIFIED KDIGO CLASSIFICATION

Stage 0

- No change or rise <0.3 mg/dl within 48hrs
- Urine output over 24 hours >1mL/kg/h

STAGE 1

- Rise in S Cr by 0.3 mg/dl within 48 hrs OR
- Rise in S Cr 150-200% of lowest previous value within 7 DAYS
- Urine output over 24 hours <1 mL/kg/h

STAGE 2

- Rise in S Cr 200-300% of lowest previous value
- URINE OUTPUT IN 24 HRS <0.5 mL/kg/h

STGAE 4

- Rise in S Cr 300% of lowest previous value or 2.5 mg/dl or receipt of dialysis
- URINE OUTPUT IN 24 HRS <0.3 mL/kg/h

COMBINED APGAR SCORE

- C-Continuous positive airway pressure
- O-Oxygen
- M- B -Mask and bag ventilation"
- I-Intubation and ventilation
- N-Neonatal chest compression
- E-Exogenous surfactant
- D- Drugs

Perfusion Index

- Perfusion index (PI) is the ratio of pulsatile to nonpulsatile blood flow in tissues.
- It is a measure of peripheral tissue perfusion.
- The normal range of PI in neonates is 1.0-2.5%.

Pleth Variability Index

- Pleth variability index (PVI) is a measure of dynamic changes in PI due to respiratory cycles.
- Seen in the wave forms of pulse oximeter
- PVI is mainly evaluated as a measure of hypovolemia and volume- responsiveness in neonates with shock.
- PVI > 14 % is considered significant

Micro ESR in sepsis screen

- Pre heparinized micro hematocrit tube (75 mm length, internal diameter of 1.1 mm and outer diameter 1.5 mm)
- Absolute value more than 15 mm at the end of one hour or more than, days of life + 3 is considered to be significant.

CSF examination POSITIVE

- A polymorphonuclear count higher than 20/ cumm should be regarded with suspicion and counts above 30 /cumm are strongly indicative of meningitis
- CSF glucose usually 70-80% (at least 50%) of plasma glucose, lower values suggest meningitis.
- In cases of documented meningitis repeat LP after 48-72 hrs to check response to therapy
- Repeated CSF studies are required till the CSF is sterile.
- Document a normal CSF routine and culture report as well as neuro-imaging prior to discharge.

CRP

1. Serial determinations 24-48 hrs after symptoms
2. Sensitivity:74-89%
3. Specificity:74-95%

Affected by

- PROM
- IVH
- Maternal fever
- Meconium aspiration
- Fetal distress

Sepsis Screen

- Presence of two abnormal parameters in a screen is associated with a sensitivity of 95-100%, specificity of 83%, positive and negative predictive values of 27% and 100% respectively in detecting sepsis
- If $\geq$2 parameters are abnormal, it should be considered as a positive screen

ICROP 2021

ZONES IN ROP

- Zone I: most posterior; retinal area within a circle

centered on the disc and with a radius of twice the estimated disc–foveal distance

- Zone II: ring-shaped retinal area extending nasally from the edge of zone I to the nasal ora serrata and with the same radius distance temporally, superiorly and inferiorly; posterior zone II is a region of 2 disc diameters peripheral to the zone I border
- Zone III: residual crescent-shaped retinal area extending beyond zone II to the ora serrata

STAGES OF ROP

- Stage 0: incomplete vascularization (no ROP)
- Stage 1: a thin, flat, sharp white line of demarcation between the vascular and avascular retina
- Stage 2: an intraretinal elevation (ridge with height and width) at the junction between vascularized and avascular retina
- Stage 3: a ridge with extraretinal neovascular extension into the vitreous (can be flat)
- Stage 4: partial retinal detachment; stage 4A, does not involve the fovea; stage 4B, involves the fovea
- Stage 5: total retinal detachment; stage 5A, optic disc is visible by ophthalmoscope (open-funnel); stage 5B, optic disc is not visible (retrolental fibrovascular tissue or closed-funnel); stage 5C, 5B findings plus anterior segment abnormalities (lens displacement, shallowing of the anterior chamber, corneal opacification, etc.)

Aggressive ROP* (A-ROP)

- Rapid development of neovascularization and severe plus disease without progression through typical stages of ROP; atypical stage 3 (flat neovascularization), dilated vascular loops, arteriovenous shunts, ill defined vascular-avascular junction

Plus disease spectrum Presence of dilated and tortuous vessels in the posterior (Zone I) retina

Pre–plus disease spectrum abnormal vascular dilation and tortuosity that are insufficient for diagnosis of plus disease

Diagnostic Criteria for Hyperinsulinism (values at the time of hypoglycaemia)

1. Insulin >2 uIU/mL)
2. β-hydroxybutyrate of <1.8mmol/L
3. FFA <1.7mmol/L
4. Glucagon stimulation test rise of ≥30mg/dL
5. IGF-BP1 ≤110 ng/mL

NEONATAL REFEEDING SYNDROME

1. Combination of high aminoacid intake with low electrolyte intake LEADS to
2. LOW phosphorus
3. Low magnesium
4. Low potassium
5. High calcium
6. High glucose
7. High sodium

What is Antimicrobial Stewardship?

A set of coordinated interventions designed to improve and measure the appropriate use of antimicrobial agents, by promoting the selection of optimal antimicrobial drug regimen including dosing, duration of therapy and route of administration to reduce or avoid their use"

Is the use of "the right antibiotic, for the right indication (right diagnosis), on the right patient, at the right time, with the right dose and route, causing the least harm to the patient and population"

CLINICAL THRESHOLD definition of hypoglycaemia

Glucose concentration low enough to cause signs and/or symptoms of neuronal brain injury

Cornblath's "OPERATIONAL THRESHOLD" Does not address threshold level for neuronal injury

- In Healthy full term infant
  - o < 24 hr of age – 30 to 35 may acceptable, but not < 45 after feeding
  - o > 24 hr threshold is 45 to 50 mg/dl
- Infants with abnormal signs or symptoms- 45 mg/dl.
- Asymptomatic Infants with risk factors- 36 mg/dl.
- For any baby if glucose is < 20 to 25 I.V glucose is needed

NEUROPHYSIOLOGICAL THRESHOLD

Based on latencies in BERA - prolonged latencies <47 mg/dl

AAP DEFINITION of hypoglycaemia

- 0-4 hours: <25 mg/dl
- 4-24 hours: <35 mg/dl
- After 24 hours: <45 mg/dl
- After 48 hours: target blood sugar- 60 mg/dl

Hypoglycemia- alternate fuels for brain - lactate, ketone bodies (produced from liver)

GLOW STUDY

- Healthy infants have completed their metabolic transition by day 4.
- Mean glucose concentrations increased over the first 18 hours, remained stable to 48 hours before increasing to a new plateau by the fourth day.

Respiratory quotient (RQ)

- CO_2 production / oxygen consumption
- If glucose supply exceeds the maximum glucose oxidation rate, glucose is converted to fat.

43 NNF Guidelines Summary

1. In neonates born at >34 weeks of gestation and with mild respiratory distress, nasal cannula with low flow rate (0.5 - 1 L/min) should be used for delivering oxygen in preference to oxygen by hood or incubator oxygen
2. In neonates being administered oxygen at high flow rate (>1 L/min) through nasal cannula, warming and humidification of the inhaled gases may be preferred over no warming and humidification. Warming and humidification may not be necessary when flow rate through nasal cannula is low (< 1 L/min).
3. In neonates on respiratory support pulse oximeters with or without signal extraction technology may be used for monitoring of oxygen saturation.
4. Prophylactic surfactant should NOT be administered to preterm neonates <28 weeks' gestation with RDS.
5. Preterm neonates with RDS should be stabilized on CPAP and if indicated selective surfactant replacement therapy should be administered.
6. Sub-group considerations: Clinicians may consider delivery room surfactant in subgroup of neonates <28 weeks' gestation who are intubated in the delivery room for severe RDS.
7. Early INSURE (within 2 hours) may be used for preterm neonates < 34 weeks' gestation with established RDS and who satisfy the criteria for surfactant administration.
8. Surfactant may be given to preterm neonates < 34 weeks' gestation with RDS stabilized on CPAP, who require a PEEP of > 6 cm H2O and a FiO2 > 0.30 to maintain SpO2 > 91%
9. LISA may be preferred over INSURE for surfactant administration in preterm neonates < 34 weeks' gestation with RDS.
10. LMA should NOT be used for surfactant instillation outside research context in preterm neonates < 37 weeks' gestation with RDS
11. Poractant-α (200 mg/kg) may be used for treating preterm neonates < 34 weeks' gestation with RDS and who satisfy the criterion for surfactant administration
12. Multiple doses of surfactant should be used in the treatment of preterm neonates < 34 weeks' gestation with RDS who satisfy the pre-determined criteria for additional surfactant doses
13. A higher threshold (MAP/ PEEP ≥7 cm H2O and FiO2 > 0.4) may be used for repeat doses of surfactant in preterm neonates < 34 weeks' gestation with RDS who are on invasive or non-invasive ventilation. Sub-group considerations: A lower threshold (any mechanical ventilation and FiO2 > 0.3) may be considered for neonates with RDS and concomitant perinatal asphyxia or sepsis.
14. Early surfactant may be used in late preterm (34-36 weeks' gestation) and early term neonates (37-38 weeks' gestation) with RDS who satisfy the criteria for surfactant therapy. (FiO2 > 0.4, PEEP ≥ 7 cm H2O
15. The guidelines panel suggests NOT using surfactant therapy in preterm neonates born at less than 34 weeks of gestation who present with respiratory distress at a referral hospital beyond 72 h of age, irrespective of prior surfactant therapy
16. Early intra-tracheal corticosteroids may NOT be used as an adjunct to surfactant in the treatment of preterm neonates < 34 weeks' gestation with RDS.
17. Bolus surfactant may be used in treating late preterm and term neonates with severe MAS requiring invasive ventilation with an oxygenation index of more than 15.
18. Surfactant may be considered in late preterm and term neonates with severe bacterial pneumonia requiring invasive ventilation with an oxygenation index of more than 15.
19. Surfactant therapy should be given only in neonatal units with availability of CPAP machine and preferably also a back-up ventilator
20. The guidelines group suggests NOT to use serum CRP routinely for the diagnosis of sepsis in neonates with suspected late onset sepsis Weak Moderate b. However, in level-2 neonatal units with no facilities for blood culture, the group suggests using serum CRP as a

screening tool to rule out sepsis in neonates with a low probability of late-onset sepsis (for example, neonates with apnea, feed intolerance, or fast breathing

21. The guidelines group suggests that there is NO advantage in using PCT over CRP as a screening test for LONS
22. The guidelines group suggests using CSF WBC count and protein estimation for diagnosis in neonates being evaluated for suspected meningitis
23. The group suggests NOT to use CSF glucose estimation for diagnosis in neonates being evaluated for suspected meningitis
24. The guidelines group suggests NOT using the various early-onset sepsis calculators (e.g., the EONS calculator by Kaiser Permanente network) developed in high income countries for the management of well-appearing, asymptomatic neonates born at or after 35 weeks with risk factors for early onset sepsis
25. The guidelines group suggests administering antibiotics in symptomatic+ neonates born at any gestation and having maternal-perinatal risk factors of early-onset sepsis.
26. The guidelines group suggests considering initiation of antibiotic therapy in asymptomatic preterm neonates born before 35 weeks of gestation and having maternal-perinatal risk factors of early onset sepsis. In the > 32 weeks' gestation group, antibiotics may be considered for any one red flag risk factor or ≥2 yellow flag risk factors; and in the ≤32 weeks' gestation group for either one red or one yellow flag risk factor
27. In case antibiotics are started, the guidelines group recommends that antibiotics may be stopped after 36 hours if the blood culture remain sterile, the baby's clinical condition remains stable, and there are no signs suggestive of sepsis.
28. For asymptomatic neonates born at or after 35 completed weeks of gestation and at risk of early-onset sepsis, the guidelines group suggests administration of antibiotics only in the presence of positive laboratory markers of sepsis (such as, CRP, PCT or hematological parameters beyond age appropriate cut-off value
29. The guidelines group suggests NOT to use a shorter course of intravenous antibiotics (typically 5-7 days) in the management of neonates with uncomplicated@ and definite (i.e., culture-positive) neonatal sepsis; these neonates may preferably be treated with the standard course of antibiotics (typically 10-14 days).
30. The guideline group suggests NOT to use a shorter course of antibiotics (typically 2-3 days) for the treatment of uncomplicated@ probable neonatal sepsis or pneumonia; these neonates may preferably be treated with the standard 5-7 days course of intravenous antibiotics.
31. The guidelines group suggests NOT to stop antibiotic therapy based on one or serial negative biomarker report(s) in neonates with uncomplicated@ probable (i.e., culture-negative) neonatal sepsis; these neonates may preferably be treated with the current standard practice of 5-7 days of intravenous antibiotics
32. The guidelines group suggests NOT to use a short course of intravenous antibiotics (typically 14 days or less) in neonates with definite or probable uncomplicated$ neonatal meningitis; these neonates may preferably treated with the standard course of antibiotics (typically 21 days).
33. The guidelines group suggests NOT to use a shorter course of antibiotics (<4 weeks) in New-born infants with complicated meningitis (ventriculitis, brain abscess); these neonates may preferably be managed with the standard longer course of antibiotics (4-6 weeks)
34. The guidelines group suggests NOT to use a shorter course of antibiotics (typically ≤10 days) in New-born infants with uncomplicated% urinary tract infection (UTI); these neonates may preferably be treated using a standard longer course of antibiotics (typically 14 days)
35. The guidelines group suggests using antifungal therapy for 14 days after documented clearance of Candida species from the bloodstream and resolution of signs attributable to candidemia (and NOT for a pre-fixed duration - typically 14-21 days)
36. The group suggests a longer duration of antifungal therapy in case of a deep seated tissue infection or metastatic complication based on the site of infection, the patient's response to treatment, and the resolution of signs and symptoms
37. The guidelines group suggests NOT to use Cefotaxime + Amikacin or higher broad spectrum antibiotics for probable sepsis or meningitis in neonates admitted to special care neonatal units (SNCUs); these neonates may preferably be treated with the WHO recommended first-line antibiotics of Ampicillin + Gentamicin.
38. All neonatal units including SNCUs and NICUs should have an active antimicrobial stewardship program. The

program should preferably be integrated with the hospital's wider antimicrobial stewardship program.

39. Doctors and nurses working in SNCUs and NICUs should be trained in principles and practice of antimicrobial stewardship.
40. Every neonatal unit should implement a facility specific empirical antimicrobial therapy policy. This should be based on the local antibiogram and should be periodically reviewed and updated at pre-decided intervals of not more than 12 months.
41. Antibiotic cycling and/or mixing may NOT be practiced in neonatal units.
42. Standard antimicrobial prescription forms (printed or electronic) mentioning the indication, dose, duration, and route of antibiotic administration should be used for prescribing antibiotics.
43. Regular auditing of antibiotic use (selection, indication, duration, dose and route) followed by feedback to the SNCU/NICU staff must be an integral part of the antimicrobial stewardship program.
44. Scheduled 'reviews' (e.g., at 48 hours, 5 days) to decide about continuation of antibiotics may be used in neonates receiving antibiotics for being at risk of sepsis due to perinatal risk factors or having culture-negative probable sepsis.
45. Microbiology laboratories should follow selective and cascade reporting of antibiotic susceptibility patterns. If the organism grown in culture is sensitive to a narrow spectrum first-line antibiotic, only that sensitivity pattern should be mentioned in the report.
46. Facilities managing neonates at risk of systemic sepsis may consider use of rapid blood culture technology, as per availability and prioritization of resources.
47. We suggest monotherapy in preference to combination antimicrobial therapy for treatment of culture-positive systemic sepsis.
48. We suggest completion of planned antibiotic course by parenteral route in preference to switching to oral antibiotics following a short course of parenteral antibiotics, in preterm and hospitalized sick term neonates
49. Systemic antibiotics should NOT be used for prevention of sepsis in neonates with indwelling central arterial/venous catheters, invasive ventilation, total parenteral nutrition, prematurity, or non-infectious morbidities (e.g., meconium aspiration syndrome).

44 Neonatal Resuscitation Program

- 85% of term New-borns does not require any intervention
- 10% require drying and stimulation
- % 5 require PPV
- 2% require intubation
- 1-3/1000 births needs chest compressions or emergency medications
- A New-born requires resuscitation because respiratory failure different from adult resuscitation where cardiac etiology is most common.
- Ventilation of the New-born's lungs is the single most important and effective step in neonatal resuscitation.

Salient changes in NRP 8th Edition

- Now The 4 pre-birth questions are: (1) Gestational age? (2) Amniotic fluid clear? (3) Additional risk factors? (4) Umbilical cord management plan?
- Change in sequence of Initial steps: Warm, dry, stimulate, position airway, suction if needed.
- Must cardiac monitor -When an alternative airway becomes necessary. a cardiac monitor is recommended for the most accurate assessment of the baby's heart rate.
- Bolus - Flush IV/IO epinephrine with 3 mL normal saline (applies to all weights and gestational ages)
- Dose of adrenaline - The suggested initial IV or 10 dose = 0.02 mg/kg (equal to 0.2 mL/kg)
- The suggested endotracheal dose (while establishing vascular access) = 0.1 mg/kg (equal to 1 mL/kg)
- If confirmed absence of HR after all appropriate steps performed, consider cessation of rhesus- citation efforts around 20 minutes after birth (decision individualized on patient and contextual factors).

What is the 4 pre birth questions asked?

1. What is the expected gestational age?
2. Is the amniotic fluid clear?
3. Are there any additional risk factors?
4. What is our umbilical cord management plan?

Every birth should be attended by at least 1 qualified individual who can initiate resuscitation and whose only responsibility is management of the newly born baby.

If risk factors are present, at least 2 qualified individuals should be present

What is closed-loop communication?

Closed-loop communication is a technique that ensures instructions are heard and understood.

For most vigorous term and preterm New-borns, clamping the umbilical cord should be delayed for at least 30 to 60 seconds.

Three questions asked after birth

1. Does the baby appear to be term,
2. Does the baby have good muscle tone, and
3. Is the baby breathing or crying

Ask if the baby is term, has good muscle tone, and is breathing or crying

The 5 initial steps include the following: provide warmth, dry, stimulate, position the head and neck to open the airway, clear secretions from the airway if needed

Use pulse oximetry and the Target Oxygen Saturation Table to guide oxygen therapy (a) when resuscitation is anticipated, (b) to confirm your perception of persistent central cyanosis, (c) if you give supplemental oxygen, or (d) if positive-pressure ventilation is required

Early (immediate) cord clamping is indicated, or may be considered, in certain cases.

1. Placenta! abruption, bleeding placenta previa, bleeding vasa previa, or cord avulsion,
2. there is currently not enough evidence to evaluate the safety of delayed cord clamping in the setting of a multiple gestation birth
3. Safety data on delayed cord clamping are limited, - fetal intrauterine growth restriction (IUGR), abnormal umbilical artery Doppler measurements, abnormal placentation

Very preterm babies less than 32 weeks' gestation because they should be covered immediately in polyethylene plastic wrap.

Tactile stimulation

Gently rub the New-born's back, trunk, or extremities

Sniffing the morning air" position

For suction -Turn the head to one side, this will allow secretions to collect in the cheek where they can be removed by bulb sucker.

If suction machine is used for suctioning use pressure not more than of 80 to 100 mm Hg

Always Suction mouth before nose

Estimate the heart rate by counting the number of beats in 6 seconds and multiplying by 1 0

In the New-born, PEA should be treated the same as an absent heart rate (asystole)

Place the pulse oximeter sensor on the baby's right hand or wrist

How do you administer supplemental oxygen?

1. Holding oxygen tubing close to the baby's mouth and nose
2. Using a flow-inflating bag or T-piece resuscitator, hold the mask close to the face but not tight
3. The tail of a self-inflating bag with an open reservoir.

Do not attempt to give free-flow oxygen using the mask of a self-inflating bag.

What are the different types of resuscitation devices used to ventilate New-borns?

A self-inflating bag fills spontaneously with gas after it has been squeezed and released.

A flow-inflating bag (also called an anesthesia bag) only fills when gas from a compressed source flows into it and the outlet is sealed.

A T-piece resuscitator continuously directs compressed gas toward the baby.

How to use a self inflating bag?

- Ventilation rate – how many times you squeeze the bag
- Inflation time – how quickly you squeeze the bag
- PIP – how hard you squeeze the bag
- PEEP – if additional PEEP valve is attached
- It cannot be used for CPAP delivery
- **pop-off valve- set to release at 30 to 40 cm H20 pressure**

How to test a self-inflating bag?

1. Block the mask and squeeze the bag
2. Feel for the pressure on hand
3. Check if manometer reads the pressure
4. Check that pop off valve release at 30-40 cm water

Advantage of self-inflating bag

1. Easier to use
2. Requires little time to set up
3. Not require a compressed gas source
4. Can be used in an emergency setting

Disadvantage of self-inflating bag

1. Large leak missed because of self-inflating nature of the bag
2. difficult to control the inflation time and pressure if no manometer is attached

T-piece resuscitators

- The device requires a compressed gas source
- Ventilation rate depends on rate of occluding the opening on the cap
- inflation time- how much time you occlude the cap
- The peak inflation pressure control knob limits the peak pressure during each assisted breath
- Maximum pressure relief control – acts a pop off valve. It is covered with a shield.
- Adjust the PEEP knob for desired peep which in on the cap. adjustable dial
- manometer measures the inflation and expiratory pressure

Testing a T-piece resuscitator

1. Block the mask at gas outlet without occluding the opening on the T-piece cap.
2. Check the peep reading
3. Now occlude the opening on the cap
4. See that the peak pressure read 20 to 25 cm H20

How to set a T piece

1. Connect the t piece tubing to outlet and cover the outlet with palm /test lung
2. Compressed gas source to inlet

3. Set flow at 10 L/min
4. Set the maximum pressure-relief control 40 cm H20 is the recommended maximum for term New-borns, 30 cm H20 is the recommended maximum for preterm New-borns) and cover the knob
5. Now Set the desired peak inflation pressure (PIP) by occluding the cap with your finger to desired pressure 20-25 cm H2O
6. Set the peep after removing your finger from the cap, adjust with peep dial

Advantage of T piece

- It provides more consistent pressure with each breath
- Leak detected easily on manometer
- User not fatigued easily compared to self-inflating bag
- More control on inflation time
- T-piece can deliver CPAP, PEEP, and free-flow oxygen.

Disadvantage of t piece

- Requires some preparation time for setup
- It requires a compressed gas source

Indications for positive-pressure ventilation?

- PPV is indicated if the baby is not breathing (apneic), OR if the baby is gasping, OR if the baby's heart rate is less than 100 bpm
- Should be started within 1 minute of birth.
- Stand at the head end of baby while delivering ppv

Neonatal masks have a cushioned or soft pliable rim

Two types of mask are available -anatomically shaped and round (mostly we use round)

The mask should rest on the chin and cover the mouth and nose, but not the eyes

One-Hand Hold of mask –

- Hold the mask on the face with the thumb and index finger encircling the rim.
- Place the other 3 fingers under the bony angle of the jaw and gently lift the jaw upward toward the mask

Two-Hand Hold With Jaw Thrust

- Use the thumb and first finger of both hands to hold the mask against the face
- Place the other 3 fingers of each hand under the bony angle of the jaw and gently lift the jaw upward toward the mask

For the initial resuscitation of New-borns greater than or equal to 35 weeks' gestation, set the blender to 21 % oxygen

For the initial resuscitation of New-borns less than 35 weeks' gestation, set the blender to 21 % to 30% oxygen

Target Pre-Ductal Oxygen Saturation (for easy recall 1-3-5-6-7-8)

1 minute	60 %
3 mimute	70 %
5 minute	80 %

10 min 85%-95%

PPV

1. Breaths should be given at a rate of 40 to 60 breaths per minute.
2. Use the rhythm, "Breathe, two, three; breathe, two, three; breathe, two, three:
3. "Breathe"- squeeze the bag
4. "Two, three":- while release
5. Start with a PIP of 20 to 25 cm H20
6. When PEEP is used, the suggested initial setting is 5 cm H20
7. The most important indicator of successful PPV is a rising heart rate.

Within 15 seconds of starting PPV, the baby's heart rate should be increasing.

AFTER 15 SEC OF PPV

Heart rate increasing	continue PPV
Heart rate not increasing but chest rise present	continue PPV
Heart rate not increasing and no chest rise	MRSOPA

MR.SO.P.A

M	Mask adjustment
R	Reposition the head and neck
Give 5 breaths and assess chest movement. If no chest movement, do the next steps.	
S	Suction the mouth and nose.
O	Open the mouth
Give 5 breaths and assess chest movement. If no chest movement, do the next steps.	

Cont...

P	Pressure increase. Increment of 5-10 cm H2O
Give 5 breaths and assess chest movement. If no chest movement, do the next step	
A	Alternative airway, insert a laryngeal mask or endotracheal tube

Maximum pressure

Max 40 cm H20 term

Max 30 cm H20 preterm

After 30 seconds of PPV - check the baby's heart rate response again.

When the heart rate is consistently greater than 100 bpm, gradually reduce the rate of PPV, observe for effective spontaneous respirations, and gently stimulate the baby to breathe

Positive-pressure ventilation may be discontinued when the baby has a heart rate continuously greater than 100 bpm and sustained spontaneous breathing

If the heart rate is at least 60 bpm but less than 100 bpm - continue to administer PPV

If the baby's heart rate remains less than 60 bpm after at least 30 seconds of PPV that moves the chest, preferably through an alternative airway, increase the F102 to 100% and begin chest compressions

Place a CO2 detector between the PPV device and mask- IF available - detector turn from purple to yellow during each exhalation

If the baby's heart rate is very low or not pumping blood, the detector may not change color because CO2 is not being carried to the lungs even though you are ventilating the lungs

What is a laryngeal mask?

- Small mask attached to an airway tube
- It makes a seal over the entrance to the baby's trachea (the glottis after inserting
- If the baby cannot be successfully ventilated with a face mask and intubation is unfeasible or unsuccessful, a laryngeal mask may provide a successful rescue airway

If baby has labored breathing or low oxygen saturation despite free-flow oxygen - CPAP may be considered

If a New-born requires CPAP or PPV for longer than several minutes, consider placing an orogastric tube.

Measure the distance from the bridge of the nose to the earlobe and from the earlobe to a point halfway between the xiphoid process (the lower tip of the sternum) and the umbilicus

Mortality was decreased among term and late-preterm babies resuscitated with 21 % oxygen compared with 100% oxygen

In preterm New-borns, there was no difference in outcomes between those resuscitated with low oxygen (21%-30%) and high oxygen (60%-100%). to start with low oxygen and titrate upward as needed using pulse oximetry

INTUBATION

Laryngoscope blades (straight Miller)*

- No. 1 (term New-born)
- No. O (preterm New-born)
- No. 00 (optional for extremely preterm New-born)

Tube has a vocal cord guide that is used to approximate the insertion depth

Endotracheal tubes are described by the size of their internal diameter (mm ID)

< 1 kg	< 28 weeks	2.5 mm ID	5 /6 F
1-2 kg	28-34 weeks	3 mm ID	6/8 F
>2 kg	>34 weeks	3.5 mm ID	8 F

Steps of intubation

- Hold the laryngoscope in your left hand with your thumb resting on the upper surface of the laryngoscope handle and the blade pointing away from you
- TO be held in the left hand by both right- and left-handed users
- Right index finger or thumb to gently open the baby's mouth
- After insertion the tip of laryngoscope blade should lies in the space between the base of the tongue and the epiglottis. This space is called the vallecula
- Lift the entire laryngoscope in the direction that the handle is pointing
- Insert the tube into the right side of the baby's mouth, outside the blade, with the concave curve in the horizontal plan
- Do not insert the tube through the laryngoscope's open channel
- The steps of intubation should be completed within approximately 30 seconds.

2 types of CO_2 detectors

Colorimetric devices - The colorimetric CO_2 detector is purple or blue before detecting exhaled CO_2. The detector turns yellow in the presence of exhaled CO_2.

Capnographs

Tube IS IN trachea but NO color change

1. Inadequate ventilating pressure
2. Collapsed lungs
3. Bilateral pneumothoraces
4. Very low heart rote
5. Low cardiac output
6. Obstructed endotracheal tube

Tube is NOT in trachea but color changes

1. Defective device changed color in package before use
2. Epinephrine contamination
3. Surfactant contamination
4. Atropine contamination
5. gastric secretion contamination

Exhaled CO_2 and observing a rapidly increasing heart rate are the primary methods of confirming endotracheal tube insertion within the trachea.

Tip is only 1 to 2 centimeters below the vocal cords

Nasal-tragus length (NTL) is a method both full-term and preterm New-borns.

Distance (cm) from the baby's nasal septum to the ear tragus

The estimated insertion depth (cm) is NTL + 1 cm

The tip of the tube should appear in the mid-trachea adjacent to the first or second thoracic vertebra on X-ray

Sudden deterioration after intubation DOPE

- D Displaced endotracheal tube
- Obstructed endotracheal tube
- P Pneumothorax
- E Equipment failure

Chest compressions are indicated when the heart rate remains less than 60 beats per minute (bpm) despite at least 30 seconds of positive-pressure ventilation (PPV) that inflates the lungs (chest movement)

Those who do not respond to ventilation have very low blood oxygen levels, significant acidosis, and insufficient blood flow in their coronary arteries

These lead to severely depressed cardiac muscle function

Improving coronary artery blood flow is the urgent need to reverse this

Depressing the sternum compresses the heart against the spine, pushes blood forward, and increases the blood pressure in the aorta. When pressure on the sternum is released, the heart refills with blood and blood flows into the coronary arteries

Chest compressions are indicated if the baby's heart rate remains less than 60 bpm after at least 30 seconds of PPV that inflates the lungs, as evidenced by chest movement with ventilation.

Only approximately 1 to 2 per 1,000 New-borns are expected to require chest compressions.

Once intubation is completed and the tube is secure, the compressor should move to the head of the bed while the person operating the PPV device moves to the side

STEPS IN CHEST COMPRESSION

- Apply pressure to the lower third of the sternum.
- Do not place your thumbs on the ribs or on the xiphoid.
- Depress the sternum approximately one-third of the anterior-posterior (AP) diameter of the chest
- TWO Thumbs technique
- The compression rate is 90 compressions per minute. To achieve this rate, you will give 3 rapid compressions and 1 ventilation during each 2-second cycle.
- Coordinated Compressions and Ventilations
- 3 compressions + 1 ventilation every 2 seconds (90 + 30 = 120 events per minute)
- One-and-Two-and-Three-and-Breathe-and; One-and-Two-and-Three-and-Breathe-and; Oneand-Two-and-Three-and-Breathe-and.
- Compress the chest with each counted number ("One, Two, Three").
- Release the chest between each number ("-and-").
- Pause compressions and give a positive-pressure breath when the
- compressor calls out "breathe-and. 1
- When chest compressions are started, increase the Fio 2 to 100%
- Wait 60 seconds after starting coordinated chest compressions and ventilation before briefly pausing compressions to reassess the heart rate.

- Stop chest compressions when the heart rate is 60 bpm or greater.

Questions to Ask When Heart Rate Is Not improving With Compressions and Ventilation (Mnemonic CARDIO)

1. Chest movement: Is the chest moving with each breath?
2. Airway: Is the airway secured with an endotracheal tube or laryngeal mask?
3. Rote: Are 3 compressions coordinated with 1 ventilation being delivered every 2 seconds?
4. Depth: Is the depth of compressions one-third of the AP diameter of the chest?
5. Inspired Oxygen: Is 100% oxygen being administered through the PPV device?

Pressure applied directly over the xiphoid could cause laceration of the liver.

Why does the Neonatal Resuscitation Program Algorithm follow A-B-C (Airway-Breathing-Compressions) when other programs follow C-A-B (Compressions-Airway-Breathing)?

- Underlying problem is respiratory failure with impaired gas exchange
- NRP focuses on establishing effective ventilation, rather than starting chest compressions because the vast majority of New-borns who require resuscitation have a healthy heart

Why does the Neonatal Resuscitation Program use a 3: 1 compression-to-ventilation ratio instead of the 15:2 ratio used in other programs?

- Neonatal animal studies have shown that the 3:1 ratio shortens the time to return of spontaneous circulation

Epinephrine is indicated if the baby's heart rate remains less than

60 beats per minute (bpm) after:

a. At least 30 seconds of positive-pressure ventilation (PPV) that inflates the lungs as evidenced by chest movement and
b. Another 60 seconds of chest compressions coordinated with PPV using 100% oxygen.

Concentration OF adrenaline: 0.1 mg/mL = 1 mg/10 mL

c. Route: Intravenous (preferred) or intraosseous
d. Intravenous or intraosseous = 0.02 mg/kg (equal to 0.2 mL/kg)
e. May repeat every 3 to 5 minutes
f. Range = 0.01 to 0.03 mg/kg (equal to 0.1 to 0.3 mL/kg)
g. Rate: Rapidly-as quickly as possible
h. Flush: Follow intravenous or intraosseous dose with a 3-mL saline flush IV /IO Flush:

Endotracheal dose of adrenaline = 0.1 mg/kg (equal to 1 mL/kg)

- Range = 0.05 to 0.1 mg/kg (0.5 to 1 mL/kg) suggested endotracheal dose is 0.1 mg/ kg (equal to 1 mL/kg).
- If no response, recommend intravenous or intraosseous for subsequent doses

Volume expansion recommendations

- o Solution: Normal saline (NS) or type O Rh-negative blood
- o Route: Intravenous or intraosseous
- o Preparation: 30- to 60-mL syringe (labelled NS or O-blood)
- o Dose: 10 mL/kg
- o Rate: Over 5 to 10 minutes (Use caution with preterm New-borns less than 32 weeks' gestation).

A reasonable period for considering cessation of resuscitation efforts is around 20 minutes after birth

How epinephrine works in NRP

It causes constriction of blood vessels outside of the heart, which increases blood flow into the coronary arteries. Blood flowing into the coronary arteries carries the oxygen required to restore cardiac function. In addition, epinephrine increases the rate and strength of cardiac contractions.

When umbilical venous access is not feasible or successful, the intraosseous route is a reasonable alternative

Endotracheal (less effective) - No flush is recommended.

Repeat every 3 to 5 minutes if heart rote remains less than 60 bpm. Endotracheal: Administer PPV breaths to distribute into lungs. No flush

The recommended crystalloid solution for acutely treating hypovolemia is normal saline (0.9% NaCl).

Intraosseous needle insertion

For term New-borns, the preferred site is the flat surface of the lower leg, approximately 2 cm below and 1 to 2 cm medial to the tibial tuberosity (the bony bulge below the kneecap)

REFERENCES WILL BE PROVIDED ON REQUEST